VOGUE

STAY YOUNG

VOGUE
STAY YOUNG

EDITOR
ALEXANDRA PENNEY

ASSOCIATE EDITOR
DIANA EDKINS

DESIGN
MIKI DENHOF

M

MACMILLAN LONDON

Associate designer: Carl Barile

First published in the United States of America 1981 by
St Martin's Press Inc

This edition first published in Great Britain by
Macmillan London Limited

First published in paperback 1983 by
PAPERMAC
a division of Macmillan Publishers Limited
4 Little Essex Street London WC2R 3LF
and Basingstoke

Associated companies in Auckland, Dallas, Delhi,
Dublin, Hong Kong, Johannesburg, Lagos, Manzini,
Melbourne, Nairobi, New York, Singapore, Tokyo,
Washington and Zaria

ISBN 0 333 35151 7

Printed in Hong Kong

CONTENTS

INTRODUCTION

With the two possible exceptions of gold and the Holy Grail, only a few quests have so beguiled the human imagination as the pursuit of everlasting youth. And none has done so more consistently; for all its intensity, gold fever comes and goes sporadically, and beyond the literary and operatic delights of the Arthurian legends, the Grail takes up only the tiniest space in our mythology. But the lure of eternal youth, in myth and in reality, continues unabated through time.

In its name, the Greeks sacrificed to Hebe, and the Spanish explorer Ponce de León raised an expedition. Not to mention Faust, who, for 24 additional years in which all pleasure and knowledge would be his, sold his soul to the devil. Even more dramatic because true: The Countess Elisabeth Batthory, an acclaimed beauty of 16th-century Hungary, was walled up alive as punishment for the unorthodox way in which she attempted to prolong her youth and good looks; it was the Countess's practice to bathe as frequently as could be managed in the blood of her servant girls.

Alas for the servant girls, the Countess was born too soon. Had she lived in our own time, her purpose would have been spectacularly better served by far less desperate measures. Nor is it likely that Faust, were he living in the 1980s, would be quite so willing to do business with the devil—why, after all, opt for drastic means when the desired ends are so conventionally accessible? And the truth of the matter is that today they are.

To begin with, medical science has made such significant advances that in many parts of the world—and surely in ours—certain diseases are all but obsolete; others have been rendered reversible or controllable; and about an impressive number of others—respiratory diseases, for instance, and heart disorders and various forms of cancer —research is already pointing the way to prevention and cure strategies. These findings aren't secret; the information is available to all of us—it's in this book, for one thing—not only knowledge of how the body functions, but of how it can function optimally at any given age, and of how dysfunction can be minimized—or even prevented —in every area of the human mechanism . . . at any age.

In the face of such progress, we almost can't help ourselves: Barring catastrophe, we are going to live longer. On the actuarial tables, we have already passed the biblical three-score-and-ten (the life-expectancy figure for men in this country is now around 76 years, for women 80-plus). But remember: Faust, understanding that simple longevity was not in itself a blessing, made a crucial stipulation; he wanted not just more years, but more good—i.e., *youthful*—years.

Simply living longer isn't the issue anymore; it's the given. Neither is the issue one of trying to look 20 when you're 50. The point is, the whole question of age is telescoping; there is no longer a vast distinction between 20 and 50. There is simply a different—a younger—concept of 50, or 40, or 70. And it has to do with how you live your inevitably longer life—how healthily, how actively, how productively, how enjoyably, and even, since strong appetites are almost by definition vigorous and young, how greedily you live this life. Or, more precisely, how you *choose* to live it.

And make no mistake, when it comes to staying young—by which we mean staying alive—choice is the key. We all know septuagenarians who live as vitally as 30-year-olds. And we have all seen grandmothers with skin almost as fine as their grandaughters', and bodies as lithe.

And we have all seen the opposite; there is no trick to burning yourself out at 40—if that's what you want. No medical policeman is going to pull you out of your chair and put you onto an exercise mat so you don't get arteriosclerosis, or pull the cigarette out of your mouth so you don't get lung cancer, or pull you out of the sun so you don't get wrinkles, or pull the salt shaker out of your hand so you don't get high blood pressure, or pull you out of a job that's driving you up the wall so you don't get hypertensive, or pull you out of a boring job so you don't get used to not using yourself fully. It's all up to you.

In other words, to a larger degree than you may have suspected, the quality of your life is your choice. Nobody is programmed to stay young, but the opportunity is there for everyone. And the purpose of this book is to help you to make the most of it.

Edith Loew Gross
New York, 1981

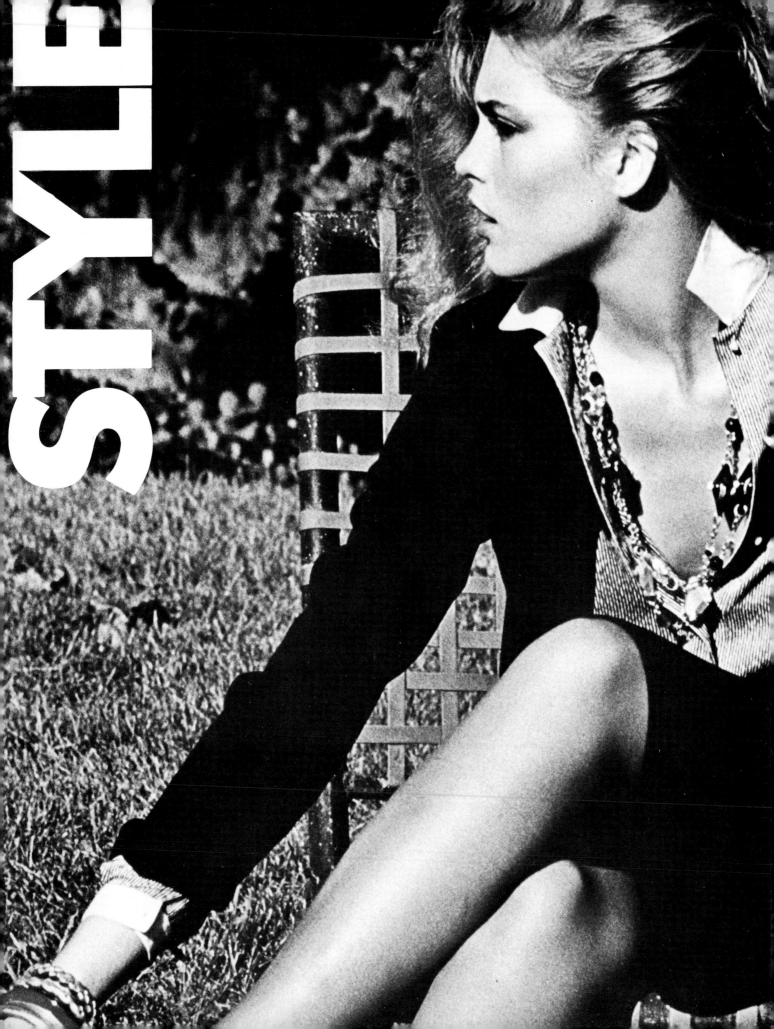

STYLE

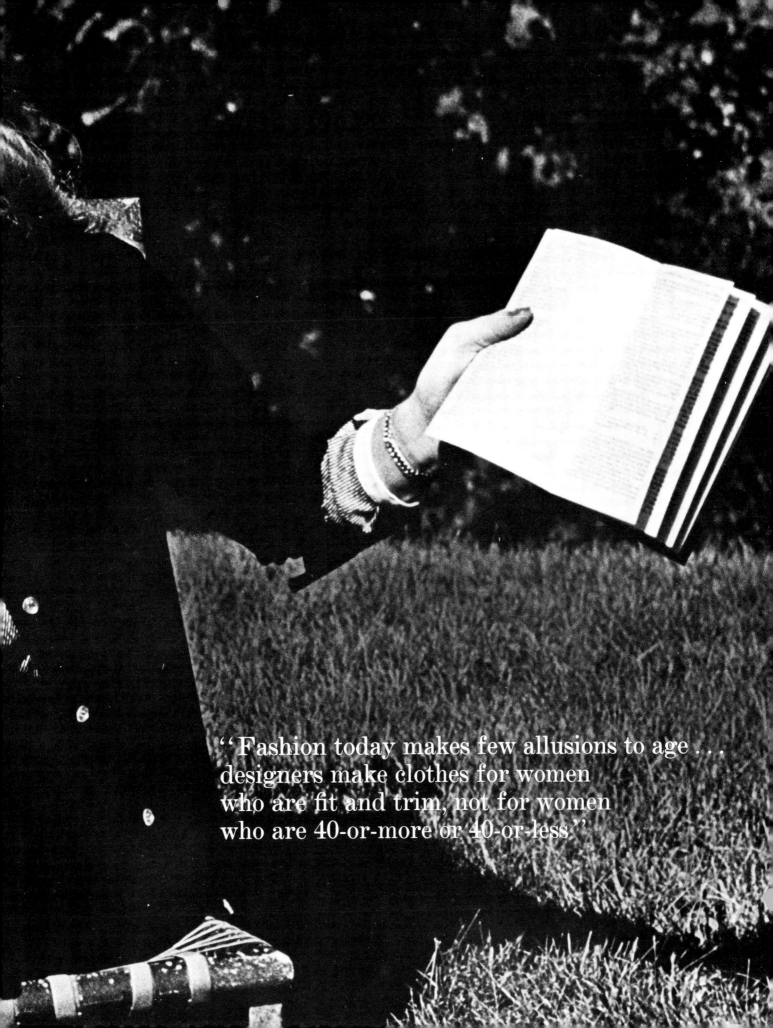

"Fashion today makes few allusions to age ...
designers make clothes for women
who are fit and trim, not for women
who are 40-or-more or 40-or-less."

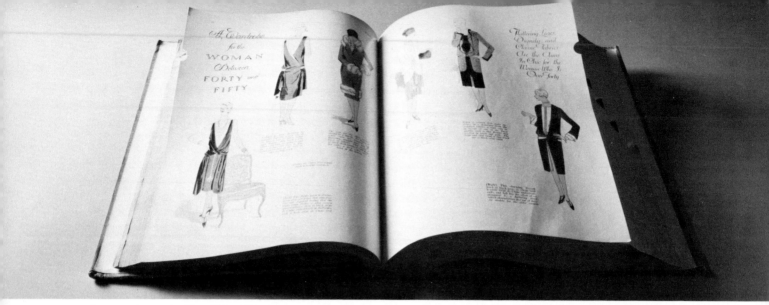

Over 40 in 1927: The Older Woman

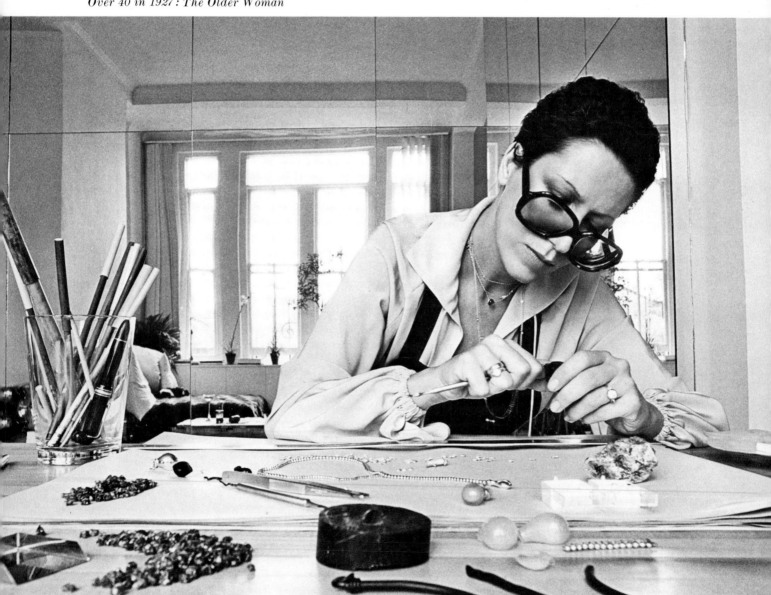

Over 40 today: jewelry designer Elsa Peretti

STYLE

by Edith Loew Gross

Fashion, for most of us, is simply what we wear—or would like to wear. We don't analyze it too deeply; on the brink of buying something new, about the only questions we ask ourselves are: Is it attractive? Is it becoming? Is it going to fill a need? Can I afford it? But there was a time when such a list would have seemed glaringly incomplete, when a crucial question would have been: Is it correct for a woman of my age? Not that any woman had to grope for the answer; it was laid out for her. Like rites of passage, each transition in a woman's life—debutante to young matron to matron to elderly woman—was marked by a different way of dressing: Different cuts, different colors, different fabrics, different accessories....

An ad in a 1911 issue of *Vogue* shows a photograph of a sweet-faced woman with short, tightly curled hair and no makeup. She is wearing —in the heyday of the toque and the turban!—a plain dark bonnet tied, Salvation-Army-style, to one side under her chin. The text, in its entirety, reads: "Holland Hats—Elderly Ladies' Hatters." It would be interesting to know who was meant

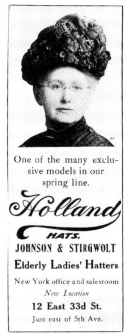

One of the many exclusive models in our spring line.

Holland

HATS.

JOHNSON & STIRGWOLT

Elderly Ladies' Hatters

New York office and salesroom

New Location

12 East 33d St.

Just east of 5th Ave.

Vogue 1911

by "elderly"; the model's age is anybody's guess—her face is not especially lined and the contours are good—but the text and the hair and the relentlessly out-of-fashion bonnet tell us that the Holland Hat people were speaking to women well out of the mainstream, women of 80 or so. Or were they?

An editorial feature in *Vogue*, January 15, 1927, is more specific. The title: "A Wardrobe for the Woman Between Forty and Fifty." Excerpt from the caption under one of the drawings: "The coat for the older woman ... No flights of fancy enter her fashions...."

And so on through the years— until 1962, in fact, when Mrs. Exeter, *Vogue*'s paragon Older Woman, whose appearances had become increasingly rare, turned up for the last time in a printed dress with matching jacket and a few tactful pleats at the front of the skirt (a woman of 40 or more might be presumed to need such devices, her muscle tone having long since given way to a soft little cushion of tummy).

It seems absurd to us—after all, who are the 40-and-over women we know? Jane Fonda, Ali MacGraw, Barbara Walters, Jacqueline Onassis, Mary Wells Lawrence, Bess

13

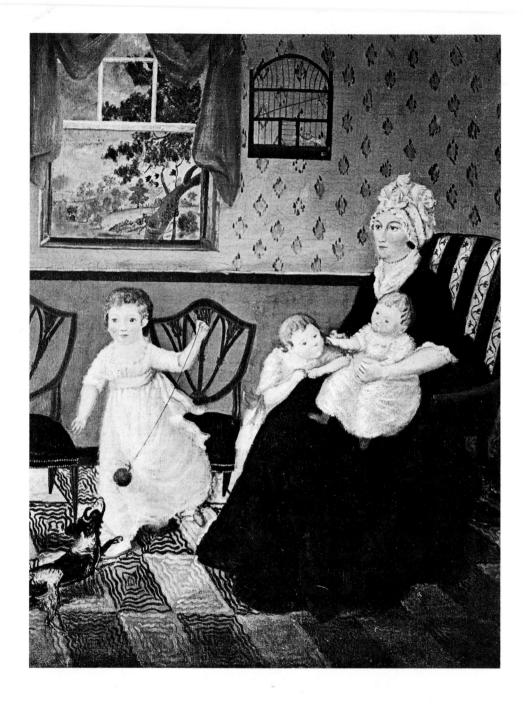

Myerson, Lauren Bacall—what have tactful pleats to do with them? For that matter, can you see 70-year-old Millicent Fenwick in an "Elderly Ladies' Hat," or 76-year-old Claudette Colbert? Or 80-plus Martha Graham, Rose Kennedy? 60-plus Katharine Graham or Lena Horne? (For the record, this is designer Calvin Klein's recent memory of Lena Horne: "Black cashmere turtleneck, black leather jeans and a trenchcoat.")

The point is less that these women look younger than their age than that we have a different mind's-eye vision of how a woman is supposed to look at any given age. In truth, our whole concept of women and aging has changed dramatically. For one thing, women are living longer: In 1920—the decade of *Vogue*'s Older Woman Between 40 and 50— the life expectancy for an American woman was only a shade over 54 years; that figure is into the eighties today. For another, they are living healthier; being well-informed on such

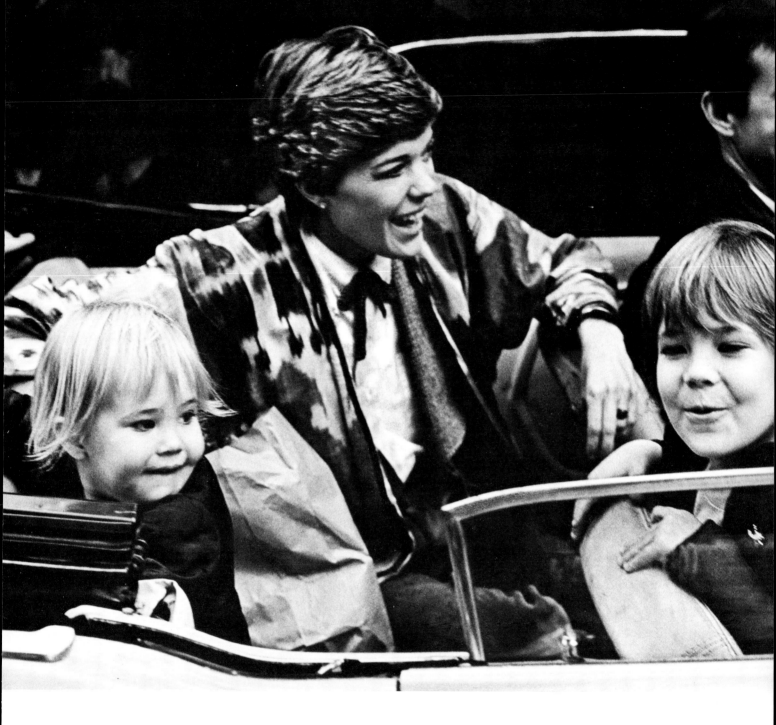

matters, they are eating better and—on the evidence of attendance rolls at health clubs, spas, exercise classes and the like—taking better care of their bodies. For yet a third thing, ours is no longer a rigidly structured society that assigns to women certain roles at certain ages. In our time, grandmothers—or women old enough to be grandmothers—are law students, congresswomen, publishers, business executives, New York Marathon runners. The fact is, in the 1980s, a woman of 40

Berry Perkins, above, and her sons, Osgood and Elvis, enjoy a vital life together. Left, the 1776 image shows a young, blooming woman, flocked with children and chores, who had an expected life span of 35.5 years— little enough time for the work of her family's survival.

1951

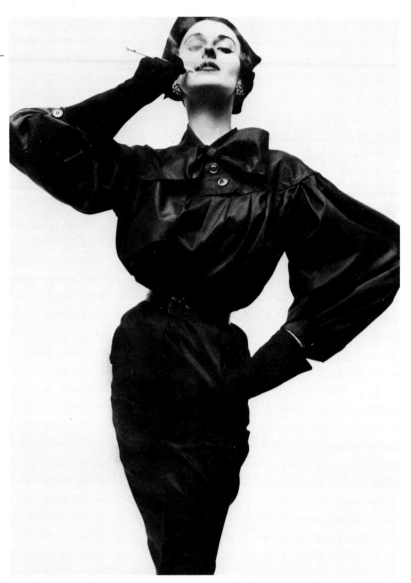

or more isn't expected to be out of the mainstream. Or out of shape. Or out of fashion.

This would seem to suggest that grandmothers, if they're in shape, should be dressing like their daughters and granddaughters. And in a general way—in the broad context of contemporary fashion—it's true. It doesn't, however, mean that a grown woman would want to get herself up in a miniskirt and a tumble of hair to the shoulders. No matter how in-shape she may be, the associations are psychologically wrong: It's how we think of little girls dressing, or cheerleaders. We associate it with extreme youth, which we're willing to concede to a 20-year-old, but much

beyond that we get into a kind of reverse illusion: Instead of a youthful-looking woman youthfully dressed, we see an adult masquerading as a teenager, and there are few deceptions more cruelly aging.

The idea of generations dressing alike is plausible—and attractive—precisely because

Models in the Fifties weren't older than the models of today. They just looked older. The characteristics of fashion in that time, in direct contrast to fashion now, define what we think of as "older."

1981

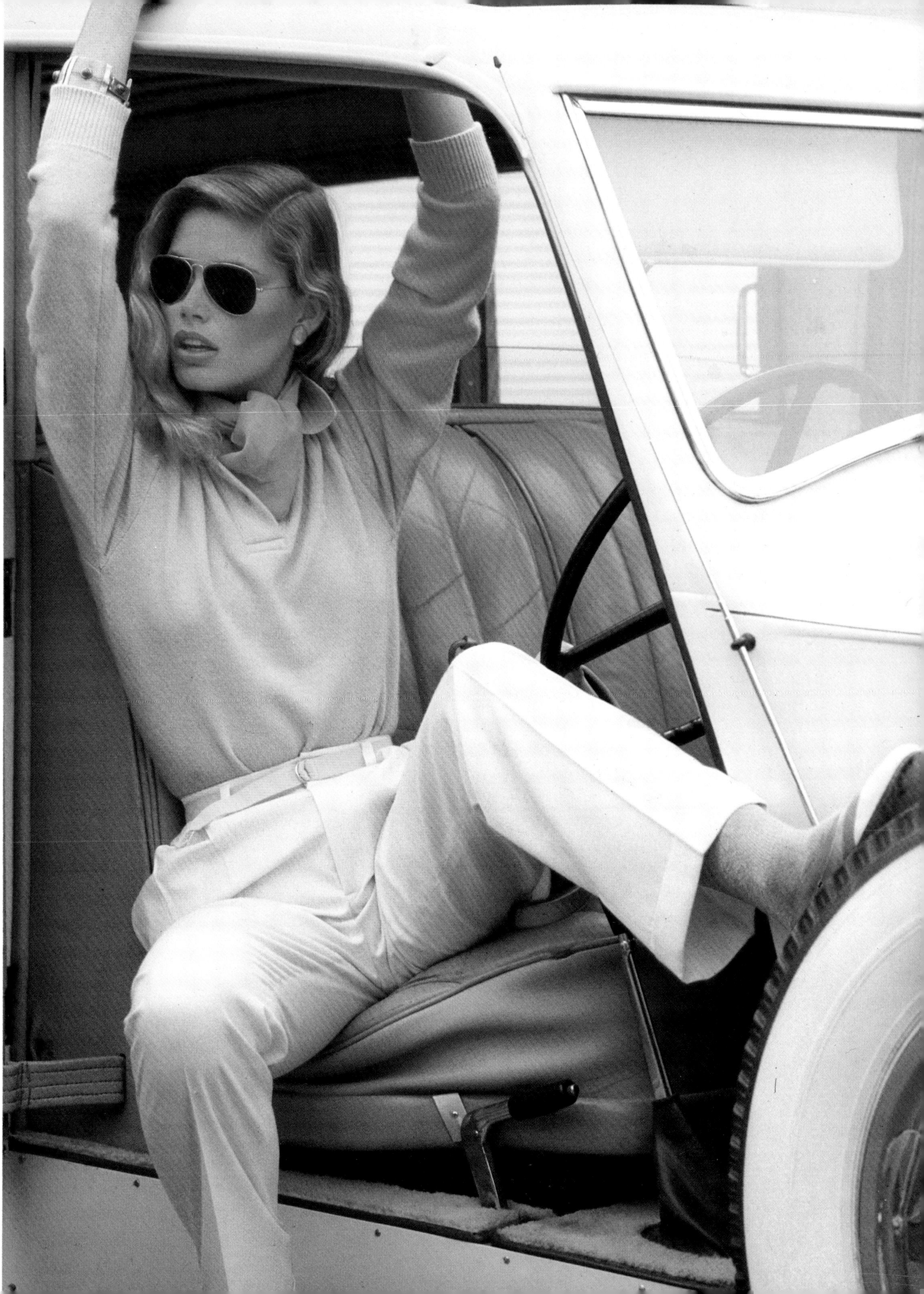

it does not mean dressing younger than one's age. Nor does it mean dressing older. The truth of the matter is that, unlike the youth-focused fashion of the sixties or the very studied (and therefore older-looking) era that preceded it, fashion today makes clothes for women who are fit and trim, not for women who are 40-or-more or 40-or-less.

Practiced fashion-observers see this not as an arbitrary change but as a classic example of fashion as a mirror reflecting major trends in society—in this case, the more active role of women and an increasingly casual style of living—and they welcome it. But some women —particularly women who use as a point of reference a more formal time, such as the 1950s—are less sanguine. They look at the magazines, see models obviously in their twenties wearing clothes that are hardly more serious than sweaters, and conclude that there is nothing in fashion for anyone over 30. They might do well to check their reference. It would reveal, for instance, that models in the 1950s weren't older than the models of today. They just looked older: their hair, set flat to the head under stiff little hats, didn't move; their faces, under heavy, opaque makeup, seemed frozen and unreal. And their clothes, made of hard, firm-bodied fabrics, and into which they appeared to be rigidly corseted, were very serious, indeed: sculptural, stylized, "important"-looking. Fashion in the fifties was in the silhouette, and every complicated dressmaking device was used to maintain it—seaming, darting, boning, facing, interfacing, interlining. On the hanger or on a human body, it was all the same: Clothes could practically stand on their own, but they could barely move across a room, except

Continued on page 25

"No matter how young or how old or what you've got on, if the grooming isn't there, forget it. It's grooming and comfort, then the clothes."

18

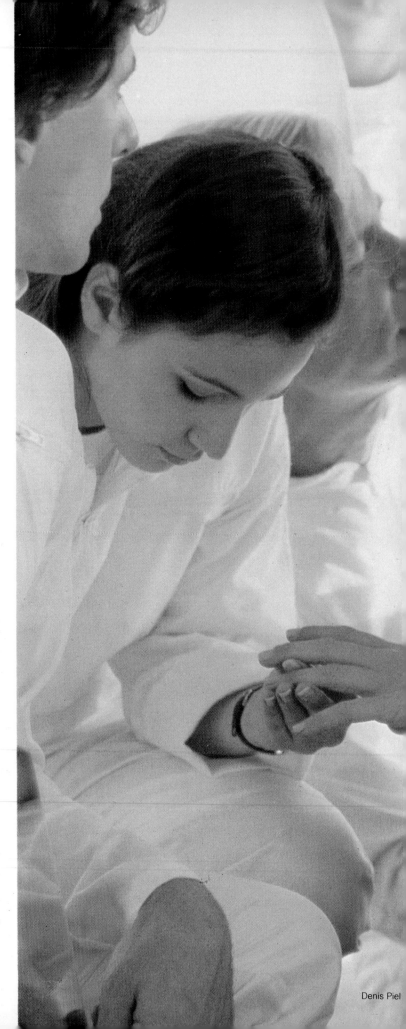

Denis Piel

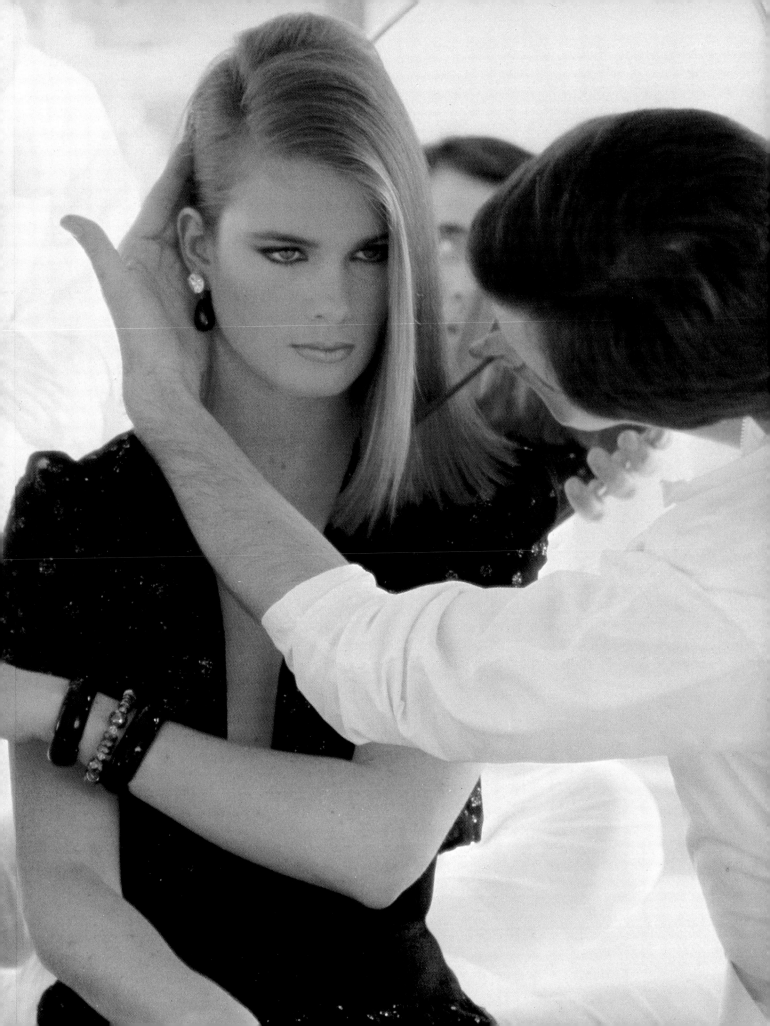

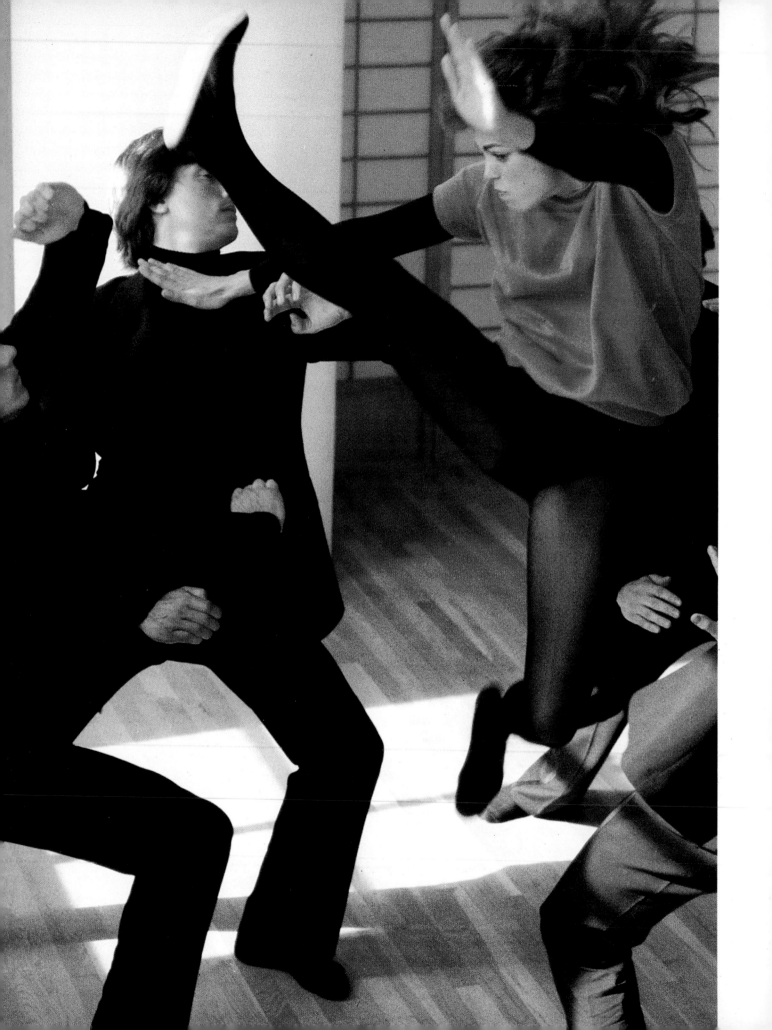

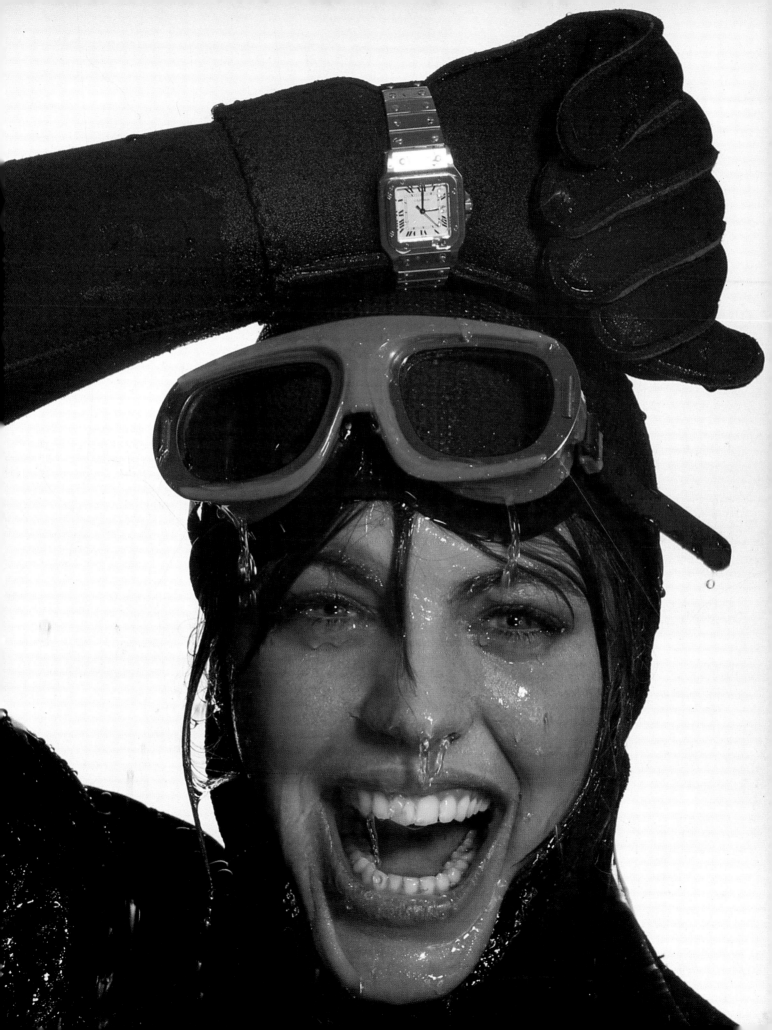

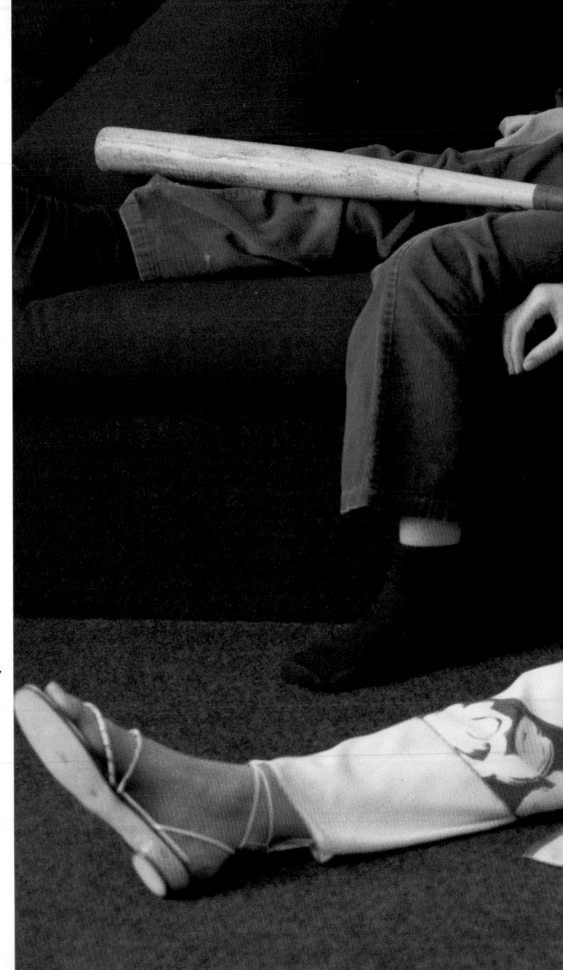

P*receding pages:*
"If you keep your
figure—if your body
is shipshape—you can
wear what's current
forever."

"Not caring about how
you look is a cop-out.
This isn't only physical,
it is also the mental
thing of keeping up
with the times, wanting
to be part of society
and in the swim of
things."

It isn't so much that a
sweater and skirt or a
caftan are "young," as
that they have nothing
to do with a particular
age. They have to do
with ease and comfort
and simplicity: They
are any-age fashion.

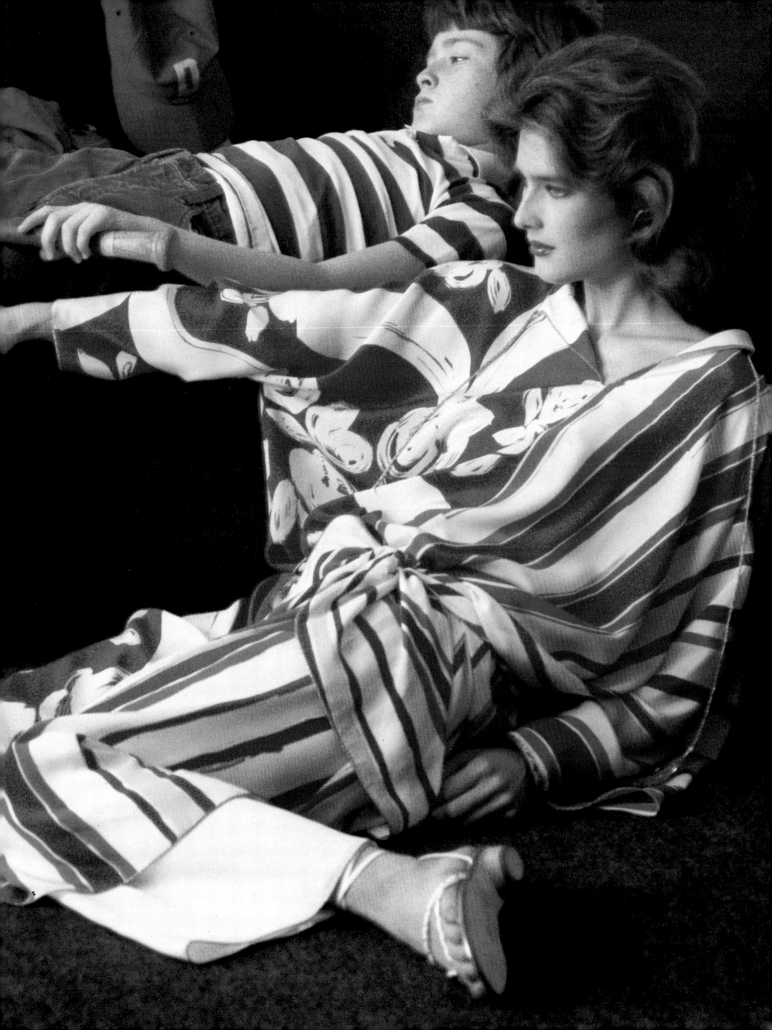

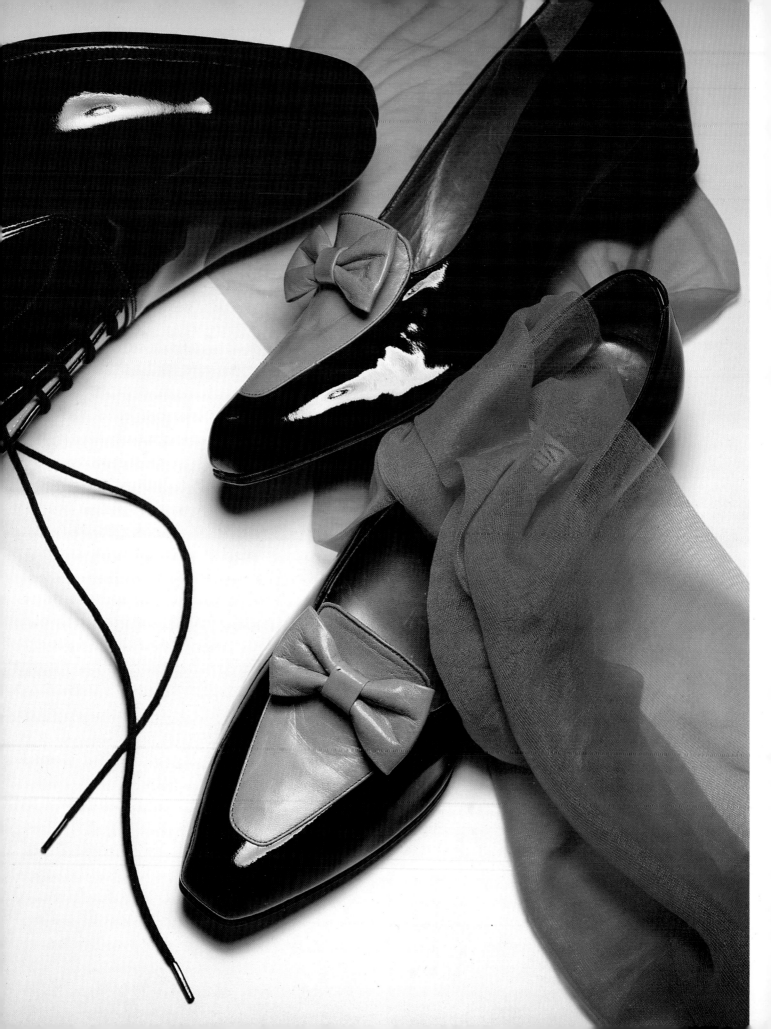

Continued from page 18

stiffly. And everyone looked older. The characteristics of fashion in that time, in direct
contrast to fashion now, define what we think
of as older: Formal is older than casual; what
doesn't move with ease is older than what
does; stiff, heavy and complicated are older
than supple, light and simple; a body in need
of corseting is older than one that isn't. . . .

Let's cross an inevitable bridge of misun-
derstanding: Is there in all of this the implication that younger is better than older? The
answer is: Not if you're talking about age—a
woman walking down the street, with a free
and easy swing to her step, unencumbered by
the clothes she wears, gives off an air of
health and fitness and well-being that we tend
to call young because they are qualities one
associates with youth. In that sense, younger
is better—at any age. The unconvinced might
take an object lesson from this description, by
designer Geoffrey Beene, of a woman he met
on a recent visit to Florida: "She's 75, white-
haired, and I've never seen anyone so alive.
She had on a blue denim skirt. She had on a
sweater (it was coral-colored, which was marvelous with her hair) with the sleeves pushed
up a bit. And she had on espadrilles. Obviously, this woman had chosen to wear these
things because she found them comfortable to
be in, and how she looked reflected how she
felt. She just looked wonderful!"

It isn't so much that a sweater and skirt are
"young," as that they have nothing to do
with any particular age. They have to do with
ease and comfort and simplicity; they are
any-age fashion. Many things are. Many are
not.

. . . . Here, from four of this country's leading designers—Geoffrey Beene, Bill Blass,
Halston and Calvin Klein—some guidelines.

*T*oo high a heel can throw
off the equilibrium and distort
the thrust of the body," states
Mr. Beene. "It's uncomfortable
and it shows."

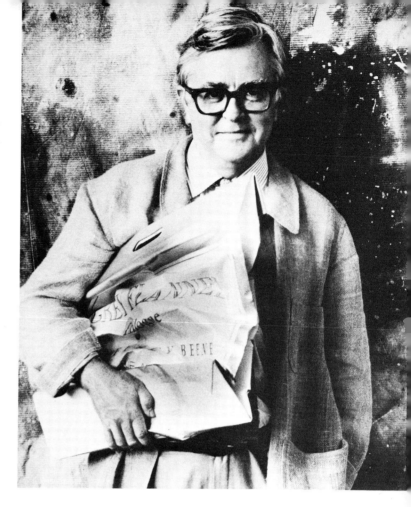

"Comfort comes first . . . more than anything else, it helps to develop personal style"
GEOFFREY BEENE

Comfort comes first—being comfortable in what you're wearing,
liking yourself in it. More than
anything else, it's what helps to
develop personal style, because
being comfortable in your clothes
means you're not thinking about them or how
you look; you feel confident and it comes
through. That's what fashion is really about.
Interestingly, I think, it's typical of a young
mentality to insist on comfort; no 20-year-old
would buy anything she wasn't comfortable
in. The only thing nearly as important is

grooming—no matter how young or how old or what you've got on, if the grooming isn't there, forget it. It's grooming and comfort, then the clothes. . . . This thing about aging, it's all a question of mentality. I know so many women that you'd call quote-older-un-quote. But their attitude is young. One woman I know never wore trousers until she was into her seventies. She said, 'I can't wear them; I'm too large.' Not 'too old,' you see, just 'too large.' And I said, 'Yes, you can wear trousers—if you wear a tunic with them,' because a tunic elongates the figure. Now, of course, she wears trousers all the time; she's an active, modern woman and trousers are active, modern clothes. . . . Once you've found a style of your own—something you're comfortable in, that makes you feel good about yourself and the way you look—you don't change it as you get older. But you can vary it. You can do it in a more sophisticated way. A woman going into her forties, say, who looks terrific in jeans—which implies a certain fitness—should stick with them. But she does not have to stick only to blue denim. She can move on to silk, to cottons, to wonderful colors. Stay with what looks best on you; just refabricate it, recolor it. . . . One thing a woman should watch as she gets older is the height of her heel. Too high a heel can throw off the equilibrium and distort the thrust of the body. It's uncomfortable and it shows. Even a young woman looks ridiculous when she walks off-balance. No matter what the fashion, don't be victimized by it! . . . I think a long dress, all the way to the floor, ages a woman. First of all, it's not modern: It's sweeping the floor, which has echoes of huge cleaning bills or personal maids. Also, it limits one to where one is going. If you have it ankle-length, you can go to a restaurant, you can go to a ball, you can entertain at home. It is just so modern. A long dress is time and place and nothing else. . . . Anything passé is by definition aging. That's why I renounced and denounced retro; it was a horrendous period. Even in their time, those things made women look older: Shoulder pads—what do they do except hinder movement? Those V-necklines! —typical of what not to wear as one ages is anything that is working the same way gravity works. And those strange little ruffles. They never had any body to them. They never rippled. They were just flat. It's always better to give some dimension to clothes. A Peter Pan collar, for instance, is usually crisp, or it stands. The Peter Pan collar is one thing that should be worn a whole lifetime, cradle to grave! It's charming, it's young. It's a question of lifting up rather than dragging down. So; an ascot, a bow, a Peter Pan collar; not a V-neckline. . . . I'd stay away from soft drapery around the face—drapery drapes, skin sags. As a woman ages, I think she should stay away from too-soft clothes, in general. More tailored clothes, neater clothes are what's wanted. There's an uplift and a crispness to tailoring that is ageless. But it should also be soft; I believe in sweatery clothes for all ages, so I use soft fabrics but I give a hard edge to the clothes. It's a matter of defining, of giving clarity to the design. . . . For the same reason, I'm a fanatic about stripes—there's a clarity about them, too. And polka dots. A dot is a dot; a stripe is a stripe. But on the whole, I'd stick to solid-colored clothes. Almost like a man's wardrobe, where we take five or six colors and build on that, and use shirts and ties as accessories to change the classic tweed into something else. . . . Accessories are major because always—at any age—you want to restrict your clothes to simple, simple lines. Forget embellishments that are sewn on or embroidered on; let accessories do the embellishing—a wonderful piece of sculptured jewelry, colored bracelets of all different textures, scarves. . . . Some people think that black is aging. I don't agree at all; with a wonderful chiffon scarf at night—or by day with a scarf of bright suede—it is just beautiful and upbeat for every age.''

"Once you've found a style of your own, don't change it as you get older—vary it—you can do it in a more sophisticated way."

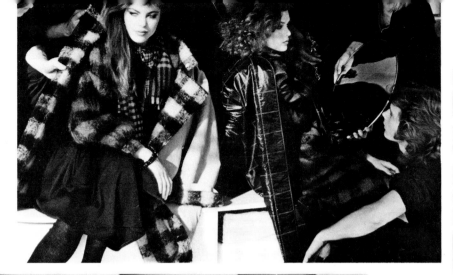

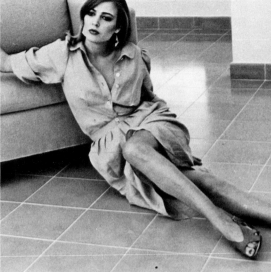

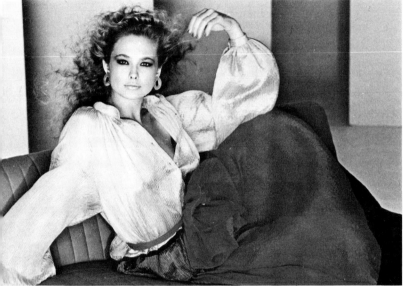

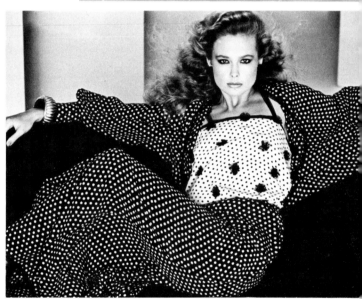

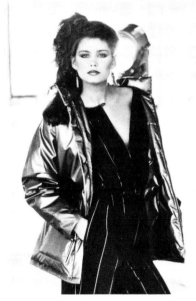

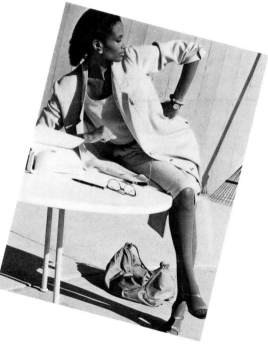

Geoffrey Beene's clothes from the pages of Vogue.

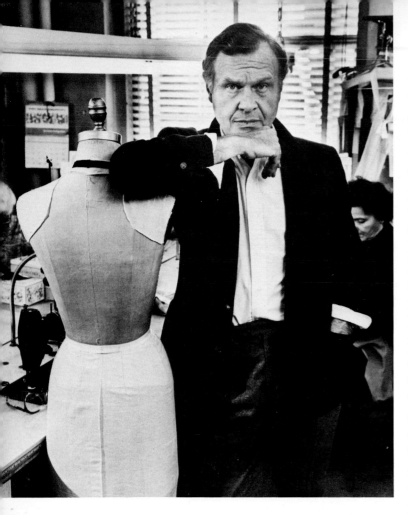

"... youthful is anything you can wear that makes you forget you're wearing clothes"

BILL BLASS

My theory has always been that if you dress in a style that is too young, it can only be aging—jumpers, pinafores, organza dresses with overly big skirts, a too-youthful hairstyle. So many American women tend to wear their hair the way it was most becoming when they were debutantes. The Duchess of Windsor is a good example of the opposite: Although she kept the basic style, she always updated it in a way that was very interesting and contemporary.... A woman who really understands fashion wouldn't wear anything trendy, whatever her age. Nor would she wear clothes that were too tight or clinging if her body wasn't absolutely firm. But first, she has to understand what she looks like; not many women do. Very few ever have an honest approach to themselves, and it's terribly important.... I don't think of a woman in terms of age as much as of figure. As long as she keeps her figure—and her skin and hair are good—her age doesn't make much difference. The fitness program that most women adhere to now is an interesting factor in fashion: When I first came into the business, the average size in America was 14, then it became 12, then 10. Now, I think, it's 8.... Realistically speaking, even a woman who takes care of herself doesn't always have the figure she had as a girl. If she's smart about herself, she wears clothes that minimize not-so-good features. That's why there's no way in the world that fashion will ever kill the chemise; it's extremely becoming to a great many women who may not have a 22-inch waistline. And with good accessories, it will look up-to-date and attractive.... Always aging is jewelry worn around the neck. Earrings are rarely aging, but unless the neck and chin are in superb condition, an elaborate necklace is aging. Also, diamonds may be a girl's best friend, but they are aging—the hardness of them in contrast to skin and facial lines. Black with a diamond necklace or pearls is aging. To look young, black needs marvelous skin color and/or a strong makeup.... Not youthful are constricting clothes, clothes that have set accoutrements, such as a bow or a pouf, or anything that makes you self-conscious.... What *is* youthful is anything you can wear that makes you forget you're wearing clothes, that makes you move easily and young. If you're fit and your hair is good and your skin is good, you can wear a classic raincoat over a dinner dress. You'll look great—and a lot younger than in yards of mink!''

"As long as a woman keeps her figure—and her skin and hair are good—her age doesn't make much difference."

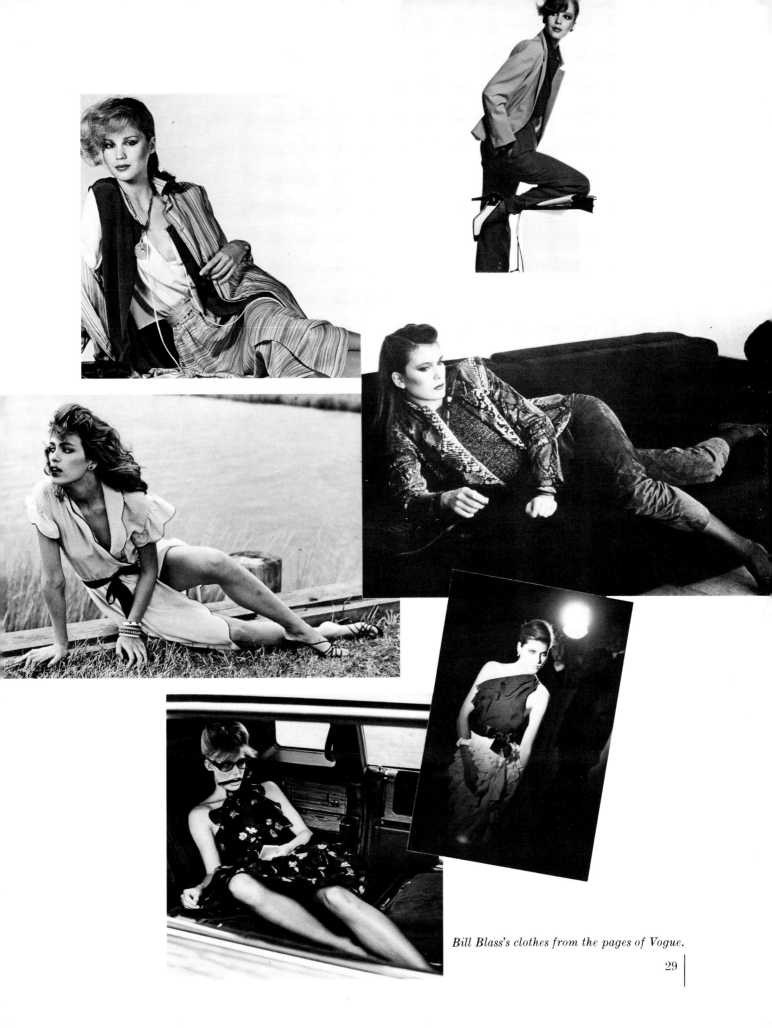

Bill Blass's clothes from the pages of Vogue.

"Simple is best, less is more."

HALSTON

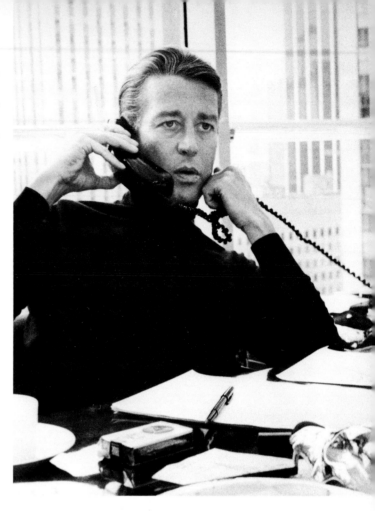

There are no old ladies in America unless they choose to be that. It's a fascinating thing. It used to be that grandmothers didn't compete with their granddaughters. Now, in a funny way, they do. I always think of Babe Paley. She had her children. Her children had children. And she'd walk into a room and turn everybody's head more than her children or grandchildren. It has to do with knowing your own style. And it has to do with change. Some women—say, a woman who grew up in the twenties—tend always to relate to that period, when they were forming their style. They carry it over. In their sixties and seventies, they have a 1920s approach. The more intelligent woman changes constantly. It doesn't mean changing one's central style; that's a matter of knowing what's basically right for you—skirt length, heel height, that sort of thing. The Duchess of Windsor, for instance. She never changed the length of her skirts very much, no matter what the fad of the day. And there are certain women who never change the height of their heel. But maybe boots are in, so they get a boot with that height of heel. And there are certain women who have always worn tailored two-piece suits. But maybe casual sportswear is in, so they get a 'suit' that's a sweater and skirt.... Always look at what's happening and adapt it to yourself. Know yourself. Look at yourself in the mirror, in the nude, and say to yourself: How do I best handle my figure to make me look attractive and fashionable? A woman who is truly interested can adapt almost anything to her needs. She can wear the great American sportwear look of a blouse and skirt. Maybe it can't be a tight-fitting body-blouse because her bosom is too substantial or her waist not too great; it might be an over-blouse instead. It still can be part of the times.... More than just knowing yourself, it's caring about yourself—caring about how you look. Not caring is a cop-out. This isn't only physical; it is also the mental thing of keeping up with the times, wanting to be part of society and in the swim of things. Martha Graham is an example—a woman who really is a grown-up woman who doesn't try to look like a kid, but she always wants to be stylish and have something on that's new and in fashion.... My mother is 73. The other day, I talked with her on the phone. I said, 'Wouldn't you like me to make you something new?' And she said, 'I'd like to have a sexy pajama to wear to play cards.' Now, that made me feel good, because I know she's still in the running. Even if it's to play cards with

"Most women probably need fewer things than they think they do, and simpler things."

30

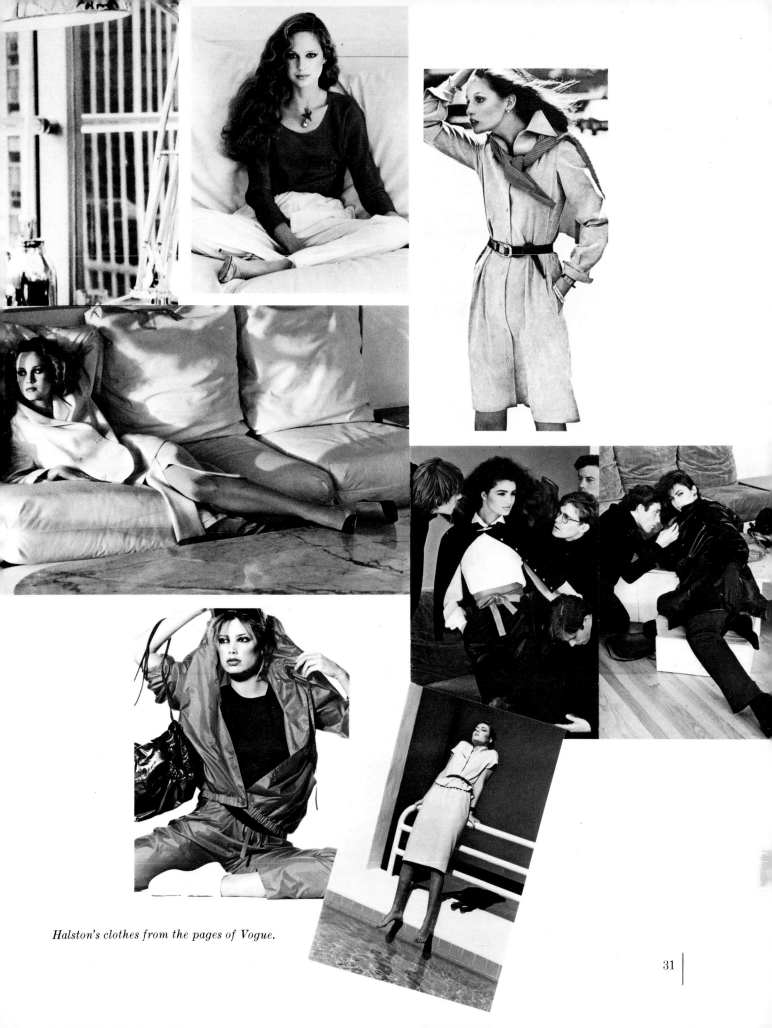

Halston's clothes from the pages of Vogue.

her friends, she wants to look a little bit provocative, just to have people comment.... A pajama, especially for older women, can bring out a youthful quality without being kid-y. It makes you look taller. It elongates the figure. Caftans do that, too. No woman has to resort to the obvious 'old-lady' things—the white-collar-and-cuff approach or the lace collar of the navy-blue dress with a zipper up the back or the princess dress with a little pin on one shoulder.... If you keep your figure—if your body is shipshape—you can wear what's current forever. But you have to take care of yourself. It's food, it's exercise, it's good grooming. Very importantly, it's balance. So often you see people walking on the street, and they're looking down—literally watching their step, because they've somewhat lost their balance and are afraid of falling. In time, it creates a curvature of the shoulders, and the head goes over—in dressmaking, it's called 'old-age hump,' but it doesn't necessarily have to do with being old. It has to do with not standing up straight; gradually you lose the strength to do it, and you lose your balance. The longer you maintain your balance, the longer you maintain your youth!... About dressing, in general: Simple is best, less is more. Most women probably need fewer things than they think they do, and simpler things—clothes that are easy to get in and out of; clothes that work for whatever their life might be; plus something a bit amusing—everyone likes to attract attention now and then.... Have things that interrelate in your wardrobe. Don't spread the color around. Let's say you're going to concentrate on beige. You buy beiges that relate to each other. You might buy a beige suit; you might buy a beige dress. And you use browns for all your accessories. In other words, limit the color, limit the accessories. Then each season, you can buy a little something that will update your wardrobe—a scarf, a new jewelry idea, a belt. But as a basic rule: Have what's of the moment, but not too much of the moment.''

"If you feel good about yourself . . . if you're active, you're bound to have a younger attitude. And it shows in everything . . ."

CALVIN KLEIN

I used to think there were rules about what looks older or what looks younger. I don't know if that's true anymore. For instance, beads on dresses might be something one associates with an older person, but it doesn't always work that way. We took beads and put them on suede and, while it's not for a teenager, it's very young. On crepe or georgette, it tended to get older. Some prints look older—little, tiny, muddy, nondescript prints are dowdy-looking—like the print Bette

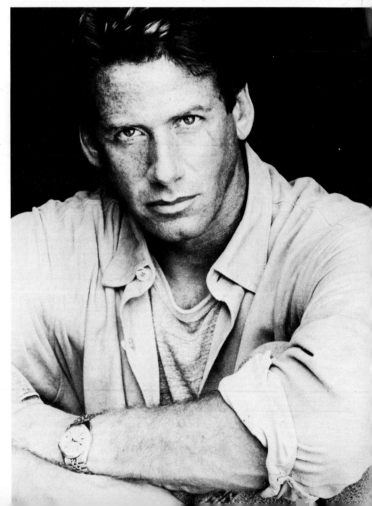

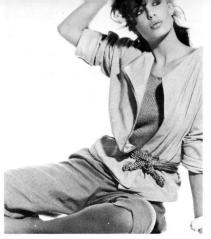

Davis wore in the first part of *Now Voyager*. Or *The Prime of Miss Jean Brodie*. When we do longer lengths—mid-calf-length skirts—

"I think youthfulness in fashion has to do with the simplicity of the clothes. Simplicity of cut, of fabric, of accessories."

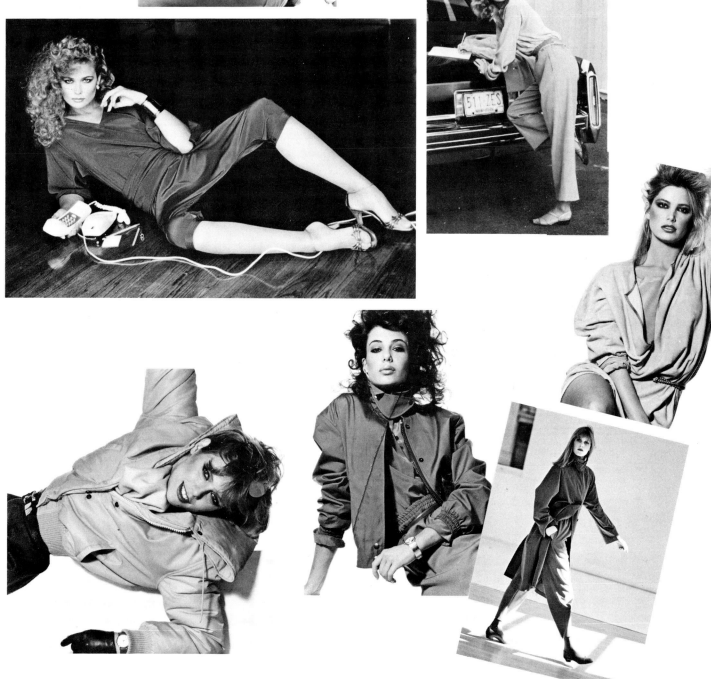

Calvin Klein's clothes from the pages of Vogue.

they're never straight. The straight skirt that is short looks great, very young. But the straight skirt that goes to mid-calf starts to look like *The Prime of Miss Jean Brodie*. But if you make it full, it's young and swingy. Gray can be aging, but gray flannel is young. Things can be made to look younger.... Sometimes a longer waistline is older, because lines that are lower tend to bring your eyes down. The more your eye goes up, the younger. If you lift the waist up—if you make a jacket about a quarter-of-an-inch shorter in front—it gives you a prettier and younger look.... While I don't so much believe in rules about clothes—like saying don't wear black because it's aging (black can be very young)—I do think there are rules about attitude. If you feel good about yourself, if you're healthy, if you work, if you're active, you're bound to have a younger attitude. And it shows in everything you do. Look at Ali MacGraw. Here is a 40-year-old woman who takes care of herself, is interested in her body and clothes and everything that's happening. She can wear anything. She looks great in jeans; she would never put on a pair of jeans and say, I'm too old to wear jeans. She would just wear what she liked.... I believe in clothes that move with the body, that relate to the body, that are soft and feminine but not in the sense that they are loaded with ruffles or feathers or have tricks all over them. If women stick with what's relatively simple—if it's a print, it shouldn't be absolutely tiny—I don't think they can go wrong. The danger is in trying to be too of-the-moment. It's safer to stick to something ... I hate to say 'classic' because I don't mean only a man-tailored jacket and a shirt ... but something pure in line, not over-designed ... clothes that are just sort of easy to wear.... Anything retro adds years. Anything that looks antiquated, anything that looks outdated should be avoided; it doesn't make sense to go back. I think that hats in general, unless it's a knitted pull-on stocking hat, should be avoided. Hair shouldn't be too

short, too pulled away from the face. It shouldn't be too long; it should be just framing the face.... There are furs one tends to associate with old ladies. I'd keep away from Persian lamb. Even if you're 20, it's aging—it's heavy and it brings you down. One always hears that mink is flattering. I'm not so sure; that very, very deep, dark shade that's supposed to be good I think is difficult for an older woman to wear.... Diamonds have the same associations for me as mink, and I'd stay away from them. On the other hand, Elsa Peretti took diamonds and made them young; her Diamonds by the Yard are young because they're not so serious-looking. It's what I try to do with clothes. I try to take wonderful, luxurious fabrics and treat them casually rather than as if they were very serious and important. Not too long ago, some European designers were putting whalebone in crepe de Chine. But the whole point of crepe de Chine is that it's thin and soft and absolutely drips on the body. So why try to give it something that has nothing to do with its character? Why make it stiff and old when it should be soft and young?... Whenever I think of Balenciaga's clothes, I think of an older person. They're so rigidly constructed they stand up by themselves. They look very serious, very important and therefore older. And then I think of Chanel, whose clothes were really soft. Even a suit jacket was very soft, almost like a sweater. Those things make a woman look younger. In constructed clothes there is no sense of the woman's body. And you can't move easily in them. You have to walk slowly, which is elderly. Young people move; clothes should move. They shouldn't have a life of their own. Constructed clothes do. So do some synthetics, such as double-knit polyesters. So do double-faced coats; buy an unlined coat instead—it's soft, it moves and it costs a lot less!... Mostly, I think youthfulness in fashion has to do with the simplicity of the clothes. Simplicity of cut, of fabric, of accessories. The more you put on—the more dressing, the more detail—the more you apply, the older it gets. It's like decoration in a house—moldings and a lot of stuff applied to the walls make it look a bit older, of another time, not modern. . . . If a woman shops in the sportswear department, as opposed to the dress department, she's got a much better chance of coming up with clothes that are modern and youthful. They're active clothes; the attitude is younger than the attitude about dresses. Dresses can be wonderful, but most that I see tend to make women look older—dresses with zippers rather than dresses that simply wrap, which would be great; too-formal dresses, too uptight, too much for the older woman. But most sportswear—most jackets, most skirts, most sweaters, most blouses—looks younger to me. . . . Most clothes that are supposed to flatter a woman's figure by camouflaging certain faults tend to have an opposite effect: You automatically assume that what's being camouflaged is more hopeless than it probably is. It's an old-lady look. So-called 'illusion' dresses are the same sort of thing. Usually, it's a dress with a slit that isn't really going

anywhere and maybe chiffon on top—if you can't wear it sheer all the way, avoid it entirely. I saw a television program recently. The star was a woman in her fifties, with a really good body. But she chose to wear a nice, obviously expensive, ladylike 'illusion' dress, and it aged her. It was a chiffon dress—one layer of chiffon, but with a slip so that the breasts were covered. It could have been just two layers of chiffon, which would have been great. If I had been dressing her, I wouldn't have put her in something that sheer—maybe crepe de Chine—because she obviously wanted to cover herself up. But in that case, she should have been covered up, period, rather than trying to create an 'illusion' of being bare. It's an old-fashioned kind of refinement, neither tantalizing nor sensual. Deceptions are out of date. To be all covered up is a younger attitude."

In the mix of texture and color—in the putting together of pieces as Calvin Klein presented them here—he turns the whole world of separates dressing in a new direction.

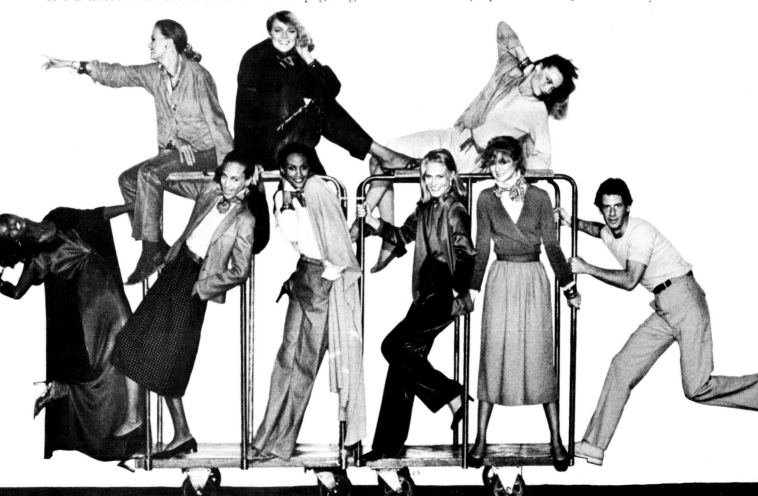

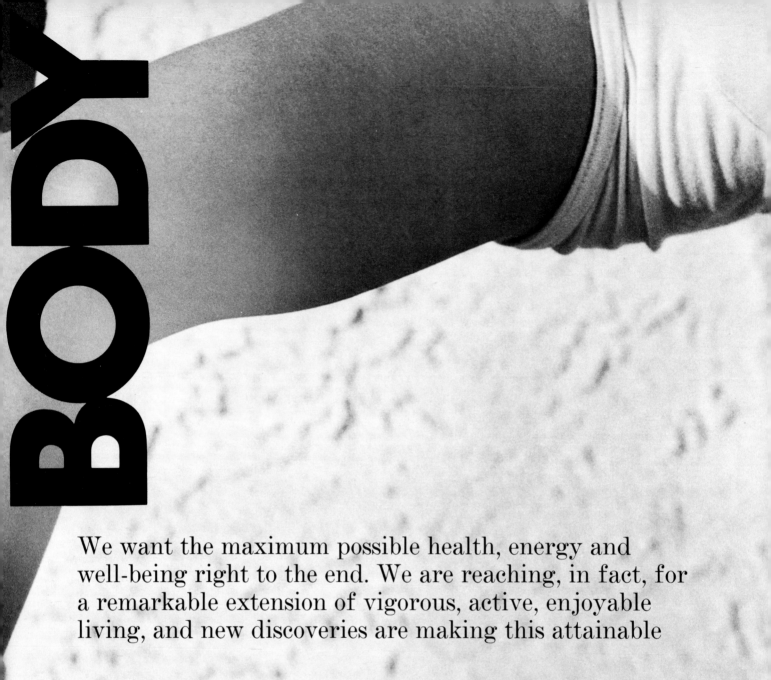

BODY

We want the maximum possible health, energy and well-being right to the end. We are reaching, in fact, for a remarkable extension of vigorous, active, enjoyable living, and new discoveries are making this attainable

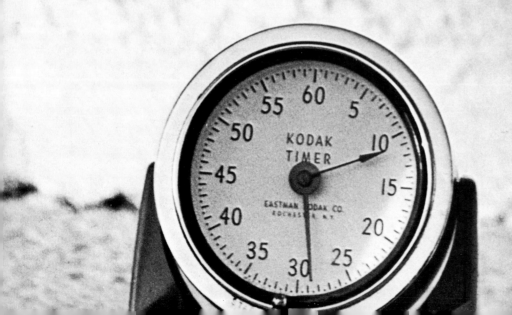

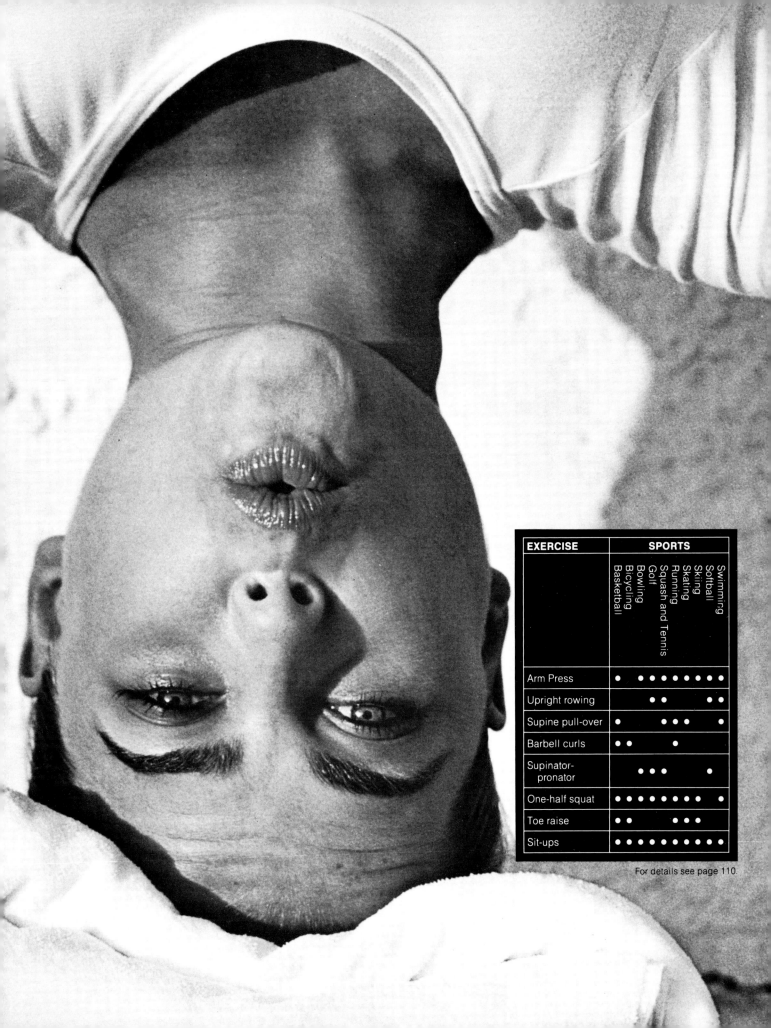

EXERCISE	Swimming	Softball	Skiing	Skating	Running	Squash and Tennis	Golf	Bowling	Bicycling	Basketball
Arm Press	●		●	●	●	●	●	●	●	●
Upright rowing			●	●					●	●
Supine pull-over	●			●	●	●				●
Barbell curls	●	●			●					
Supinator-pronator			●	●	●					●
One-half squat	●	●	●	●	●	●	●			●
Toe raise	●	●			●	●	●			
Sit-ups	●	●	●	●	●	●	●	●	●	●

For details see page 110.

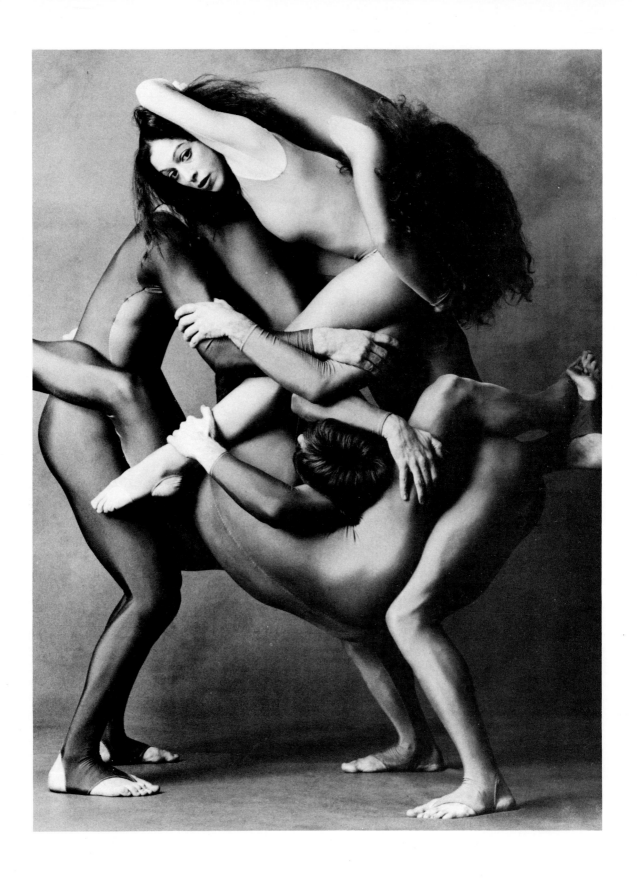

BODY

by Melva Weber

Corporeal; of the body. Each one of us has an aging body—infant, schoolboy, bride, executive, grandparent. With time's passing, changes occur—in cell, organ, total body.

Discard at once the old fuzzy notion that bodily aging processes are all bad, all breakdown and deterioration. Many people are physically more comfortable as they grow older, are less prone to infectious diseases—probably from having acquired a wealth of antibodies. The wise ones have learned to take care of their health, have outgrown poor habits and body neglect. They also know that physical well-being is the single most important key to rewarding, worthwhile living. And many find a growing intensity and sense of adventure, from the maturing years right into advanced age. For them, life gets more exciting with each passing day.

The present era, in which persons past 65 make up the fastest-growing segment of our population, brings with it some new insights on body aging. Medical investigators are finding out that many body conditions attributed to aging—and neglected because they have been considered inevitable—are instead highly treatable, often reversible. They may also be largely preventable.

Pilobolus dance group demonstrates the extraordinary flexibility of the body.

Lewis Thomas, M.D., president of Memorial Sloan-Kettering Cancer Center in New York City, as well as a renowned writer on biology, sets up a goal for us as we consider our bodies and the time we have for living. Our model, writes Dr. Thomas, is found in a poem by Oliver Wendell Holmes, ''The Deacon's Masterpiece, or, the Wonderful One-Hoss Shay.'' In it, the deacon sets out to build a carriage, or chaise, in which each part is as strong and enduring as every other part—in short, no weak places that could bring about a premature breakdown.

The chaise was built to last—and did last—for 100 years. Then—a carriage, like a human body, must wear out some time—the old one-hoss shay simply fell apart, all at once. ''No grief,'' comments Dr. Thomas, ''just, in the way of the world, total fulfillment.''

> . . . it went to pieces all at once—
> All at once, and nothing first—
> Just as bubbles do when they burst.

Dr. Thomas continues: ''This is, in high metaphor, what happens when a healthy old creature, old man or old mayfly, dies. There is no outside evil force, nor any central flaw. The dying is built into the system so that it can occur at once, at the end of a pre-clocked, genetically determined allotment of living.''

If we accept the possibility that our bodies

39

are programmed to wear out at the end of a lifespan—and this is only one of several theories about aging—we are still vitally interested in achieving that full lifespan; we don't want to die earlier than necessary. We also want the maximum possible health, energy and well-being right to the end. We want more than to merely prolong age or relieve some age-related disabilities. We are reaching, in fact, for a remarkable extension of vigorous, active, enjoyable living.

Let us briefly examine the normal aging process as it affects various parts of the body —never forgetting that we are reviewing only what has happened in the past, not what is becoming possible. New biological discoveries and ever-improving health care can be expected, even in our own time, to prevent, reduce in severity, or greatly postpone many of the problems of aging as they have been known in the past.

KEEPING THE HEART YOUNG

A remarkable fist-shaped organ, the heart beats about three billion times during an average lifetime—but is certainly not preset to stop at the three-billion-and-first beat. In the absence of circulatory disease, such as high blood pressure or clogged blood vessels, the heart is built to last a great deal longer. And, indeed, this nation's hearts are getting healthier all the time; heart disease deaths have dropped by 20 percent in the past decade. Health experts believe good changes in the American lifestyle have brought about the improvement—more exercise, better weight control, earlier attention and treatment for high blood pressure.

The heart does undergo changes as age advances. There is a gradual loss of muscle fibers, and granules of protein and fat accumulate to replace muscles. The aged heart pumps less blood; at 90, it may be pumping about half the amount it pumped at 20. But the change is highly individual. Many over-80

persons have hearts that work better than those of many 40-year-olds.

Blood vessels gradually lose elasticity. The walls of the larger vessels become a little thicker, with slowly increasing connective tissue. The connective tissue gets stiffer. These changes could, but don't necessarily, cause blood pressure to rise.

Build-up of fatty plaques inside the blood vessels, or atherosclerosis, is a disease, not an inevitable condition of aging. Kept disease-free, the heart and circulation can more than meet the demands of vigorous living for a very long time. In response to physical exercise, for example, the amount of blood being pumped can be doubled or tripled, although with aging the maximum possible output of the heart is less, as is its reserve capacity, and recovery from a burst of activity will be slower.

Blood pressure rises with age, usually gradually and moderately. Thus at age 25, one's systolic pressure (at the peak contraction of the heart) might be around 116–125, and the diastolic pressure (during the dilated stage of the heartbeat) between 73 and 76. When the same person reaches his or her seventies, the systolic pressure may be 150–160, while the diastolic pressure hovers around 80. Clearly, the systolic or contraction pressure increases with age at a faster rate than does the dilated pressure. The blood pressure usually stops rising as one enters the seventies, and after the age of 80 both men and women commonly experience a drop in blood pressure.

Since it happens to most people in the industrialized world, the age-related rise in blood-pressure is considered "normal." But is it? In other cultures—for example, among natives of New Guinea—blood pressures do not normally rise with age, but may even gradually decline in the elderly. Studies in some African areas have shown generally lower systolic pressures throughout life, and very slight changes with aging.

What can we do to stay literally, physically, young in heart?

HOW AEROBICS BURN OFF CALORIES

According to Dr. Cooper, by combining an aerobics program with a reduced-calorie diet, you burn up 100 percent fat. Without exercise, you burn up 50 percent fat, 50 percent muscle and wind up with sagging tissues.

● Exercises Burning 100–149 Calories	Walk 1½ miles in 30 min. Walk/jog 1 mile in 12 min. Run 1 mile in 8 min. Swim 900 yards in 30 min. Cycle 3 miles in 12 min.
● Exercises Burning 200–249 Calories	Walk 3 miles in 45 min. Walk/jog 2 miles in 24 min. Run 2 miles in 16 min. Swim 1,350 yards in 45 min. Cycle 6 miles in 24 min.
● Exercises Burning 350–399 Calories	Walk 5½ miles in 1 hour, 36 min. Walk/jog 3 miles in 36 min. Run 3½ miles in 28 min. Swim 1,350 yards in 36 min. Cycle 9 miles in 36 min.
● Exercises Burning 450–500 Calories	Walk 7 miles in 2 hours 20 min. Walk/jog 4 miles in 48 min. Run 4 miles in 32 min. Swim 1,800 yards in 48 min. Cycle 12 miles in 48 min.

From Aerobics For Women, © 1972 by Mildred Cooper and Kenneth H. Cooper, M.D. Reprinted by permission of the publisher, M. Evans and Co., Inc., N.Y.

Exercise, certainly. Physical action produces better circulation and improved well-being, as well as protection from heart attacks. "Vigorous, regular activity reduces an individual's risk of heart attack by as much as 35 percent," declared Ralph S. Paffenbarger, Jr., M.D., of Stanford University.

Let it be aerobic exercise, specifies Kenneth H. Cooper, M.D., M.P.H., president and founder of the Aerobic Center in Dallas. This means activity demanding a large amount of oxygen over a fairly long period, making the heart and lungs produce a sustained effort.

Along with the decreasing incidence of heart disease, American *diet patterns* have changed—largely for the better.

In America, controlling weight is virtually a national obsession. Weight-loss methods fill countless magazine pages, books, TV programs—and also fill the coffers of a host of related businesses and manufacturers. And, it appears, this pays off not merely in profits for purveyors but in better condition for the person who stays slim. Since obesity is related to higher blood pressures, keeping off unnecessary pounds can mean erasing one more health risk factor. The Baltimore Longitudinal Study of Aging has found, however, that mild to moderate obesity does not seem to shorten the average lifespan in the population studied—although, as we'll discuss later, animal experiments indicate that controlled food intake may greatly extend the lifespan.

Although the improving patterns of diet and exercise are definitely benefiting heart and circulatory health for more and more people, we still have some distance to go regarding some food habits. We are eating *too much salt* for the state of our blood pressure, and *too much fat* for our blood vessels.

No smoking is a cardinal rule for health of the heart and circulatory system, as well as dozens of other bodily sites and functions. Smoking impairs heart performance, as shown in study after study. Significantly increased heart rates taken one minute after test exercise have been found in smokers of all ages and in both sexes. The heart works harder, faster, but less efficiently. In his *Healthy People* report, Surgeon General Julius Richmond states that smoking is the largest single preventable cause of illness and premature death in the United States. Smokers, he says, have a 70 percent greater death rate from all causes. Tobacco is associated with 320,000 premature deaths each year and with 10 million cases of debilitating chronic disease. If Americans stopped smoking, says the Surgeon General, coronary deaths alone would drop by 30 percent, a saving of more than 200,000 lives per year.

Significant lifestyle changes now going on in America are resulting in improved health, well-being and life expectancy in more and more of our people. One important item in the brightening health picture: More than 30 million Americans have quit smoking.

THE DIGESTIVE TECHNOLOGY

Built to last, the digestive system tends to change very little as years go by. There is a gradual decrease in the stomach's secretion of hydrochloric acid and other enzymes, but most nutrients should continue to be absorbed as well in the elderly as in younger people. Studies show some impairment in fat absorption with advancing age, and this may be why we notice that most people in their mid-eighties and nineties are relatively thin. Nutritional practices of the future may postpone the aging process in the digestive system until well into the second century of life.

What is most important, when we consider the effects of aging on the digestive system, is proper maintenance and nutrition. By and large, the digestive problems of older people are not caused by age; many can be corrected and even reversed.

Start with teeth. Problems of digestion often begin with inadequate chewing of food because teeth are missing or need repair, a situation that can be allowed to start quite early in life.

The dental handicap to good digestion is likely to diminish with today's improved dental care and the reduction of tooth decay in the young due to fluoridated water and dentrifrices. Dental experts predict that we'll soon see the first whole generation of school youngsters in whom tooth decay will be virtually nonexistent. Growing older, those children probably will be spared many "digestive" complaints whose source today is dental.

The intestinal tract is an ever-busy, self-regulating, beautifully coordinated system. It receives liquefied food from the stomach and, using at least four kinds of muscular movements, it mixes, kneads, processes, squeezes and moves the contents along to colon and rectum, whose job it is to signal the owner and assist in expelling the residue, or feces.

Much more in the past generation than at present, people have mistreated, overdosed and generally abused their intestines through a combination of bad habits and misguided use of laxatives. A great many people still are living with a kind of intestinal Catch-22: While eating a diet of largely refined, low-residue foods, they are still under the delusion that a daily bowel movement is an absolute

THE ADEQUATE MEDICINE CABINET				
Basic equipment	For minor injuries	For short-term mild discomfort	For prevention or treatment of skin woes	Emergency phone numbers
Toothbrush Dental floss Toothpaste Thermometer	Bandage strips Gauze Cotton Adhesive tape Hydrogen peroxide or styptic pencil (to check minor bleeding)	(not for continuous use) Aspirin Nasal decongestant Diarrhea medication Laxative Antacid Liniment	Petroleum jelly Hand lotion Sunscreen Lip balm Calamine lotion Talcum powder or cornstarch Fungicidal cream or powder	Doctors treating family members Local emergency service (911 in many areas) Local hospital emergency room Private ambulance service (choose one that can give cardiac emergency care, if possible) Poison control center All-night drugstore

must; if they don't have one, they believe they are constipated and must take a laxative. Older persons, more likely to have these impressions, may also believe that faulty bowel function is part of growing older, and may therefore dose themselves regularly with laxatives.

THE FACTS:

Both the amount and frequency of bowel movements depend on the undigested material that is left after the digestion process. A diet with a good deal of bulk and fiber produces more stool, more often, compared with a smooth, concentrated, low-bulk diet.

Simple constipation, which can happen to anyone, usually is best handled by adding some bulk, such as a daily serving of bran cereal, to the diet. Plenty of fluid, such as an extra two glassfuls of water in addition to other beverages, is essential. Finally, good bowel habits may need to be established. People who habitually have postponed or ignored the urge to defecate run the risk of dimming the urge signal, weakening the defecation reflexes. With prompt attention to the bowel movement urge, the intestinal system tends to become regulated. Children ordinarily produce bowel movements following meals; adults may develop individual scheduling. Perfectly normal bowel frequencies range from three times a day to once in three days —and in some people, either more or fewer can be within normal limits.

Use of a laxative may be justified, according to medical advisors, on the infrequent occasions when you've eaten unwisely and have had an upset that produced difficult or hard, dry stools. But regular laxative use may aggravate constipation, rather than relieve it, and can interfere with nutrient and vitamin absorption.

Above all, reject the idea that the intestinal tract runs down or wears out with age. It doesn't, but it can do either with misuse.

75,000 (±) MEALS OVER YOUR LIFETIME

Could you get along on less than two-thirds of what you're eating now? What if it meant a dramatic increase in your lifespan, and during nearly all of that lifetime you would keep the muscle tone and strength of youth, maintain high resistance to infections, kidney disease and cancer, have the cholesterol and blood fat levels of a youngster, and stay slim and lively into advanced old age?

It's being achieved in experimental rats. At the University of Texas Health Science Cen-

> **" New biological discoveries . . . can be expected, even in our own time, to prevent, reduce or greatly postpone many of the problems of aging "**

ter in San Antonio, physiology department chairman Edward J. Masoro, Ph.D., conducts research into metabolic changes that occur with aging as they affect the physiology of the laboratory rat. Rats' bodies have similarities to humans'; they metabolize foods and other substances in similar ways, and they have an average lifespan of only about two years, so they are important experimental subjects for scientists trying to unravel the mysteries of aging.

With colleagues Helen Bertrand, Ph.D., and Byung Pal Yu, Ph.D., Dr. Masoro placed on tests two groups of rats; one group was fed a well-balanced nutritious diet which they were allowed *ad libitum,* or as much as they liked. The other group of rats received similar food, but were only given 60 percent of what rats normally eat when allowed to feed freely.

The freely fed animals, well cared-for by all rat standards, had a median 23½ months of life, with the oldest reaching 32 months. The restricted-diet rats had a median life length of 35 months. Their maximum length of life was not known, Dr. Masoro said, because as the study was being reported some of them were still alive at a venerable 44 months. The oldest lived to 47½ months.

Comparing rat lives with human lives (which scientists hesitate to do because it may lead to imprecise conclusions) and assuming the rat's two-year life is comparable to the human three-score-and-ten, then the well-fed rats achieved, on the average, about a 70-year lifespan and their oldest member had died at about 93.2 human years. But the average life of the underfed rats was comparable to about 105 years, and the old-timers still alive at the time of reporting were, by human standards, around 132 years old.

Beyond remarkable delays in metabolic aging, the Texas scientists observed that food restriction delayed age-related loss in muscle mass and function; in other words, it took much longer for muscles to become shrunken and weak. Other studies have found earlier that breakdown of the immune system, which provides resistance to infections, also is greatly delayed in food-restricted test animals.

Achieving the ultimate step the Texas team aims for—translating our rat knowledge into a workable diet lifestyle for people—is still some distance down the road.

" A great many people are still living with a kind of intestinal Catch-22 "

Dr. Masoro and his colleagues believe delays in the body aging process, produced by restricting the diet, are themselves the reason thin rats live longer, through retarding the development of conditions that allow breakdown and result in death. This means being slower to get old, not merely slower to die. If this holds true, it may help answer the important question: "Why extend our lives for more years merely to be old, weak and ailing for a longer time?" The hopeful answer: Ex-

tending the years would be a by-product. The primary aim—continued vigor and well-being inside the framework of those years—would mean becoming, in a sense, larger than life.

KEEPING THE LUNGS YOUNG

Three hundred million alveoli, tiny air sacs, are alloted to the average adult pair of lungs; a generous endowment clearly designed for many years of effective work.

Lung functions diminish very gradually with aging. The total amount of air you can draw into the lungs may be somewhat less at 45 or 50 than at 20. The amount of air you can push out after filling the lungs as much as possible—a measure called vital capacity—also becomes less with aging. This means the amount of air left behind in the lungs is proportionately greater.

Nobody can say whether these or many other "aging processes" are natural for human beings. Age-related effects as observed and measured by western-world scientists reflect the changes that happen to most people, not what must inevitably happen.

Far greater threats to respiratory health than the aging process are smoking, other air pollutants, infections and allergies. The greatest of these is smoking. Besides being directly related to lung cancer—100,000 deaths each year, 80 percent of them attributed to smoking—smoking also is associated with disabling and fatal lung diseases including emphysema and chronic bronchitis.

Even when it doesn't set off disease, smoking accelerates the aging process in lung tissues. If you smoke, say lung specialists, your lungs may be physiologically older than you are.

But the lungs are forgiving: When cigarette smokers quit smoking, lung tissues immediately start to recover, and lung function measurements begin to improve. Long-term heavy smokers between 50 and 60 years old have returned to normal, healthy lung performance within a year or two after they stopped smoking.

What should be done to keep the lungs "young"? Will deep-breathing exercises help? Can exercise increase lung capacity?

Conscious deep-breathing exercises are pointless, say pulmonary authorities; at best they may bring on hyperventilation, which makes you dizzy. Sonia Buist, M.D. an expert in research on respiratory function at the University of Oregon's Health Sciences Center, explains why: "Control of your breathing is automatic and unconscious," she says, explaining that the body has a chemical sens-

❝ Many over-80 persons have hearts that work better than those of many 40-year-olds ❞

ing and feedback system, with sensors that detect the smallest changes in carbon dioxide. "Suppose you now hold your breath. The chemical receptors sense it and immediately send a message to the brain: 'For heaven's sake, take a breath.' When you take the breath, sensory receptors in muscles, chest wall and diaphragm get somewhat stretched and send back a message saying, 'You've breathed in enough; breathe out now.' So breathing is quite complex, but it is quite automatic."

Lung tissue has no muscles of its own, so exercise does not expand lung volume, Dr. Buist explains. Even athletic conditioning does not expand the lung capacity. But what exercise (swimming, running, walking, bike riding, dancing) does do is tune up the muscles, heart and circulatory system, which in turn helps the whole body.

The major concern with age and lung health is not that lungs get old, but that accumulated, repeated assaults by pollution and infection can bring on impairment over time. Steps to take, as suggested by specialists, include:

- *Tests of breathing capacity, called spirometry. These should be routinely done in physical examinations, believes Dr. Cooper of the Aerobics Center, to provide early detection of emphysema, a lung-damage condition that affects 1.3 million Americans and kills 18,000 each year. Doctors can do much to stop or slow down the progress of this disease, in which the breather had trouble emptying the lungs.*

- *Older people in particular should guard against influenza. It's suggested that persons with mild breathing impairment or in the older age groups should consult their physicians before flu season begins each year, for a decision on whether health risks warrant flu prevention treatment by vaccination or anti-viral drugs.*

- *Doctors agree that outdoor exercise in badly polluted air has dubious value, and may be hazardous to those with chronic bronchitis or other lung conditions. Even for people with healthy lungs, Dr. Cooper says, "My strong recommendation is don't exercise outdoors if there's a smog alert. People with any pulmonary problems should limit outdoor activities even without a smog alert, if the pollution is considerable."*

- *Exercises can help emphysema—not breathing exercises, but whole-body exercises to strengthen muscles.*

HEALTH CHECKUPS YOU NEED

To watch model Michelle Stevens in action is to take a lesson in fitness—what it is, how to live it. We chose her to demonstrate the process because she is an average, young, healthy working woman and because her plan for staying healthy and looking her best is one she's worked out with the expert advice of doctors. (Prerequisite for being good to yourself: being well informed about what's good for you.) While Michelle asked the experts

```
- - - - - - - - - - - - - - - - - - - - - - - - - - - - - - - - - - - - -
        12 YOUR RISKS IN DESCENDING IMPORTANCE
    A RISK FACTOR OF 1.0 IS AVERAGE. A RISK FACTOR LESS THAN 1.0 CARRIES LESS THA
    AVERAGE RISK. A RISK FACTOR ABOVE 1.0 CARRIES GREATER THAN AVERAGE RISK.
- - - - - - - - - - - - - - - - - - - - - - - - - - - - - - - - - - - - -
12A ARTERIOSCLEROTIC HEART DISEASE          {HEART ATTACK}

    13 AVERAGE     RISK        1,344   **********
    14 YOUR CURRENT RISK       3,494   ****************************    { 2.6 X AVG
    15 YOUR ACHIEVABLE RISK      968   *******                        {  .7 X AVG
```

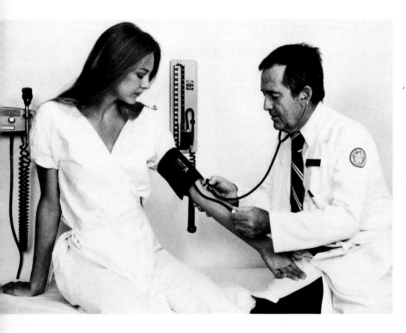

questions about how to improve on her own routine, we asked them about the basic premises of fitness and health—and good looks—for any woman. Their answers follow. Their consensus on what makes fitness work as a way of life: exercise that's fun, common-sense eating, an intelligent approach to preventing disease.

Left: Before starting an exercise program, one good check is a blood pressure reading. John H. Laragh, M.D., director of the Hypertension and Cardiovascular Center at the New York Hospital-Cornell Medical Center, measures blood pressure. "In the early stages of high blood pressure, there are no symptoms. This is why it's important to check annually," he says.
Right: Thomas C. Pickering, M.D., associate professor of Medicine at New York Hospital-Cornell Medical Center, administers a stress test. Michelle ran for 12 minutes on the treadmill, while Dr. Pickering continually increased the gradient, monitored her blood pressure, and kept close watch on the cardiograph for signs of strain, extra beats, or shortness of blood supply. At test's end, he pronounced Michelle's cardiovascular system normal and fit for vigorous exercise.

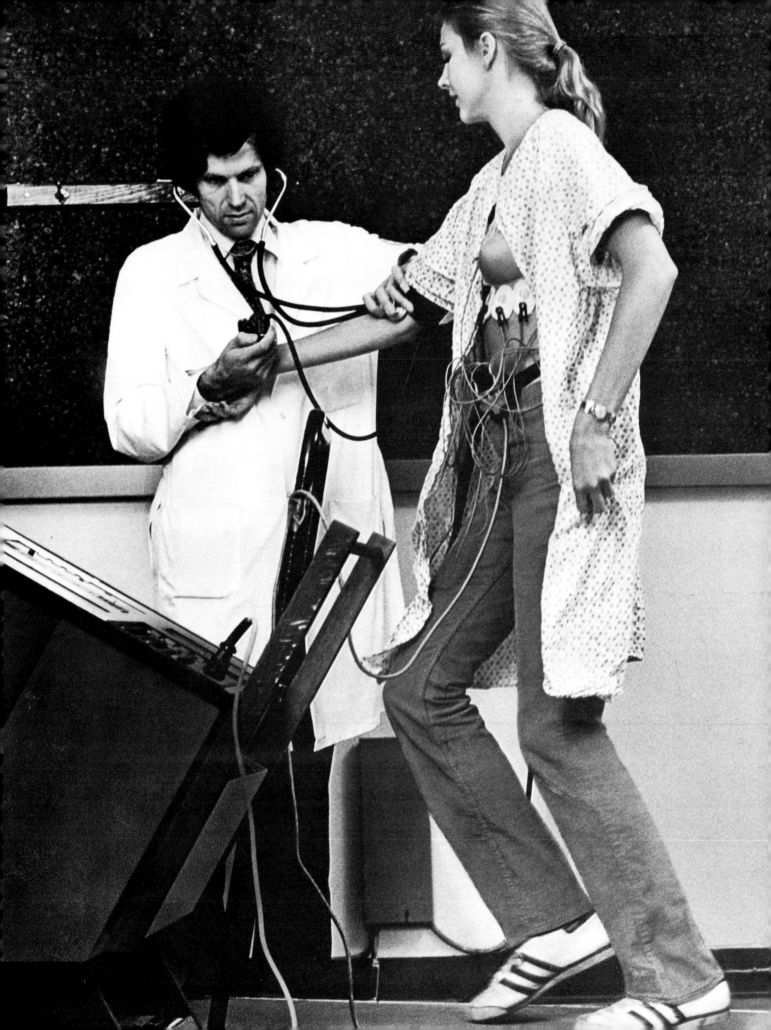

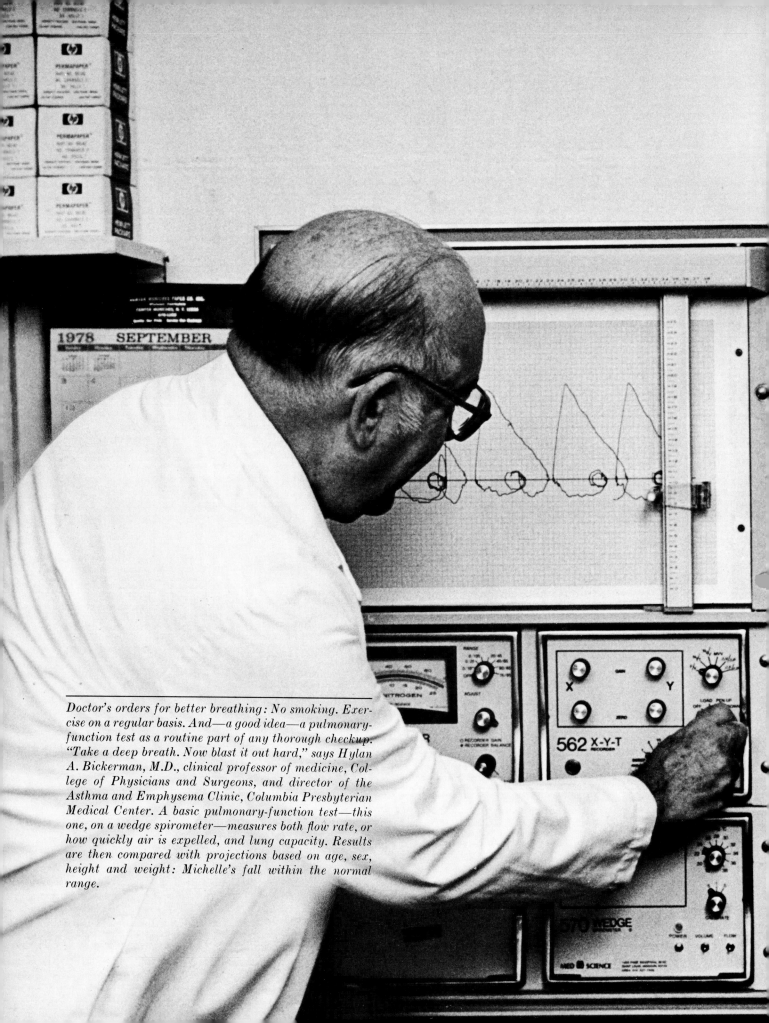

Doctor's orders for better breathing: No smoking. Exercise on a regular basis. And—a good idea—a pulmonary-function test as a routine part of any thorough checkup. "Take a deep breath. Now blast it out hard," says Hylan A. Bickerman, M.D., clinical professor of medicine, College of Physicians and Surgeons, and director of the Asthma and Emphysema Clinic, Columbia Presbyterian Medical Center. A basic pulmonary-function test—this one, on a wedge spirometer—measures both flow rate, or how quickly air is expelled, and lung capacity. Results are then compared with projections based on age, sex, height and weight: Michelle's fall within the normal range.

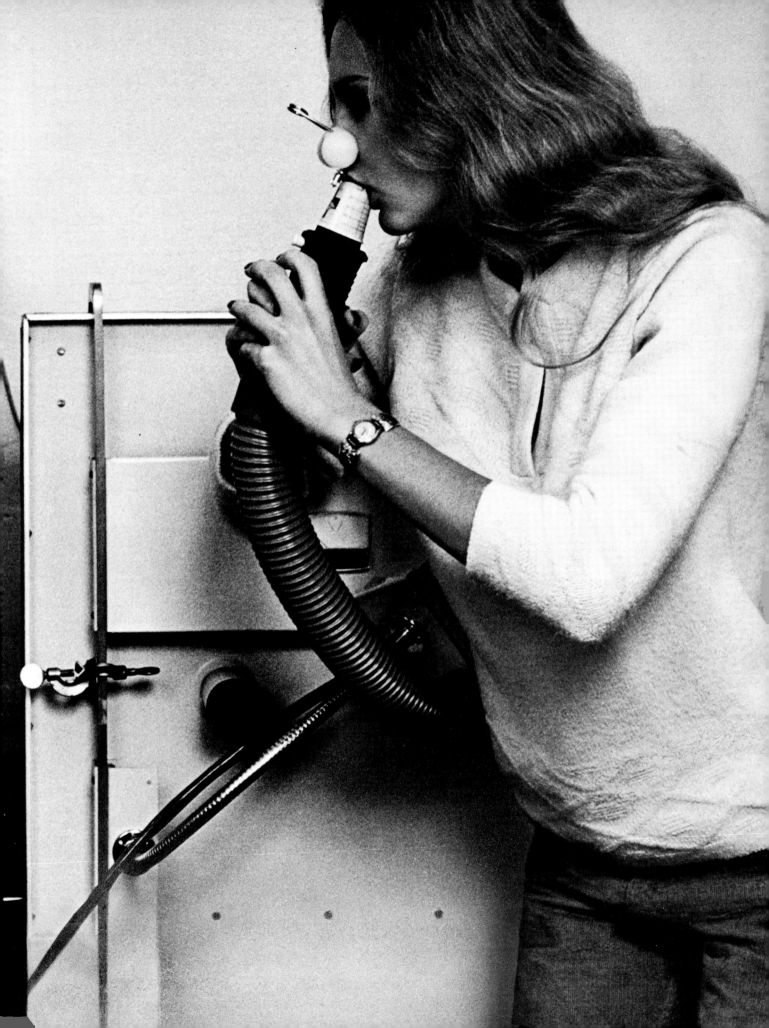

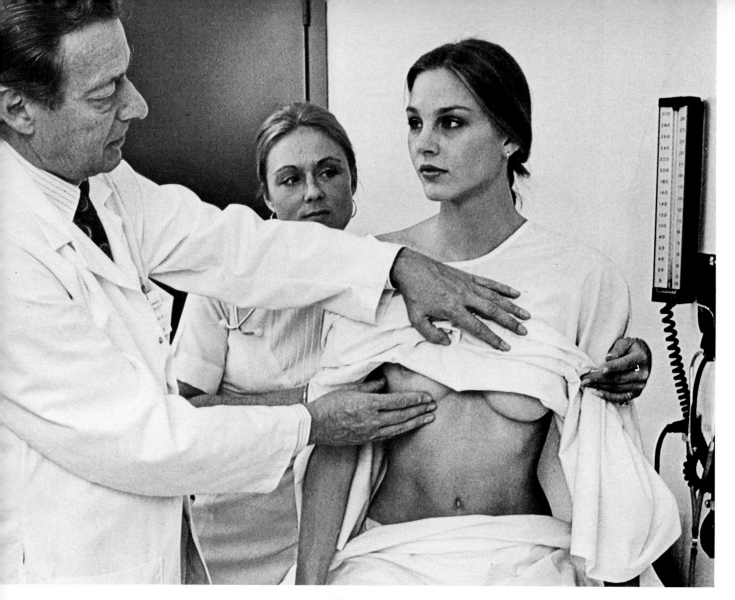

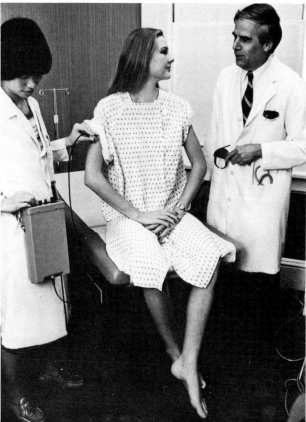

Above: Fritz F. Fuchs, M.D., Harold and Percy Uris professor of reproductive biology at the New York Hospital-Cornell Medical Center, does a breast exam, once a year, in a visit that includes thorough breast, pelvic and rectal examinations and a Pap smear. Dr. Fuchs advises against relying on your gynecologist as a general practitioner—or on a general practitioner as a source of gynecological advice. It is best to have both.

Left: Theodore B. Van Itallie, M.D., chief and director at the Obesity Research Center, St. Luke's Hospital, New York City, discusses weight history with Michelle while his assistant measures her skinfold thickness with ultrasonic waves. The reading is then compared to standards grouped by age and sex to estimate how much of the patient's total body weight is actually fat. Michelle's skinfold thickness: 11 millimeters, a bit below the normal range for her age. Because obesity is so widespread in the United States, weight control is one of the most important reasons to establish healthy eating habits early. Dr. Van Itallie stresses the role of regular exercise: Studies show that physical activity can curb appetite. "Though women seem to be less harmed by obesity than men as far as longevity is concerned, the effects on one's overall state of health are considerable," he says.

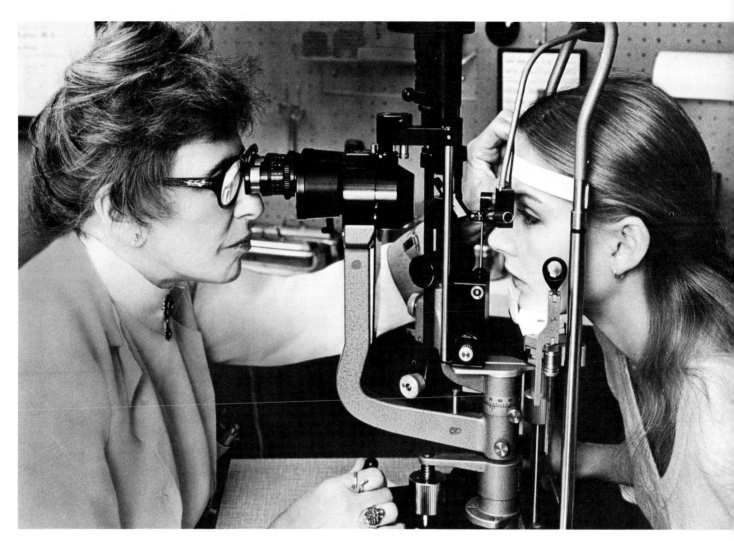

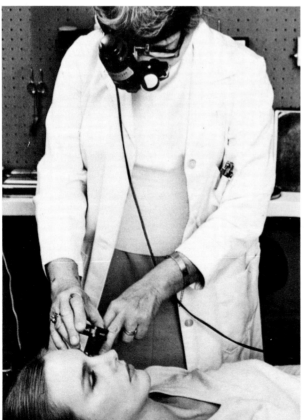

Above: Routine check for glaucoma: Virginia L. Lubkin, M.D., associate clinical professor, Department of Oph- thalmology, Mount Sinai School of Medicine, checks Michelle's intraocular tension by tonometry, which mea- sures pressure inside the eye. In its early stages, glau- coma rarely exhibits symptoms—and so goes undetected by the victim. Dr. Lubkin advises a test once every two years if you're under 40, yearly if you're older.

Left: "When we look into the eyes, we actually see into an organ. We can detect some 200 diseases by changes in the interior of the eye," says Dr. Lubkin. Here she ex- amines Michelle's ocular fundus (the interior of the eye) with an ophthalmoscope for evidence of any of the dis- eases—from diabetes to brain tumors—that produce signs or symptoms there. "In any other part of the body, only an autopsy would give information at so detailed a level," she says.

SIGHT AND SOUND: THE BODY'S RADAR

It's an almost universal experience. Around one's 40th birthday, newspapers and telephone directories become difficult to read. It becomes necessary to hold small objects and printed materials farther away from the eyes in order to focus clearly.

The condition is presbyopia, which almost literally means "old eyes." What has happened is a stiffening of the crystalline lens of the eye, a process that has gone on very gradually since about age 10. This decreases one's ability to focus on nearby objects. One becomes progressively more "farsighted." After age 55, for most people, there is little further presbyopic change.

Most people past 50 develop some degree of presbyopia, and many need reading glasses. Some people who have been severely nearsighted all their lives find the extended distance vision of presbyopia a happy surprise —they can see across the room or down the street more clearly than ever before.

Age-related eye problems most commonly include cataract and glaucoma. These diseases can be treated medically or surgically, and success rates are high.

Cataract, clouding of the lens inside the eye, can be treated only by surgery for removing the clouded tissues. The condition can happen to people at any age, even infants. Some cataracts are congenital—they run in families. Other causes include infectious diseases, rheumatoid arthritis, diabetes. Cataracts blind more than 5,000 people each year in this country—a toll, eye experts believe, that can be reduced to near zero. Properly conducted cataract surgery is successful in over 95 percent of cases.

Glaucoma is increased pressure inside the eyeball. Fluid circulating between the lens and the cornea, or outer transparent coating, can't escape through the eye's fine drainage canals. Growing pressure can damage the optic nerve and, if untreated, lead to blindness. Glaucoma can run in families and the risk of getting it increases as one ages.

Developing glaucoma doesn't hurt. The only way to detect it before visual impairment sets in is through an eye test called tonometry, which eye specialists conduct routinely in full eye examinations. The test doesn't hurt, either. If a too-high pressure is found, it usually is treated by drugs given as eyedrops, or in a continuous-release dosage in the form of a very small oval wafer placed inside the lower lid. It can't be felt and it releases its pressure-lowering medication steadily for a week.

A less-common form of glaucoma is caused by a structural defect and needs correction by surgery. To stay on the alert for glaucoma, it is recommended that people past 40 have annual eye examinations, including tonometry.

Presbycusis and presbyacusia are medical terms for hearing loss attributed to aging. For purposes of everyday living, *hearing doesn't change much with age*. After one reaches 50, very high frequency tones may become less perceptible; only a few persons above 65 can hear frequencies above 10,000 cycles per second. But these losses seem to handicap most older persons very little; for one thing, many develop adaptation, adding visual and auditory clues so that understanding of conversation remains far better than measuring tone thresholds would predict.

What does grow more important as years go on is proper care of the ears. Wax deposits can be washed out by a physician or by oneself, using wax-softening drops followed by careful syringing with warm water. Avoiding excess noise (such as amplified rock and disco music), which can cause deafness, may be insurance against hearing loss later in life. Smoking or excessive use of aspirin can aggravate tinnitus, or ear sounds of ringing, buzzing or crackling, another problem more frequent in older people. Tinnitus may strike at any age, however, and may develop from noise exposure or follow a viral infection.

BONES

Thinning and wasting of bone—osteoporosis —can be a distinct threat with age, especially to women and most particulary to those of slender skeletal frame. Mineral material, notably calcium, disappears, leaving thin, frail bones that are likely to break. Broken hips, or more often fractures of the thigh bone near the hip, occur too often in elderly women, as do spontaneous crush fractures of the spine, which leave the bent-over back traditionally

Nutritional Help For The Endocrines

A well-known endocrinologist prescribes a Gland Cocktail to ensure that his patients get nutritional help for their endocrines. Here it is:

1 egg	for protein
1 squeezed orange or lemon	for vitamic C
1 cup of mixed vegetable juice (V-8)	for A and other vitamins
1 pinch of sea salt or kelp powder	for its iodine and magnesium
1 tablespoon powdered milk	for calcium and protein
1 tablespoon brewer's yeast	for the entire B complex
1 teaspoon wheatgerm oil	for its vitamin E

Blend together in an electric blender or beat with a rotary beater until smooth. If too thick for your taste, add more vegetable juice. Kept in refrigerator, this will last for several daily doses.

associated with extreme age.

Like other age-associated problems, osteoporosis should not be considered unavoidable or a ''natural'' part of aging. It isn't. Some population groups, such as black people, seem virtually free from osteoporosis, even at bone densities matched to those of the osteoporosis-prone population.

Though some men get osteoporosis, it is largely a disease of women past menopause. Deprivation of estrogen, occurring as ovulation ceases, is believed to be the triggering event causing calcium metabolism to falter. Women past menopause who also smoke are said to be at excessively high risk of osteoporosis, especially those who have slender skeletal frames. Inadequate calcium in the diet may accelerate the problem. Other possible factors are inadequate supplies of vitamins D

and K, both of which assist in calcium metabolism. Accordingly, clinical researchers have sought to treat the condition by replacing the missing or poorly absorbed ingredients, also including fluoride. In varying degrees, these treatments have been found to stop osteoporosis or slow its course. Some patients have shown evidence of rebuilding thinned bones under a vigorous doctor-supervised nutritional program.

Preventing osteoporosis is well worth the effort. A diet supplying generous amounts of calcium and vitamins, exposure to the small amount of sunshine required to produce adequate vitamin D, plus exercise to maintain and increase bone strength, are all recommended, both for the bones' health and one's general health.

- *More important than the net amount of calcium in the diet, say bone experts, is the ratio of calcium to phosphorus, which is also involved in forming bone. These two minerals should be supplied to the body in approximately equal amounts, or with slightly more calcium.*

- *The problem: The average American diet provides a great deal more phosphorus than calcium. Meat, chicken, seafoods, all excellent protein sources, have many times more phosphorus than calcium, a situation that calls for bringing them into balance by supplying calcium from other sources. Difficult to do; though calcium-rich, milk and other dairy foods have only about one-fourth to one-sixth more calcium than phosphorus. But green leafy vegetables may have two to three times as much, and oranges and pineapples twice as much calcium as phosphorus. Many nutritionists believe it's wise to take supplemental calcium along with the daily vitamins.*

MUSCLE TONE AND HOW TO KEEP IT

Our voluntary muscles diminish in size and strength as we grow older; witness, in self and others, the thinner look of older legs compared with the same legs of earlier years.

Now being intensively studied, in long-term research backed by the National Institute on Aging, is the body's capacity for performing muscular work. The strength of the handgrip, the force that arm and leg muscles can apply to testing machinery, other muscles tests, all are carefully measured along with heart and lung functions to help scientists—and all of us—understand the aging process with the full intention of controlling, postponing and detaining body aging just as much as possible.

It comes as no suprise that continuing to exercise the muscles is the primary way to prevent loss of muscle tone. Part of the reduction in muscular strength is believed to result not from aging, but from disuse. It's easy to see this demonstrated in the excellent muscular condition and appearance of people who stay very active well into advanced years; and it's demonstrated in the negative when a young, strong person is immobilized with an injury. In a very brief period of inaction, muscles will become noticeably smaller. Fortunately, they regain their former size and strength after activity is resumed.

THE SUM-UP

How long can we expect to live? Beyond the factors over which we have little control, such as good genes and good luck, the historical period in which one lives has much to do with the average lifespan of people. In recorded history, one of the low points in life expectancy took place during the great plague that swept the world in the mid-14th century. In that period, life expectancy was calculated at about 17–18 years. When the plague passed, the figure gradually climbed to about 30 years. In the United States in 1900, life expectancies were 47.9 years for men, 51.1 for women. In 1975, the figure for men had reached 69.5 and for women 75.8. Several other nations have higher life expectancies, but in this country the expected lifespan is continuing to rise.

In a massive, six-volume study for the National Science Foundation, the Futures Group of Glastonbury, Connecticut, projected the ways population age groups might be distributed, under varying conditions, in years to come. The percentage of older persons in the population, as we know, is increasing, to some extent because of improved living conditions and successful conquests of several diseases.

Even if no medical advances were made at all, the present over-65 age group, now numbering about 22 million, would be replaced by a crowd of 56 million by the year 2025. But since medical and other progress, or "span extension technologies" almost certainly will occur, the Futures Group projections take into account the very real possibility that people will tend to live to almost twice today's average lifespan, and will not begin to drop off until ages 100, 165 or 180.

"It used to be the common wisdom that the living body was a vulnerable, essentially ramshackle affair," remarked Lewis Thomas in *The Medusa and the Snail*. It's a myth Dr. Thomas accepts not at all, for, he says, "the most impressive aspect of life is its sheer, tough power."

The possibilities for prolonging bodily health right now, and for living longer and more vigorously than any other generation, are real and within our grasp.

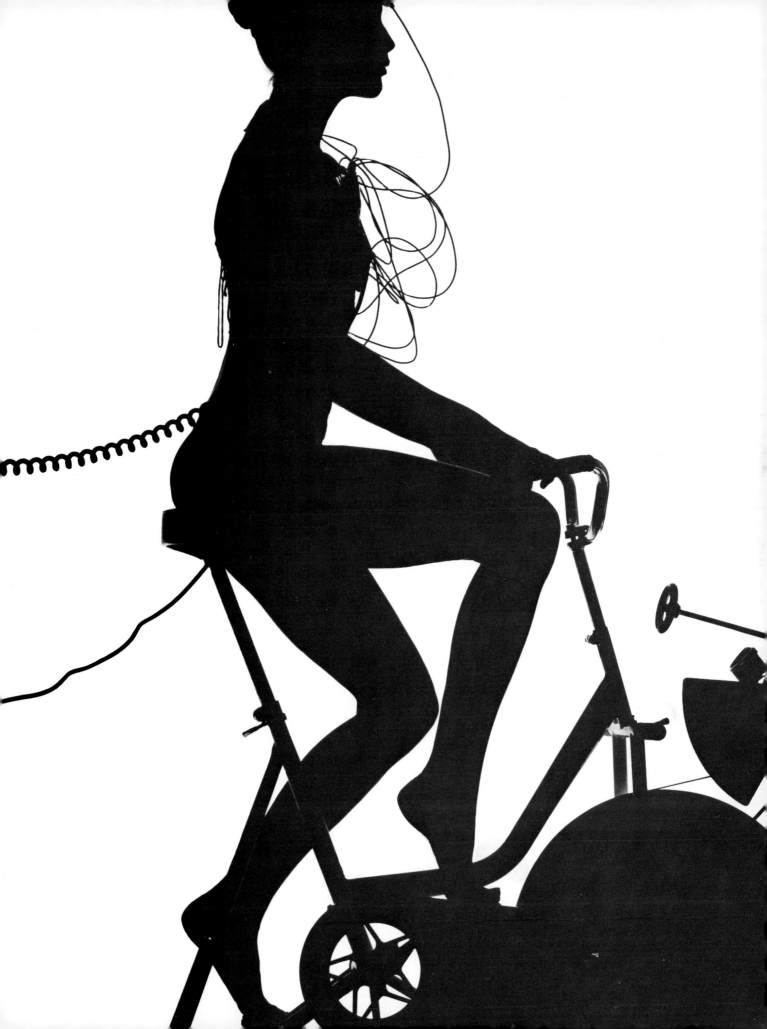

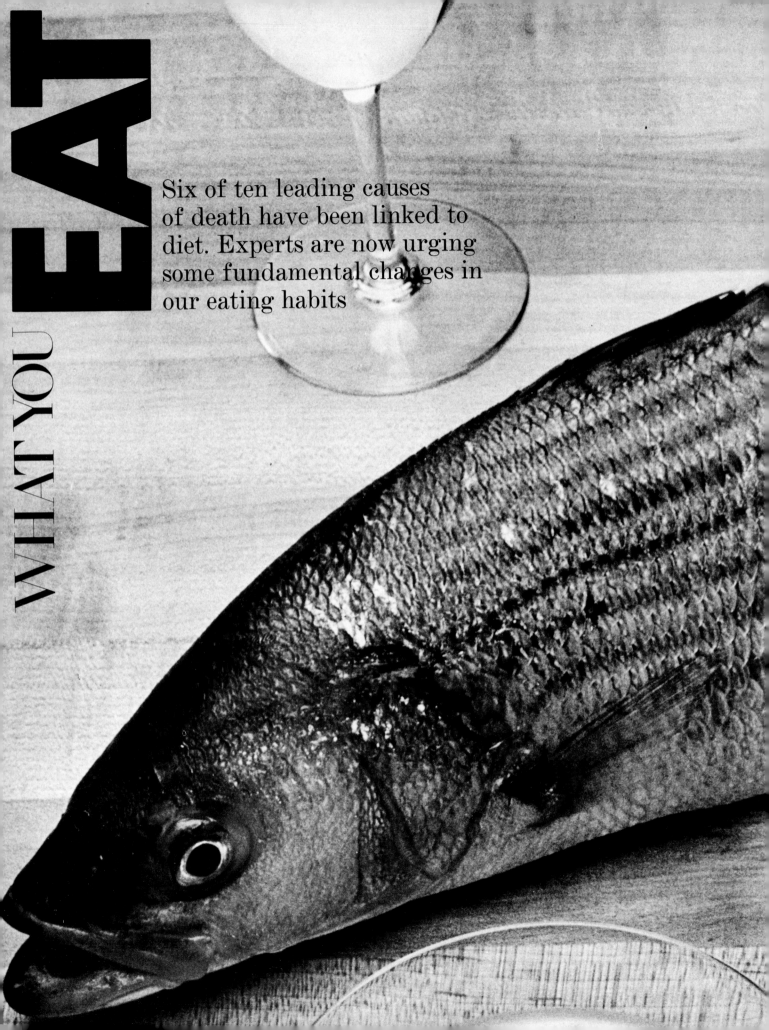

EAT
WHAT YOU

Six of ten leading causes
of death have been linked to
diet. Experts are now urging
some fundamental changes in
our eating habits

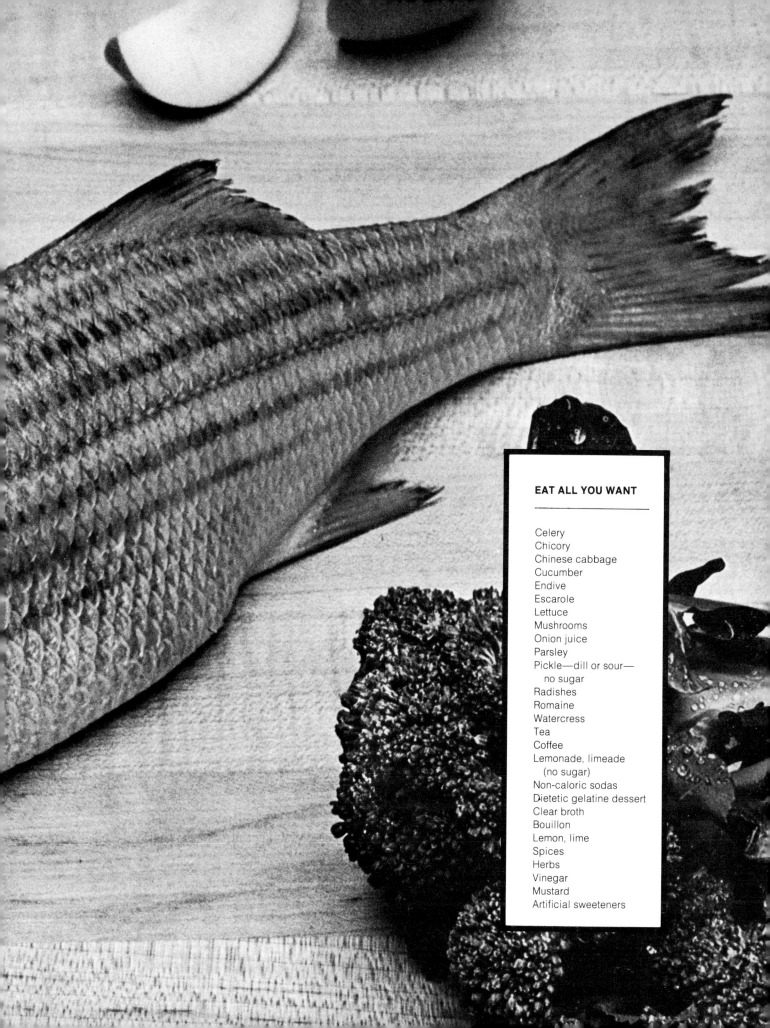

EAT ALL YOU WANT

Celery
Chicory
Chinese cabbage
Cucumber
Endive
Escarole
Lettuce
Mushrooms
Onion juice
Parsley
Pickle—dill or sour—
   no sugar
Radishes
Romaine
Watercress
Tea
Coffee
Lemonade, limeade
   (no sugar)
Non-caloric sodas
Dietetic gelatine dessert
Clear broth
Bouillon
Lemon, lime
Spices
Herbs
Vinegar
Mustard
Artificial sweeteners

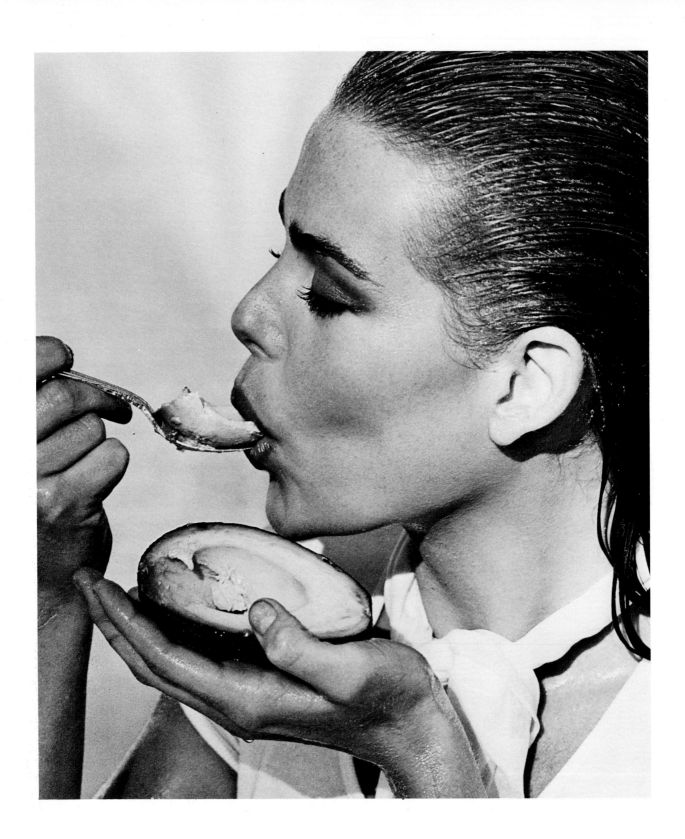

DIET AND NUTRITION

by Phyllis E. Lehmann

Evidence is overwhelming that, indeed, you are what you eat. With the abundance of food in this country, virtually all Americans have a choice: to eat their way to ill health and perhaps a shorter life span, or to seek a diet that offers the best chance for many active, healthy years. There is nothing mysterious—or even difficult—about eating right. Basically, good nutrition is just good common sense.

NUTRITION
A LIFELONG PROCESS

Nutrition is not something to consider only when you want to shed a few pounds or after you read the latest scare article on diet and disease. It's a lifelong process. One of the most important things is to start early (parents, take heed), because how you will fare in the last third of life depends on how you eat during the first two-thirds, says E. Neige Todhunter, Ph.D., visiting professor of nutrition at Vanderbilt University Medical School and an expert on age and diet. But, she stresses, it's never too late to start eating better. You may not reverse some of the damage done early in life, but studies indicate that

Margaux Hemingway, left, enjoys an element in the new scheme for dietary success and continued health—nutrient density is the name; avocado, a winner.

you may at least reduce the risk of diet-related illness.

Everyone needs to be aware of both the quantity (calories) and quality (nutrient content) of the foods he or she eats. The way to think of foods, says Dr. Todhunter, is in terms of their "nutrient density"—the ratio of calories to nutrients. Soft drinks, for example, are all calories and no nutrients and therefore have a low nutrient density, while milk, which contributes a wealth of nutrients in relation to calories, is considered of high nutrient density.

The same nutrients—protein, fat, carbohydrates, vitamins and minerals—are needed by all humans, whatever their age, but the amounts vary with age, sex, level of physical activity and degree of stress. It is well documented that physiological stress, such as pregnancy or illness, affects nutrient requirements. But according to Dr. Todhunter, several studies also show that intense emotional stress—anger, worry, even great joy—alters chemical reactions in the body so that nutrients are not used as efficiently.

HEALTHY EATING
AT ANY AGE

The U.S. Senate's Select Committee on Nutrition and Human Needs, in its 1977 report,

LIFETIME NUTRITION

	TEENS	TWENTIES
CALORIES (depending on body size and activity level)	2100 to 2400 per day	2000 to 2100
FOODS meat/poultry/fish (servings per day)	2	2
eggs (per week)	4 to 5	3 to 4
milk/milk products (servings per day)	4	2
cereals and grains (servings per day)	4	4
fruits and vegetables (servings per day)	4	4
PROTEIN	Greater-than-ever requirement to fuel teenage growth spurt.	Requirement diminishes slightly.
FATS	Only a problem if it is the source of too many calories or if too much of the fat is saturated. Ideally, no more than 30 percent of calories should come from fat.	Begin calorie cutbacks with fats.
CARBOHYDRATES	Reduce intake of sugar and refined foods and increase consumption of complex carbohydrates such as whole grains, fruits and vegetables.	
MINERALS	Calcium and phosphorus needs are at a high point.	Calcium and phosphorus requirements decrease by one-third.
	Iron needs increase with onset of menstruation and remain constant. Supplements may be needed.	
VITAMINS	If premenstrual water retention is a problem, avoid excessive salt intakes before period begins.	
	Lack of vitamin A may be a problem if junk foods take the place of dark green and yellow vegetables and if vitamin A- and D-fortified milk is replaced by other beverages.	

Dietary Goals for the United States, reached the grim conclusion that too much fat, sugar, salt and alcohol are linked directly to heart disease, cancer, obesity and stroke. "In all," the committee said, "six of the 10 leading causes of death in the U.S. have been linked to our diet." In light of accumulating evidence, nutrition experts and the U.S. government now urge some basic changes in eating habits:

EAT LESS

"By all odds, the most important thing is to maintain your weight at close to an ideal level," says Helen Guthrie, Ph.D., professor of nutrition and head of the nutrition program at Pennsylvania State University.

To lose one pound of body fat, you need to burn 3500 more calories than you consume. A healthy way to burn those calories is to increase physical activity. Simply walking more or taking the stairs instead of the elevator can make a difference. Besides, regular exercise is the surest way to stay looking and feeling young.

THIRTIES	FORTIES	FIFTIES AND OVER
1900 to 2000	1800 to 1900	1800
2 3 to 4 2 4 4	2 3 to 4 2 4 4	2 2 to 3 2 4 4
Requirement remains constant. Calorie cutbacks should not interfere with protein intake.		
	Decreasing estrogen levels diminish body's ability to handle cholesterol.	May be harder to digest fats. After menopause, women are more vulnerable to heart disease; total fat (particularly saturated fats and cholesterol) intake often limited.
Calcium and phosphorus requirements remain constant.		Calcium and phosphorus are essential to prevent bone problems. If milk or milk products are hard to digest, supplements may be needed.
		Iron needs decrease after menopause; supplements are not needed.
	Sodium (particularly salt) may be restricted if high blood pressure is a problem.	
Adequate vitamin C is essential since it aids in iron absorption.		Vitamin C needs remain constant despite drop in iron requirement.
Supplements of fat-soluble vitamins such as A and D not advised unless prescribed by a physician.		

EAT A WIDE VARIETY OF FOODS

Diversity in the diet, says Audrey Cross, coordinator, Human Nutrition Policy, of the office of the secretary of the U.S. Department of Agriculture, serves two purposes: "One, it assures that you get a nice mix of the 40 or so essential nutrients; and, two, it keeps you interested in food. People who get into tight little patterns of eating are likely to get bored and stick in things like snack foods."

A well-balanced diet means choosing foods each day from several major categories:

1 *FRUITS AND VEGETABLES;*
2 *CEREALS, BREAD AND GRAINS;*
3 *MEATS, POULTRY, EGGS AND FISH;*
4 *DRY PEAS AND BEANS, WHICH ARE GOOD VEGETABLE SOURCES OF PROTEIN;*
5 *MILK, CHEESE, AND YOGURT.*

It is wise to get some variety within each food group and even to choose foods from different geographical areas—apples and oranges, for example—because the amount of trace minerals present depends on the soil composition in the areas where food is grown.

CUT DOWN ON FATS

The link between saturated (or animal) fats and cholesterol in the diet and increased risk of heart disease has been clearly established. Since fat contains more than twice as many calories per gram than protein or carbohydrates, it also contributes to obesity. High-fat diets also are suspected of adding to the high incidence of breast and colon cancer in the United States.

```
      H H H H H H H H H H H H H H H H H
HC-C-C-C-C-C-C-C-C-C-C-C-C-C-C-C-C-COOH
      H H H H H H H H H H H H H H H H H
```

Sometimes two adjacent carbon atoms hold both hands, leaving two hydrogen spots vacant. Then the fatty acid in monounsaturated:

```
      H H H H H H H H       H H H H H H H
HC-C-C-C-C-C-C-C-C = C-C-C-C-C-C-C-C-COOH
      H H H H H H H         H H H H H H
```

If four or more hydrogen spots are empty, the fatty acid is polyunsaturated:

```
      H H H H H     H H H   H H H H H H H
HC-C-C-C-C-C = C-C-C = C-C-C-C-C-C-C-C-COOH
      H H H H       H       H H H H H H
```

If you say a particular fat, such as butter, is "saturated," this means it has a predominant amount of saturated fatty acids. If you say a fat is "monounsaturated"—olive oil, for instance—this means most of the fatty acids are monounsaturated. If you say it is "polyunsaturated"—one of the other vegetable oils such as safflower or corn oil, perhaps—it means the fatty acids are mainly polyunsaturated. Here is a list of foods that are mainly saturated or monounsaturated or polyunsaturated:

SATURATED		
Meats that are high in fat.	Hydrogenated shortening. Coconut or palm oil.	Butter, whole milk, cheese, and other whole-milk products.
MONOUNSATURATED		
Peanuts, peanut butter, and peanut oil.	Olives and olive oil. Almonds, cashew and Brazil nuts.	Avocados. Fish.
POLYUNSATURATED		
Safflower and corn oil.	Soft margarine. Walnuts. Soybeans.	Sunflower and sesame seeds and oils made from them.
Saturated dietary fat raises harmful forms of blood cholesterol, monounsaturated fat is neutral, and polyunsaturated fat lowers them.		

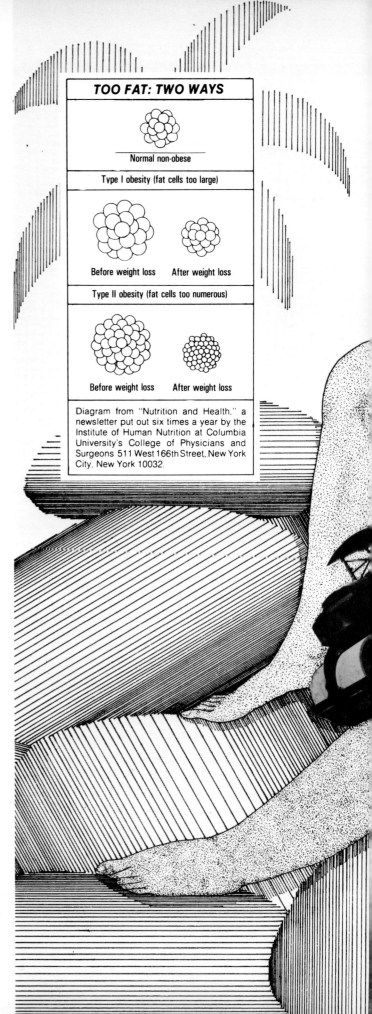

TOO FAT: TWO WAYS

Normal non-obese

Type I obesity (fat cells too large)

Before weight loss   After weight loss

Type II obesity (fat cells too numerous)

Before weight loss   After weight loss

Diagram from "Nutrition and Health," a newsletter put out six times a year by the Institute of Human Nutrition at Columbia University's College of Physicians and Surgeons 511 West 166th Street, New York City, New York 10032.

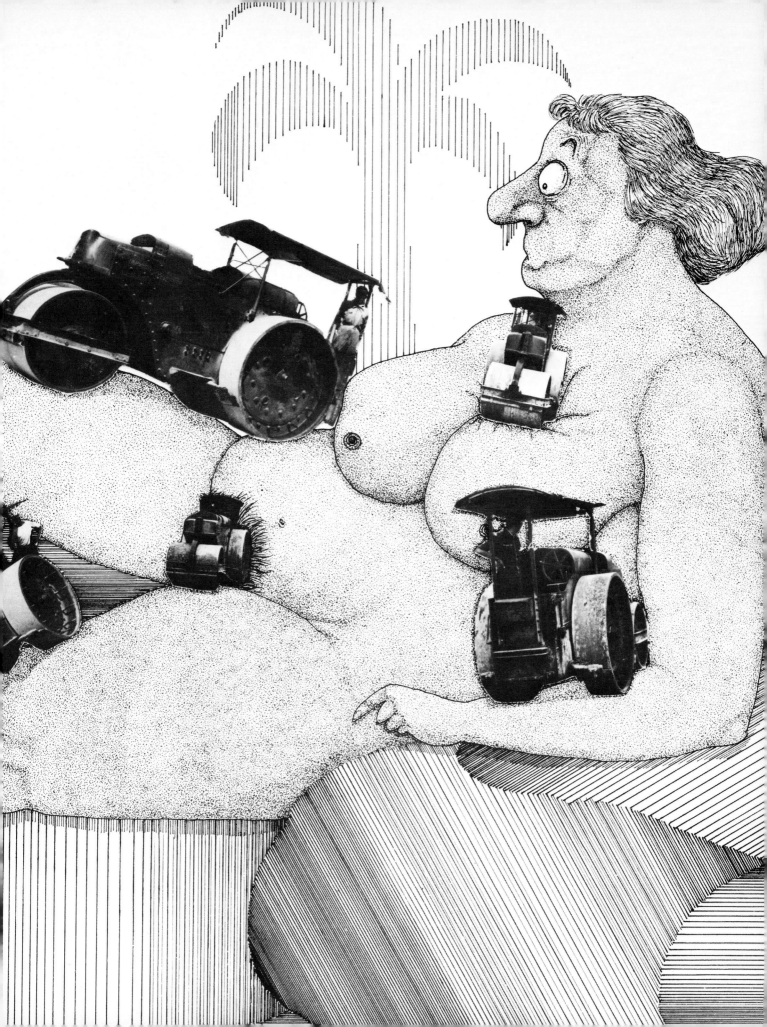

INCLUDE MORE FIBER IN YOUR DIET

Intestinal diseases such as appendicitis, diverticulosis (a painful ballooning of the intestinal wall), polyps and colon cancer are relatively rare in parts of the world where people eat large amounts of fiber. Though research is not conclusive, scientists think that fiber may reduce the risk of cancer by speeding up the movement of food (and carcinogens) through the digestive tract or by binding or diluting some of the breakdown products of fat that might cause cancer. An important recent discovery is that a high-fiber diet also aids in treating diabetics by improving their glucose tolerance and preventing them from absorbing as much glucose from the intestine, says Robert A. Levine, M.D., professor of medicine and chief of gastroenterology at the State University of New York Upstate Medical Center in Syracuse.

The average person should at least double the amount of fiber in the diet, Dr. Levine recommends, by eating more dark breads, bran cereals, fruits and vegetables. But don't go overboard. Too much fiber can hinder absorption of nutrients in the intestines.

EAT LESS SUGAR AND MORE COMPLEX CARBOHYDRATES

Sugar is not poison. It adds flavor to foods and makes possible some tasty combinations. But it contains no protein, vitamins or minerals and is extremely high in calories. It contributes to obesity and causes tooth decay when bacteria in the mouth act on it to produce an acid that dissolves tooth enamel. Despite the arguments of some scientists, the U.S. Departments of Agriculture and Health and Human Services report there is no convincing evidence that sugar causes heart attacks, blood vessel diseases or diabetes.

Use less sugar of all kinds, including brown sugar, honey and syrups. Cut down on soft drinks, sugar-coated cereals, fruits canned in syrup and processed foods whose labels list sugar as a primary ingredient. At the same time, increase your consumption of complex carbohydrates, such as whole grains, potatoes, rice and starchy vegetables like corn and lima beans. These contain a number of vitamins and minerals and are high in fiber.

AVOID TOO MUCH SALT

The average American probably consumes two to three times the amount of sodium needed, and this excess is a recognized factor in high blood pressure. Reduce your salt intake by going easy with the salt shaker while cooking and at the table. Avoid salty processed foods, such as potato chips and other snacks, pickled foods, sandwich meats, cheese spreads, condiments and sauces. A good way to control the amount of both salt and sugar in the diet is to eat more fresh fruits and vegetables.

WHAT IS FIBER?

● *Fiber, found in varying amounts in fruits, nuts, grains, and vegetables, is the part of the plant that you cannot digest and is made up of such complex compounds as cellulose, hemicellulose, pectins and lignins. Whole-grain cereals such as bran, for example, contain up to 12 percent fiber, cooked lentils up to 1.5 percent, and roasted nuts about 2.6 percent. Most fruits contain 0.5–1 percent fiber. Meat, fish and poultry, on the other hand, do not contain any fiber. All plant foods contain some fiber as long as they are not overly processed. Refined foods tend to have less fiber than unrefined foods. Brown rice is 0.9 percent fiber, while polished rice is 0.3 percent; whole-wheat bread is 1.6 percent, while white bread is only 0.2 percent. Sugar, whether white or brown, has no fiber.*

● *If your physician recommends a sodium-restricted diet, the first step is cutting down on sodium chloride, or table salt. But, to be effective, your low-sodium diet must exclude other sources; be sure to read food labels and steer away from items that list one or more kinds of sodium. Snack foods and many "convenience," highly processed, ready-to-eat foods often contain a good deal of sodium in their preservatives and flavoring. Soft drinks may have a lot of sodium (after all, they're called sodas), though seltzer water without added sodium is available. Don't forget to check for sodium content on labels of any nonprescription drugs you regularly use. Antacids, for example, commonly carry considerable sodium, though low-sodium antacids also are sold.*

ADD FIBER TO YOUR DIET
● *One way is to use bran in your cooking. Add a few tablespoons to your favorite meat-loaf recipe, add it to bread if you bake your own. You can even add bran to sauces in limited quantities. Substitute whole-grain breads for white bread. Cut down on sugar, meats and carbonated drinks, and add more foods of plant origin. Try to eat between 10 and 15 grams of fiber daily. Although an apple a day may not always keep the doctor away, several apples a day can go a long way to keeping you healthier.*

WHAT SHOULD YOU DRINK?

Do adults need milk? Is mineral water really beneficial? Should you give up alcohol? Here is the latest advice on liquids in the diet:

ALCOHOL

If you drink alcohol, do so in moderation, advises the government in recently issued dietary guidelines. There is some evidence that an ounce or two of alcohol a day may protect against heart disease, but research also shows that heavy use of alcohol, especially in combination with smoking, may lead to cancer of the mouth, throat, esophagus, larynx and stomach. Alcohol also is high in calories and low in nutrients, which makes it a bad choice for anyone trying to control weight. Two glasses of wine, for example, account for 200–300 of your total daily calories, and remember that red wine has more calories than white.

MILK

"Milk is not a baby food, it's a human food for all ages," Dr. Todhunter stresses. Milk throughout life is especially important for women, who become susceptible to osteoporosis (a decrease in mineral matter producing softening of the bones) after menopause. Skim milk is just as nutritious as whole milk and better for you—there's hardly any fat. If you don't like to drink milk, use it in cooking or eat yogurt or cottage cheese. Other cheeses and ice cream also have the food value of milk but are high in fat.

MINERAL WATER

It may be chic, but bottled mineral water is no different nutritionally than the water that comes out of your tap, because minerals occur naturally in all water.

COFFEE AND TEA

"As far as we know, caffeine does not interfere with metabolism of essential nutrients," says Audrey Cross, "so people have to make choices based on what their nervous systems can handle." Coffee and tea should not, however, replace beverages that do contain nutrients, such as milk and fruit juices.

PROTEIN: AN EXPENSIVE WAY TO GET CALORIES— FACTS AND FALLACIES

Most nutrition experts now agree that Americans do not need all the protein they consume and that its importance in the diet is overemphasized. In fact, protein is an expensive form in which to get your calories. "A gram of protein contains four calories—the same as carbohydrates—but the cost of that gram of protein is three to four times higher than for the carbohydrate," says Audrey Cross. The body makes much of its own protein and any excess from the diet is used for energy, just like fats and carbohydrates. Protein not needed for energy is converted to body fat.

Nor is protein a *better* source of energy. That theory developed among athletes because protein, with its nitrogen bonds, is more difficult than carbohydrates or fats for the body to break down and therefore was thought to produce a more sustained level of energy.

Quick weight loss on a high-protein or a low-carbohydrate diet is more apparent than real, says Richard S. Rivlin, M.D., chief of nutrition at both Memorial-Sloan Kettering Cancer Center and New York Hospital-Cornell Medical Center. A low-carbohydrate diet, he says, results in the loss of a lot of salt and water, but not necessarily fat, so weight loss is usually temporary.

VITAMINS AND MINERALS: FACTS AND FALLACIES

To maintain life, the human body requires 13 vitamins—A, B₁ (thiamine), B₂ (riboflavin), niacin, folic acid, B₆, B₁₂, pantothenic acid, biotin, C (ascorbic acid), D, E, and K—and approximately 17 minerals (scientists do not yet agree on some). The "macro-minerals," which occur in relatively large amounts in the body and the diet, are calcium, phosphorous, chlorine, sulphur, magnesium, sodium and potassium. The rest, including iron, zinc, chromium and copper, are called "trace" minerals because they are needed in small amounts. Still others, such as nickel, tin and vanadium, are essential for animals, but their role in humans has not been established.

One of the most persistent and potentially most dangerous nutritional myths is that vitamin and mineral supplements can increase vitality, lengthen life, offer magic cures and generally promote good health, regardless of diet. Nutrition experts agree that such claims are so far unsubstantiated.

Too little of an essential vitamin or mineral produces a specific deficiency disease, such as scurvy from lack of Vitamin C or goiter from lack of iodine. So many foods are not fortified with nutrients that the average American gets adequate nutrition from a reasonably well-balanced diet. Still, some 60 million people in the United States take dietary supplements they don't need, according to Stephen Barrett, M.D., senior editor of *The Health Robbers,* a guide to the various forms of health quackery. This vitamin mania is, at best, a needless drain on the pocketbook and, at worst, a hazard to health.

Here is a quick guide to some common fallacies about vitamins and minerals:

NUTRIENT	FUNCTION	FOOD
● **Vitamin A** (Retinol)	Helps repair body tissues and skeletal growth; promotes good eyesight; helps keep skin in good condition	Deep yellow foods such as apricots, butter, carrots, cheese, eggs, mangoes, papayas; liver, kidney; dark green vegetables like kale and broccoli, watercress, alfalfa sprouts
● **Vitamin B-1** (Thiamine)	Necessary for the conversion of carbohydrates into glucose for energy; important for nervous system, heart and liver	Poultry, lamb's liver, Brazil nuts, sunflower seeds, wheatgerm and wholewheat grains, rolled oats, brown rice
● **Vitamin B-2** (Riboflavin)	Helps to break down food for nutrition and energy; necessary for cell respiration and good vision	Milk, cheese, eggs, brewer's yeast, wheatgerm, wild rice, poultry, liver, kidney, almonds, avocado
● **Vitamin B-3** (Niacin)	Assists in the entire digestive process; important to mental health and the nervous system; most beneficial working in a team with the other B vitamins	Chicken, chicken liver, lamb's liver, kidneys, halibut, mackerel, sardines, peanuts, whole grains and bread
● **Vitamin B-5** (Pantothenic acid)	Involved in the metabolism of fatty acids; helps free energy from foods; essential for balanced functioning of the adrenal gland	Flesh foods, kidneys, lamb's liver, egg yolk, bran, brewer's yeast, whole grains, nuts
● **Vitamin B-6** (Pyridoxine)	Connected with growth and important in regulation of the nervous system; aids in metabolic breakdown of foods; helps form antibodies and red blood cells	Bananas, poultry, lamb's liver, mackerel, nuts, wheatgerm, whole grains and bread
● **Vitamin B-12** (Cyanocobalamin)	Essential for normal functioning of body cells, particularly those of bone marrow and the nervous system	Cheese, eggs, milk, poultry, fish, meat, liver, soybeans
● **Biotin** (Vitamin B complex)	Helps to form fatty acids, burning them up with the carbohydrates for energy; necessary for healthy skin	Raw egg yolk, liver, kidney, black currants, molasses, rolled oats
● **Choline** (Vitamin B complex)	Aids fat distribution from the liver; assists nerve transmission	Fish, heart, lentils, wheatgerm, whole grains, beans, lecithin granules
● **Folic acid** (Vitamin B complex)	Helps form red blood cells and nucleic acids, essential for reproductive process	Liver, oysters, cabbage (raw), watercress, almonds, walnuts
● **Inositol** (Vitamin B complex)	Together with choline, inositol forms lecithin, which keeps the liver free of fats	Bran, nuts, oats, sesame seeds, wheatgerm, lecithin granules
● **PABA** (Vitamin B complex)	Enables other Vitamin B elements to function properly	Broccoli, cabbage, kale, kidneys, liver, meat, poultry
● **Vitamin C** (Ascorbic acid)	Maintains level of collagen necessary for the formation of connective tissue, bone, skin and cartilage; claimed to help some virus infections	Cabbage, cauliflower, broccoli, Brussels sprouts, green peppers, watercress, alfalfa sprouts, citrus fruits, black currants, strawberries
● **Vitamin D** (Caleiferol)	Essential for healthy teeth and bones as it helps take the calcium and phosphorus to the necessary building tissues	Exposure to sunshine, eggs, cod-liver oil, halibut oil, mackerel, sardines, cheese
● **Vitamin E** (Tocopherol)	Needed for normal metabolism, believed to improve circulatory system; used to increase fertility	Carrots, cabbage, cheese, eggs, olive oil, rolled oats, sunflower seeds, wheatgerm, whole-wheat cereals and bread
● **Vitamin K**	Prevents hemorrhaging and aids the normal blood-clotting process	Broccoli, cabbage, potatoes, eggs, oats, wheatgerm, whole-wheat grains

MINERALS

NUTRIENT	FUNCTION	FOOD
● Calcium	Necessary to build and maintain bones and teeth; important for heart regulation and nerve transmission	Milk, cheese, almonds, olives, kelp and other seaweeds, sesame seeds, molasses, broccoli
● Chlorine	In conjunction with sodium, is important in cell metabolism	Celery, lettuce, spinach, tomatoes, kelp, salt
● Chromium	A trace mineral, helps regulate blood-sugar levels: believed to help keep the cholesterol level down	Bran, brewer's yeast, poultry, fruits, green vegetables, nuts
● Cobalt	A trace mineral, necessary for function of vitamin B-12	Fruits, green vegetables, meat, whole-grain cereals
● Copper	Significant in the production of red blood cells for the utilization of iron	Poultry, liver, kidney, shellfish, nuts, whole-grain cereals, lettuce, cabbage
● Fluorine	Strengthens bones and teeth by helping to deposit calcium; counteracts tooth decay	Seafood, fish, tea
● Iodine	Important for the proper functioning of the thyroid gland	Shellfish, seafood, sea salt, seaweeds, kelp
● Iron	Very important mineral involved in oxidizing cells and forming hemoglobin	Offal—kidney, liver; shellfish, egg yolk, dark green leafy vegetables, watercress, soya and sunflower seeds, whole-grain breads and cereals, molasses
● Magnesium	Important in cell metabolism: necessary as a catalytic agent for other minerals and vitamins and for the nerve and muscle systems	Almonds, barley, molasses, nuts, seafood and sea salt, olives, molasses
● Manganese	Activates enzymes; influences blood-sugar levels and helps maintain reproductive processes; a trace mineral	Kidneys, parsley, watercress, spinach, cabbage, apricots, lentils, nuts, wheatgerm
● Phosphorus	The most active of all minerals, important for growth and maintenance; together with calcium, provides hard structure for bones; passes on genetic hereditary patterns	Meat, fish, eggs, cheese, wheatgerm, whole-grain cereals
● Potassium	Often in partnership with sodium, maintaining a balance of fluids and important in muscle and nerve reactions	Seafood, potatoes, green-leaf vegetables, soya beans, lima beans, bananas, apricots, figs
● Selenium	Not exactly known, but related to vitamin E in function, a trace mineral	Kidney, liver, nuts, seafood, whole-grain cereals
● Sulfur	Helps in the formation of body tissue; necessary for activity of vitamins thiamine and biotin; a trace mineral	Milk, cheese, eggs, poultry, fish, beans, nuts, soya beans
● Zinc	A trace mineral, influences the enzyme and protein pattern in digestion	Eggs, nuts, onions, shellfish, sunflower seeds, wheatgerm, bran

FALLACY:

If some is good, more is better.

FACT:

The body needs vitamins and minerals in minute amounts—only milligrams (one thousandth of a gram) or micrograms (one millionth of a gram) a day. Whatever the intake, the body uses only what it needs. Extra amounts of water-soluble vitamins, such as vitamin C, are simply excreted in the urine. (Nutritionists say that Americans have the richest urine in the world.) Surpluses of fat-soluble vitamins, such as A and D, are stored in the liver. There is absolutely no evidence that extra amounts of these nutrients produce any health benefits.

FALLACY:

Vitamins and minerals are harmless, so there's no reason people shouldn't take them if they wish.

FACT:

In large doses, they are *not* harmless. The toxicity of vitamins A and D is well documented, and evidence is mounting against other commonly abused vitamins, such as C and E. Effects include liver and kidney damage, gastrointestinal disturbances, and retarded growth in children. Likewise, large doses of trace minerals can be quite toxic. Just four to six times the required amount of selenium, for example, can be fatal to laboratory rats.

FALLACY:

Specific vitamins or minerals will prevent or cure certain diseases.

FACT:

There is some exciting research regarding the role of vitamins in certain chronic diseases. Vitamin C interacts with nitrites in food and saliva to inhibit formation of nitrosamines, known cancer-causing agents. In work at the National Cancer Institute, vitamin A and its synthetic analogs, known as retinoids, appear to protect against cancer of the lung, stomach, intestine, kidney, bladder and uterus. Chromium, a trace mineral, appears useful in treating diabetes. As yet, however, there are not enough data to support taking excess amounts of any nutrient in hopes of preventing or curing disease.

Nor is there reliable evidence that vitamin C prevents the common cold; that vitamin E enhances sexual powers (in large amounts it has exactly the opposite effect); that vitamin B_6 prevents kidney stones; that thiamine is beneficial in the treating of multiple sclerosis, cancer or impotence; that vitamin A is useful in combatting acne, stress ulcers or dry skin; or that vitamin D lowers blood cholesterol or prevents or cures osteoporosis. Likewise, there is no indication that calcium and magnesium supplements, often sold as bone meal and dolomite, cure hyperactivity in children or eliminate leg cramps or sound sensitivity. And no one has proved that selenium prevents cancer, though scientists are sure that too much can *cause* it.

THE RIGHT WAY TO LOSE WEIGHT

Though Americans have become more weight-conscious in recent years, the average person in this country still is 20 pounds overweight. At any given time, an estimated 12 percent of adults in the United States are on a diet, 28 percent are "watching what they eat," and another 12 percent are switching back and forth between diets and binges. The bad news is that 95 percent of those who manage to lose weight on a diet gain it back. They are doomed to fail because "going on a diet is essentially avoiding the issue," says Dr. Henry A. Jordan, director of the Institute for Behavioral Education in King of Prussia, Pennsylvania, and clinical associate professor of psychiatry (School of Medicine) at the University of Pennsylvania. "People try to give up the foods they like instead of learning how to deal with them. Yet the craving is still there. Sooner or later, they come into contact with a favorite food, and their will power cracks. They overeat, often rapidly, sometimes secretly, and then feel guilty as the devil and ashamed for having failed to control themselves yet one more time. The approach I take is that it is okay to eat the foods you like. You just have to learn to eat them in moderation.''

Dr. Jordan cites four major strategies for modifying eating behavior:

BECOME AWARE OF HOW, WHAT, WHEN AND WHERE YOU EAT

There are a number of techniques: Slow down your rate of eating; keep records of everything you eat, and especially note the time and place where you eat; eat in only one place in the house; always sit down to eat; make eating a singular activity (no munching in front of the TV).

ALTER EXPOSURE TO TEMPTING SITUATIONS

Recognize that there are particular rooms in the house or social events where you will be tempted to eat. Stay out of the kitchen as much as possible. Go to another room to talk on the phone, write letters or socialize. Arrive at cocktail parties an hour later than usual so you will have less time to resist the hors d'oeuvre. Conduct more business in the office instead of at lunch.

REDUCE YOUR SUSCEPTIBILITY TO ENVIRONMENTAL CUES

Probably the most important technique, says Dr. Jordan, is to look ahead at food situations, predict what's going to happen and devise a plan of action. Make a shopping list before you go to the supermarket and stick to it. Find out in advance what is on the restaurant menu and make your selection before you get there. When faced with an enticing smorgasbord, survey what is there before you pick up a plate and decide.

CHANGE YOUR RESPONSE TO EATING URGES

When the urge to eat strikes, do something to take your mind off food: Take a walk, do a chore, or get involved in a favorite hobby (but make sure in advance that whatever you need is within as easy reach as the food).

YOUR DESIRABLE WEIGHT

women 25 years of age and over*, without clothing

Height	Small Frame	Medium Frame	Large Frame
4'8"	89–95	93–104	101–116
4'9"	91–98	95–107	103–119
4'10"	93–101	98–110	106–122
4'11"	96–104	101–113	109–125
5'0"	99–107	104–116	112–128
5'1"	102–110	110–119	115–131
5'2"	105–113	110–123	118–135
5'3"	108–116	113–127	122–139
5'4"	111–120	117–132	126–143
5'5"	115–124	121–136	130–147
5'6"	119–128	125–140	134–151
5'7"	123–132	129–144	138–155
5'8"	127–137	133–148	142–160
5'9"	131–141	137–152	146–165
5'10"	135–145	141–156	150–170

* If you are between 18 and 25, subtract one pound for each year less than 25. Adapted from Metropolitan Life Insurance.

THE WHIZZ DIET

The hardest part about dieting is getting started. It's simple . . . toss a few ingredients in your blender and within seconds, you're ready. It's only 225 calories per serving, and, most important, it allows no substitution.

WHEN TO WHIZZ

- *1 To help you get started . . . the longer you wait, the harder it gets.*
- *2 If you've been dieting faithfully for weeks and reached a plateau.*
- *3 If you just have 2 or 3 pounds to lose.*

HOW TO WHIZZ

- *1 For breakfast, lunch, dinner whip up either Whizz #1 (with yogurt) or Whizz #2 (with skim milk).*
- *2 At lunch and dinner, make sure to have carrot, celery, or cucumber sticks for roughage to keep your system working.*
- *3 You may have as much coffee or tea (without sugar or cream), water, mineral water, sugar-free diet soda, or unsweetened club soda as you like.*
- *4 Take a balanced vitamin/mineral pill daily.*

Even if you have all the willpower in the world, don't stay on the Whizz for more than a week . . . and check with your doctor before you start.

The big things are exercising the right way, eating the right way—and having a plan—so you are sure to get the variety and balance you need, with plenty of good fresh vegetables and fruit.

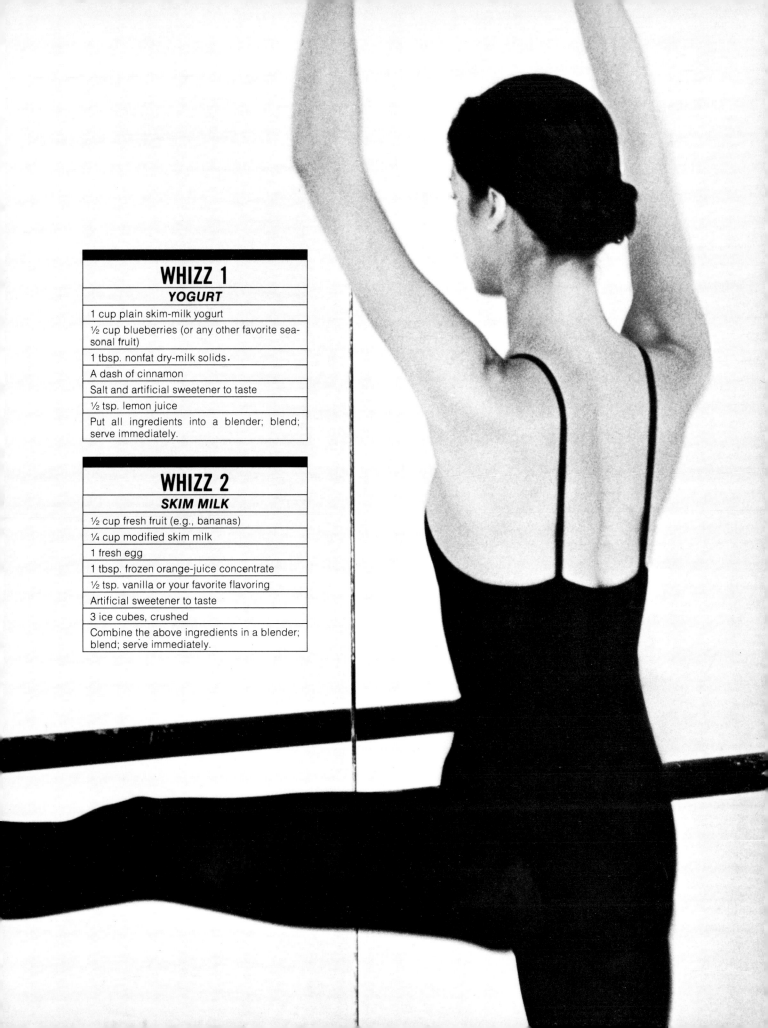

WHIZZ 1
YOGURT

1 cup plain skim-milk yogurt
½ cup blueberries (or any other favorite seasonal fruit)
1 tbsp. nonfat dry-milk solids.
A dash of cinnamon
Salt and artificial sweetener to taste
½ tsp. lemon juice
Put all ingredients into a blender; blend; serve immediately.

WHIZZ 2
SKIM MILK

½ cup fresh fruit (e.g., bananas)
¼ cup modified skim milk
1 fresh egg
1 tbsp. frozen orange-juice concentrate
½ tsp. vanilla or your favorite flavoring
Artificial sweetener to taste
3 ice cubes, crushed
Combine the above ingredients in a blender; blend; serve immediately.

NUTRITION AND LIFESTYLE IN THE 1980s

The way we live today, say nutrition experts, presents us with a number of nutritional booby traps. Some to look out for:

EATING ON THE RUN

With more women working outside the home and kids and parents involved in countless activities, family meals have pretty much gone the way of the Model T. Americans eat nearly half their meals outside the home, often in places where vegetables are not served at all or are prepared in advance and kept on warming tables so long that they lose most of their vitamins and minerals. If you eat on the run, make sure you get some fresh fruits and vegetables along the way.

NIBBLING

Food is so ubiquitous in our society that we tend, as one nutritionist put it, to "forage" all day. The availability of food in office coffee shops, vending machines and on the streets makes it very easy to become an unconscious eater. The result is that we often bypass regular meals where we would more likely have such foods as vegetables.

"NIGHT EATING"

People on the go often skip breakfast, eat rather lightly during the day, and then go home at 5:00 and start eating nonstop. They end up, says Dr. Guthrie, with a higher calorie intake than they think and probably miss out on nutrients by eliminating such "morning" foods as cereal and citrus fruits.

PROCESSED FOODS

In our passion for convenience, we have sacrificed the basics for additive-laden, low-fiber, over-salted and over-sugared packaged products. "Americans don't know how to taste anymore," declares Audrey Cross. "We have lost our sensuous attachment to food that the French, for example, still have. There's a myth that food preparation is extremely time-consuming, which it's not. It's just as easy to put a slice of whole wheat bread in the toaster as it is a frozen waffle. It only takes several minutes longer to prepare a dinner from scratch than from frozen dinners, and the one from scratch costs less, tastes better and is better for you."

INACTIVITY

Even with the physical-fitness craze, most people spend the majority of their time sitting or using labor-saving devices. Yet we continue to eat like our grandparents did. Our calorie consumption just a decade ago was only 180 calories a day below that in the early 1900s.

On the positive side, we know far more about nutrition today than ever before, and our choices for a varied diet are almost endless. Eating well is really quite easy, and it should be fun as well. "Food is intimately related to all our emotions and feelings and our joy of life, as well as being nutrient material," says Dr. Todhunter. "Fear of disease is a poor approach to nutrition and life. Food should be for enjoyment as well as for health."

Experts agree that it is never too late to start eating better.

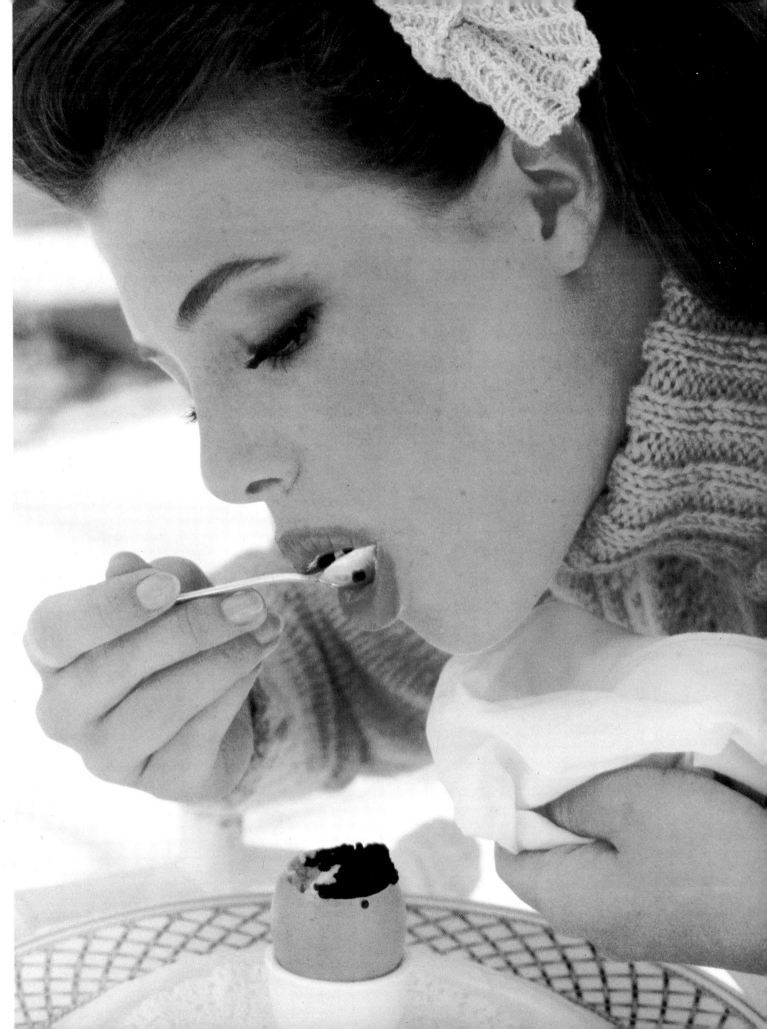

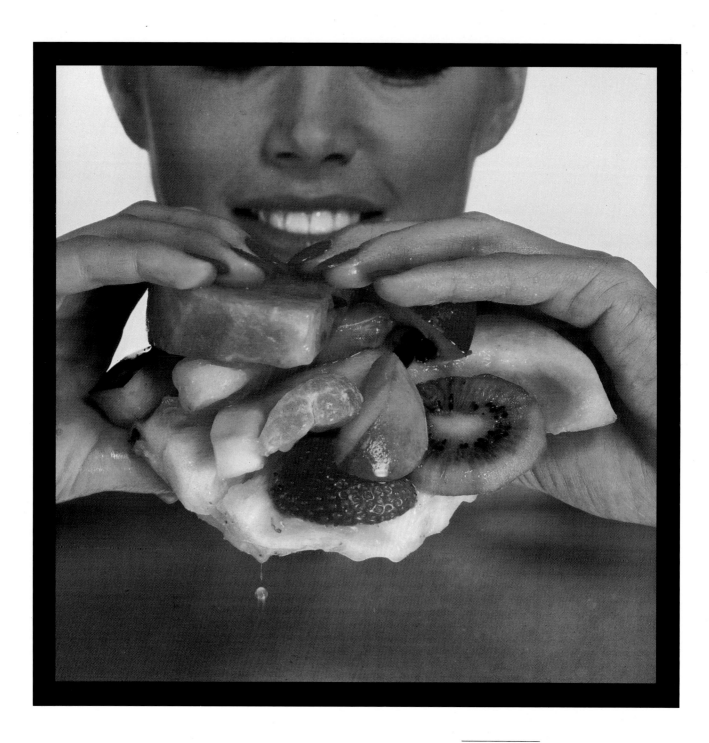

Most nutrition experts now agree that Americans do not need all the protein they consume and that its importance in the diet is overemphasized. High-protein foods such as hamburger and steak are an expensive form in which to get your calories.

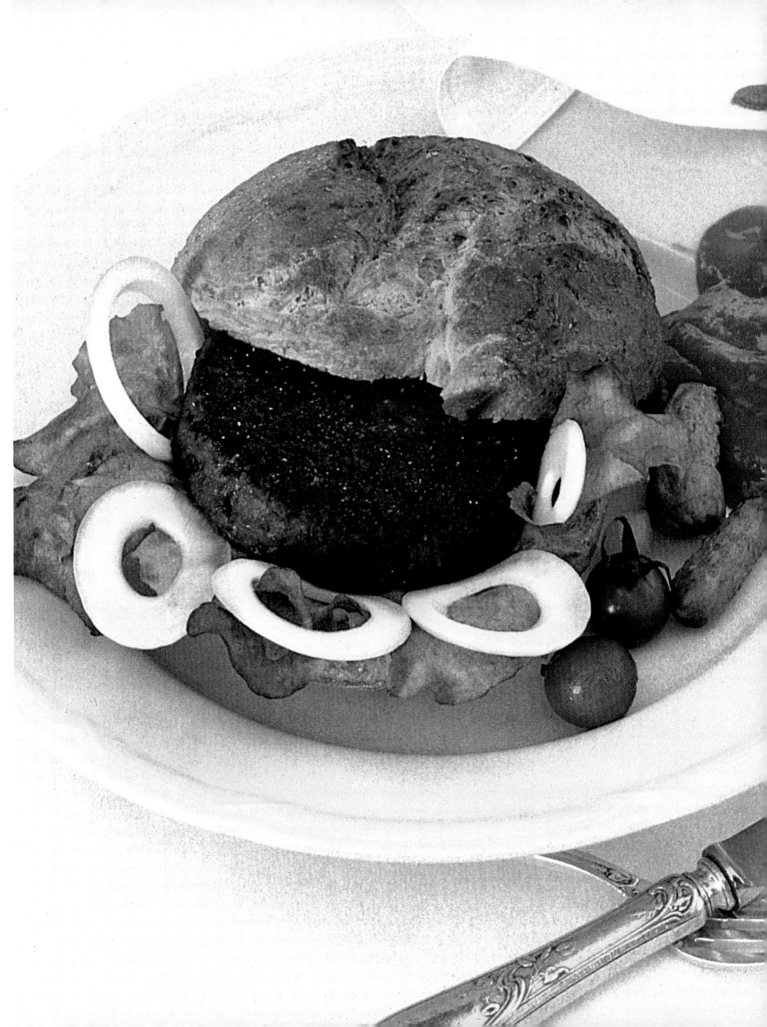

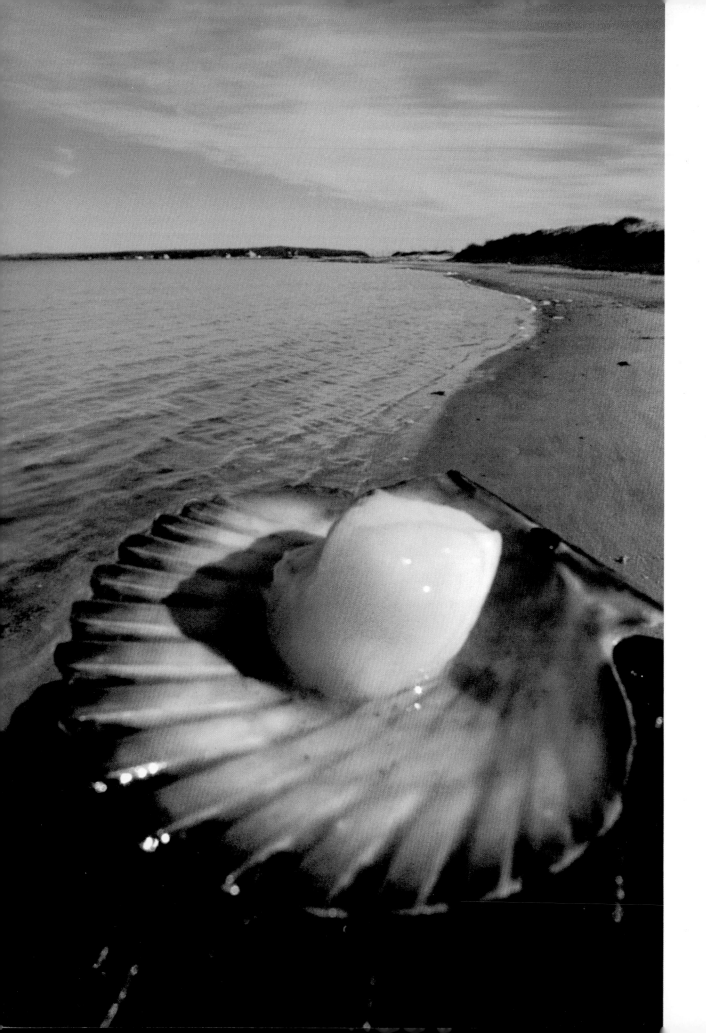

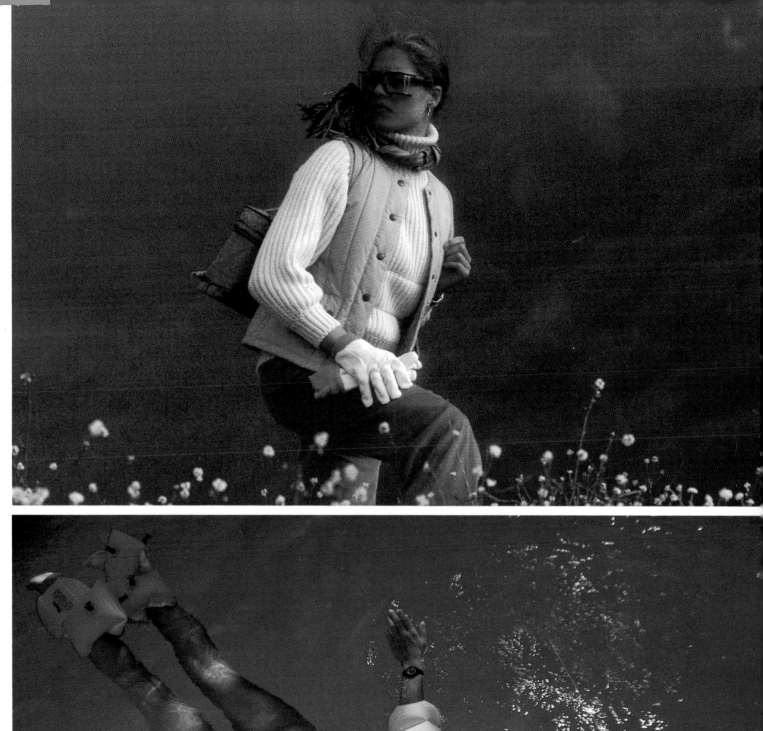
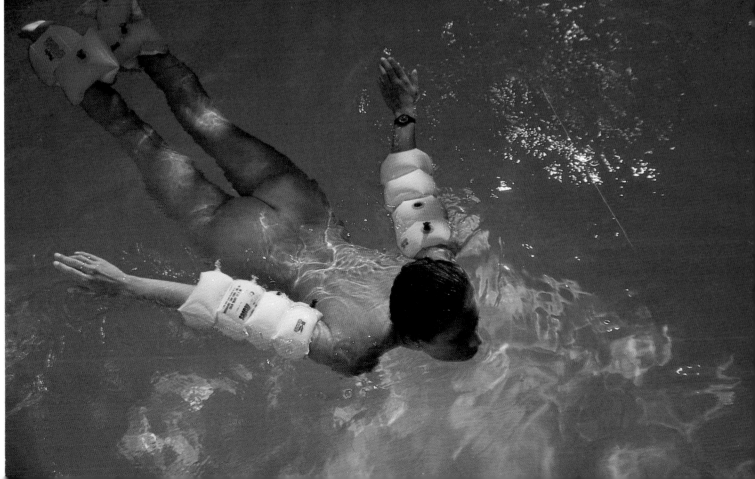

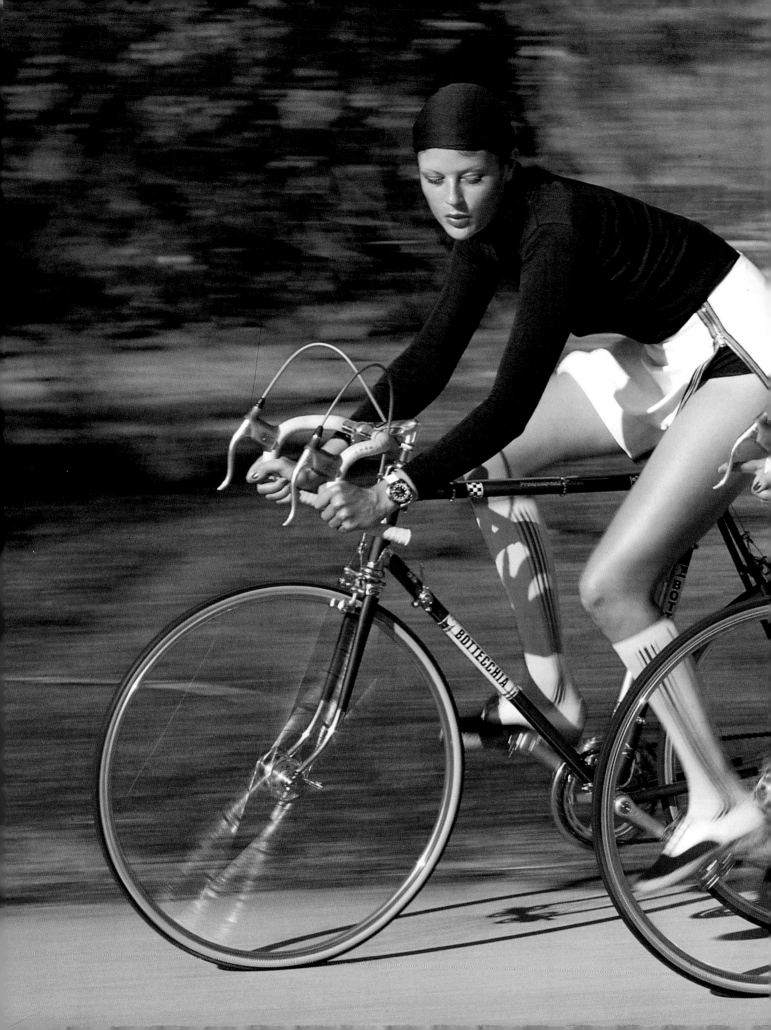

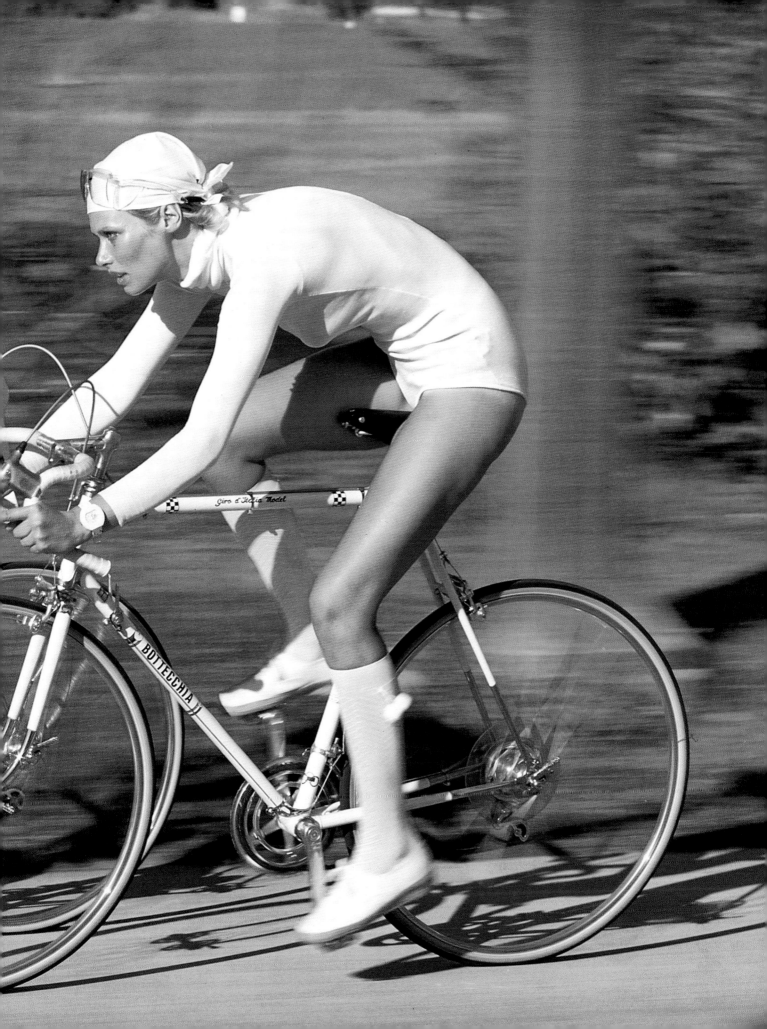

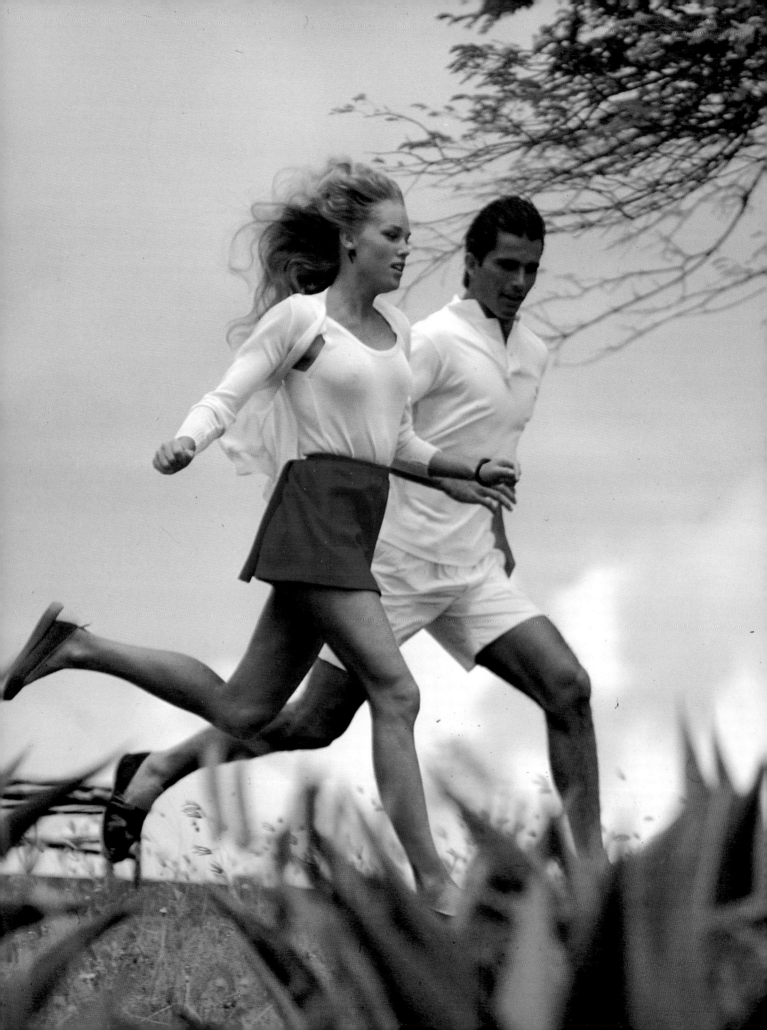

Preceding pages:
The American passion for
convenience has led to the
sacrifice of basic natural foods in
our diet. We often turn to frozen
dinners and pre-packaged foods,
forgetting that it takes only
several seconds to sauté some-
thing as nutritious and elegant
as a scallop.

Inactivity is one of the most
important nutritional booby
traps. Even with the emphasis
on physical fitness, most people
spend the majority of their time
sitting or using labor-saving
devices.

To lose one pound of fat you need
to burn 3,500 more calories than
you consume.

The great summer free style—
the active summer life—
always ready to move.

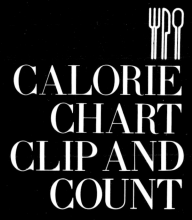

CALORIE
CHART
CLIP AND
COUNT

CALORIE COUNTING

Counting calories can be difficult to judge unless you are careful to weigh all your portions, and check them against a detailed calorie chart. For most of us, though, it is enough to understand something about how the different foods measure up in an average calorie count. Remember that the foods here are listed by portion and weight, to help you count your calories quickly and easily; portions and sizes vary so much it is really impossible to give accurate measures—a 'small' apple can be 3 oz., 4 oz., or 5 oz., depending on the type and season.

A green apple contains less sugar than a ripe one, too. If you want to be more precise, buy a pamphlet or paperback book which lists *all* the calorie values, by ounce, and buy an accurate kitchen scale. Make sure your book includes manufactured foods; they vary quite a lot from one brand to another.

FOOD	AMOUNT	AVERAGE CALORIES
Almonds, dried & unblanched	12–15 nuts	90
roasted & salted	1 oz.	176
Artichoke, raw	1 lg. bud	88
hearts, frozen	3½ oz.	26
Asparagus, cooked	⅔ cup, cut	20
in butter sauce, frozen	1 cup	81
Avocado	half	191
Bagel	1	165
Bamboo shoots, raw	1 cup	36
Beans		
green, raw	1 cup	32
green, frozen, cut	3½ oz.	25
lima, cooked	½ cup	110
wax, yellow, cooked	1 cup	22
Bean sprouts, Mung, raw	1⅔ cup	35
Beef		
hamburger, lean, cooked	1 patty	140
sirloin, lean, broiled	1 slice	128
steak, T-bone, lean only, broiled	1 steak	116
rib roast, lean only	2 slices	70
rib roast, lean & marbled	2 slices	302
Bologna	1 slice	90
Bouillon	1 cube	10
Bran	1 tbsp.	32
Bread		
French & Vienna, enriched	1 slice	58
high-protein, light or diet type	1 slice	50
rye, American	1 slice	56
wheat	1 slice	56
white, enriched	1 slice	62
Broccoli, cooked	1 lg. stalk; ⅔ cup	26
w/Hollandaise, frozen	1 lg. stalk; ⅔ cup	107
Broth, consommé	1 cup	30
Butter or margarine	1 tbsp.	100
Cabbage, raw	½ cup	10
coleslaw w/ mayonnaise	1 cup	173
Cakes		
angel food	1 piece	150
cheese, frozen	1 piece	160
chocolate, devil's food w/chocolate icing from mix	1 piece	184
Candy, chocolate	1 oz.	150
hard	1 oz.	110
Carrot, raw	1 lg.; 2 small	42
cooked	⅔ cup	30
w/brown sugar glaze, frozen	1 serving	82
Cauliflower, cooked, drained	⅞ cup	22
Celery, raw	1 lg. stalk	5
Cereals		
cooked	½ cup	65
oatmeal w/honey	6 tbsp.	72
ready-to-eat	½ cup	55
Cheese		
Brie	1 oz.	94
cream	2 tbsp. (1 oz.)	110
creamed cottage & farmer	1 cup	239
hard (American, Swiss)	1 oz.	105
pot or low-fat cottage	1 cup	163
ricotta, part-skim	½ cup	171
Chicken		
meat, fried	3½ oz.	209
meat & skin, fried	3½ oz.	250
meat, roasted	3½ oz.	183
meat & skin, roasted	3½ oz.	248
salad	½ cup	127
Chicory	1 cup	10
Chow mein	1 portion	430
Coffee, black	1 cup	0
w/cream	1 cup	30
w/cream & sugar	1 cup	50
Cookies	1 lg.; 2 small	100
Corn, cooked	½ cup	75
cornbread	1 2" square	120
Crackers	4 saltines	50
Cream, heavy	2 tbsp. (1 oz.)	110
light	2 tbsp. (1 oz.)	75
Cucumber, raw	½ med.	8
Danish pastry	3 oz.	360
Doughnut, sugared	1	153
Duck, roasted	3½ oz.	310
Egg		
boiled	1 med.	78
fried w/1 tsp. margarine	1 med.	108
scrambled	1 serving	86
Eggnog, Christmas-type	1 punch cup (4 oz.)	335
Egg roll	1	300
Fish		
anchovy	3 thin fillets	21
caviar, pressed	1 round tsp.	32
cod, lean	1 oz.	40
flounder, lean	1 oz.	40
halibut, broiled	1 serving	214
mackerel, fat	1 oz.	65
salmon, canned	1 oz.	55
sardines, canned	1 oz.	55
sole, broiled	1 serving	80
trout, lake, raw	3½ oz.	214
brook	3½ oz.	101
tuna, canned	1 oz.	55
Flour, white & whole grain	1 tbsp., unsifted	35
Frankfurter	1 average, cooked	124
Fruit		
apple	1 med.	87
baked w/2 tbsp. sugar	1 med.	188
applesauce, sweet	⅓ cup	91
unsweetened	½ cup scant	41
apricots, dried	3 med.	65
fresh	2–3	51
banana, raw	1 med.; 1 cup sliced	127
blueberries	½ cup	45
cantaloupe	½ med.	55
cherries	15 lg.; 25 small	70
dates	3 med., pitted	82
figs	2 lg.; 3 small	80
grapefruit	½ med.	41
grapes	22 med.	69
honeydew melon	½ small	66
orange	1 med.	73
peach	2 med.	80
pear	½ med.	61
plum	3	80
prunes	5 med.	127
raisins	2 tbsp.	65
raspberries, red	¾ cup	57
strawberries, unsweetened	1 cup	56
tangerine	1 med.	55
watermelon	10" x 16" wedge	234
canned fruit, syrup-packed	½ cup	100
Gelatin dessert, plain	½ cup	70
Grapefruit juice, unsweetened	½ cup	55
Honey	1 tbsp.	61
Ice cream	½ cup	130

Item	Amount	Calories
Ice milk	½ cup	100
Jam	1 tbsp.	50
Jelly	1 tbsp.	50
Lamb		
lean & marbled, roasted	2 slices	192
Lettuce	1 cup	10
Liquor		
beer	12 oz.	170
Daiquiri	1 cocktail glass	122
gin	1½ fl. oz.	110
rum	1½ fl. oz.	110
vodka	1½ fl. oz.	110
whiskey	1½ fl. oz.	110
Liver		
calf's, fried	3½ oz.	261
chicken, simmered	3½ oz.	165
paste (pâté de foie gras)	1 tbsp.	69
Liverwurst	1 slice	139
Macaroni	½ cup, cooked	80
Matzoh	1 square	130
Mayonnaise	1 tbsp.	100
Milk		
buttermilk	8 oz.	115
chocolate	8 oz.	208
evaporated skim (undiluted)	4 oz.	90
evaporated whole (undiluted)	4 oz.	170
liquid skimmed	8 oz.	105
nonfat, dry	⅓ cup	95
whole	8 oz.	160
Muffins		
blueberry	1 average	112
bran	1 average	104
corn	1 average	140
English	1 whole	138
Mushrooms, fresh, raw	4 lg.; 10 small	28
w/butter, frozen	3½ oz.	55
Noodles	½ cup, cooked	105
Oil	1 tbsp.	125
Olives, ripe, green	2 lg.	37
Orange juice, unsweetened	½ cup	55
Pancakes, buttermilk w/ butter & maple syrup	1 serving	578
Peanut butter	1 tbsp.	95
Peanuts	1 oz.	165
Peas		
blackeyed, frozen	3½ oz.	130
cooked, drained	¾ cup	88
in cream sauce, frozen	3½ oz.	156
dried	½ cup, cooked	115
frozen	3½ oz.	68
split pea soup	1 cup	145
Pies		
custard	1 piece	285
fruit	1 piece	418
lemon chiffon	1 piece	335
pecan	1 piece	334
Pizza, cheese	5½" section	185
Popcorn		
plain w/out fat or salt	1 cup (1¼ oz.)	54
sugar-coated	1 cup (1¼ oz.)	135
Pork		
fresh or frozen	1 oz.	90
loin chop, lean & fat, cooked	1 chop	314
loin chop, lean only, cooked	1 chop	170
bacon	2 slices	90
ham, fresh or frozen	1 oz.	80
ham, cured, lean & marbled, cooked	3½ oz.	348
ham, boiled	1 oz.	70
Potatoes		
baked w/out skin	1, 3¼" diam.	139
baked w/sour cream	1	243
boiled in skin	1 med.	76
chip	1 oz.	170
French-fried	3½ oz.	220
mashed w/milk & margarine	½ cup	94
sweet, baked in skin	1 med.	141
Pretzels	1 oz.	120
Radishes	4	5
Rice		
brown, cooked	1 cup	178
fried	1 cup	353
white enriched long grain—parboiled, cooked	1 cup	159
wild, frozen	1 cup	91
Rolls		
hamburger & frankfurter	1	120
hard	1 lg.	155
Salad dressings		
blue/Roquefort	1 tbsp.	71
French	1 tbsp.	57
Italian	1 tbsp.	77
Russian	1 tbsp.	74
Salami	1 oz.	90
Shellfish		
clams, raw	5 lg.; 10 small	80
lobster	1 oz.	25
oysters	5–8 med.	66
shrimp	1 oz.	25
Sherbet	½ cup	120
Soda, carbonated, sweetened	12 oz.	150
Sour cream	2 tbsp. (1 oz.)	50
Spaghetti	½ cup, cooked	80
Squash		
butternut, baked, mashed	1 cup	139
Hubbard, baked, mashed	1 cup	103
summer, boiled, drained	½ cup	14
winter, acorn, baked	half	86
Sugar		
brown, crude	1 tbsp.	14
white, granulated	1 tbsp.	50
Tomato	½ med.	20
juice	1 cup	55
soup	1 cup	85
Turkey		
dark meat, roasted	3½ oz.	203
light meat, roasted	3½ oz.	176
Tetrazzini, frozen	1 serving	282
Veal		
cutlet, round, lean & fat, cooked	3½ oz.	277
cutlet, round, lean only	3½ oz.	194
fresh or frozen	1 oz.	65
Vegetable soup	1 cup	85
Waffles, plain	1	209
Walnuts, black	8–10 halves	94
Wine		
dry	3½ fl. oz.	85
sweet	3½ fl. oz.	140
champagne, dry	4 oz.	90
sherry	1 oz.	40
Yogurt		
fruit-flavored	8 oz.	285
plain	8 oz.	135
vanilla & coffee	8 oz.	200

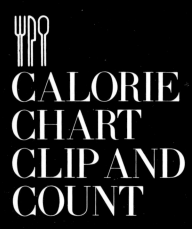

CALORIE
CHART
CLIP AND
COUNT

FASTING

Fasting has become a popular means of "cleansing" the body physically and mentally, either as part of a reducing diet or in preparation for a more healthful eating regimen.

Psychologically, a one- or two-day fast can give you an opportunity to reassess your relationship with food. And rapidly shedding a few pounds can give you the boost you need to continue reducing. Fasting, however, will do little to change your basic eating habits in ways conducive to permanent weight loss. In fact, you will likely feel so starved that you will be tempted to go on an eating spree at the end of the fast.

As for the notion of fasting to cleanse your body of accumulated toxic materials, there is no evidence that one has to stop eating in order to remove wastes. Eating a normal diet with plenty of liquids and adequate amounts of fiber should do the job perfectly well. Certainly, no one should fast for longer than a day or two without a doctor's supervision. After that time, the body's protein begins to break down, increasing the likelihood of some serious health problems.

VEGETARIANISM

In their quest for better health, more and more Americans are turning to a vegetarian diet, and scientific evidence suggests that they might have the right idea. Studies show that long-term vegetarians, such as the Seventh Day Adventists religious group, are less likely to develop heart disease, high blood pressure and high cholesterol levels.

But the strict vegetarian—one who shuns eggs and milk products as well as meat—must be especially careful to get a varied diet, nutrition experts say. Important minerals, such as calcium and iron, are much less easily absorbed from vegetables than from milk and meat. It is also difficult to get a complete balance of essential amino acids, the building blocks of protein, from vegetable sources alone. By carefully combining foods, such as beans and corn or beans and wheat, however, it is possible to achieve the balance your body needs. One vitamin, B_{12}, is present only in animal tissues, so the strict vegetarian will most likely need B_{12} supplements. Those who eat milk and eggs get plenty of B_{12}.

	FOODS TO HAVE	FOODS TO AVOID— OR GO EASY ON
● MILK	Skim milk Skim-milk buttermilk Low-fat yogurt	Whole milk Cream Cream substitutes
● EGGS	Whites only— unlimited amount Yolks—limit to 3 or fewer a week	
● MEAT	Lean, well-trimmed beef, lamb, veal, pork, ham Chicken, turkey Dried chipped beef Fish	Luncheon meats Sausages, bacon Poultry skin Regular ground beef Fatty meats Meat stock with fat Frozen and packaged dinners
● CHEESE	Skim milk pot cheese, cottage cheese and other cheeses	Cheese made with whole milk Cream cheese Creamed cottage cheese unless substituted for meat (¼ cup equals 1 ounce meat)
● POTATOES PASTA	Potatoes, white and sweet; rice, macaroni, spaghetti, noodles	Commerically prepared potatoes
● VEGETABLES	Any vegetables cooked without saturated fat Include at least 1 green or yellow vegetable daily	Buttered, creamed or fried vegetables unless prepared with the amount of fat allowed
● FRUITS	Any fresh, frozen, canned or dried fruit or juice Include at least 1 citrus daily Avocado may be used in small amounts	Fruits in sauces
● BREADS AND CRACKERS	White, whole wheat, or rye bread Crackers Graham Matzoh Melba toast Rye-Krisp	Biscuits Commercial muffins Rolls, sweet or hot Cornbread Pancakes Waffles French toast Corn and potato chips Flavored crackers

Before going on this or any other diet, consult your doctor.

MINI-MIDI-MAXI DIET

A new way to think about food

This diet is based on a daily allowance of 1500 calories. Most women use up 2000 calories a day—if you have a calorie deficit of 500 a day, or 3500 a week, you should lose weight at a rate of one pound a week. During the first week on this diet you can expect to lose considerably more, say five pounds, because initially your body gets rid of surplus water as well as surplus fat. At the end of six weeks you should have lost 10 pounds. The flexibility of this diet comes about because you can decide for yourself which meals you eat and when you eat them. It is called the Mini-Midi-Maxi plan because each day you can have: a Mini-meal—about 200 calories, a Midi-meal—about 500 calories, a Maxi-meal—about 800 calories.

GROUP A (about 5 calories an ounce)	
Apricots	Celery
Grapefruit	Chicory
Lemon	Cucumber
Melon	Eggplant
Raspberries	Lettuce
Red currants	Mushrooms
Rhubarb	Onions
Strawberries	Parsley
Tangerines	Radishes
Artichokes	Rutabaga
Asparagus	Salad greens
Beans, green	Spinach
Broccoli	Summer squash
Brussels sprouts	Tomatoes
Cabbage	Turnips
Carrots	Watercress
Cauliflower	Zucchini

GROUP B (about 10 calories an ounce)	
Apples	Pears
Blackberries	Pineapple
Black currants	Plums
Cherries	Bean sprouts
Gooseberries	Beets
Grapes	Leeks
Oranges	Parsnips
Peaches	Peppers

GROUP C (more than 20 calories an ounce)	
Bananas	Corn
Prunes	Peas
Beans, baked	Potatoes
Beans, lima	Avocado pear

MINI-MEALS

BREAKFASTS	CALORIES
1 oz. cereal	100
½ cup milk	80
	180
2 slices lightly buttered toast	200
2 tsp. marmalade	35
	235
4 oz. unsweetened fruit juice	50
1 egg, poached	90
1 slice lightly buttered toast	100
	240
½ grapefruit	40
2 oz. lean ham	135
1 small tomato	20
	195
2 oz. lean bacon grilled (4 strips)	200
1 small tomato, grilled	20
	220
1 egg, boiled	90
1 slice lightly buttered toast	100
	190

MINI-MEALS

LUNCHES OR DINNERS	CALORIES
1	
1 poached egg	90
1 slice lightly buttered toast	100
	190
3½ oz. smoked salmon, 2 pieces melba toast	200
2 oz. lean ham, grilled	135
1 small tomato, sliced	20
1 slice toast, plain	65
	220
2	
2 oz. Edam cheese	160
1 small apple	60
	220
8-oz. carton plain yogurt	130
medium orange	70
	200
2 oz. white-meat turkey sandwich on 1 piece pumpernickel with lettuce, 1 sliced tomato, mustard	200
3	
1 cup soup	100
1 roll	100
	200
8 oz. beer or 4 oz. dry white wine	100
10 potato chips	100
	200
1 plain omelet	210

MIDI-MEALS

BREAKFASTS	CALORIES
1 oz. cereal	100
½ cup milk	80
1 poached egg	90
2 strips lean bacon, grilled	100
1 medium banana	125
	495
8-oz. glass unsweetened fruit juice	100
1 hard-boiled egg	90
2 slices lightly buttered toast	200
2 tbsp. marmalade	110
	500

½ grapefruit	40
3½ oz. pickled herring	225
2 slices lightly buttered toast	200
	465

1 small orange, sliced	50
1 oz. cereal	100
½ cup milk	80
3½ oz. poached salmon	180
1 slice lightly buttered toast	100
	510

¾ cup Cream of Wheat	100
½ cup milk	80
3 oz. sausage, grilled (3 3-in. links)	300
	480

1 medium banana	125
1 oz. muesli	110
½ cup milk	80
1 slice lightly buttered toast	100
1 egg, scrambled	100
	515

MIDI-MEALS

LUNCHES OR DINNERS	CALORIES

1

1 cup soup	100
2 oz. grated cheese	220
2 slices lightly buttered toast	200
	520

5 oz. grilled sirloin steak, well-trimmed	320
4 oz. group A vegetables	20
1 medium banana	125
10 large strawberries	35
	500

6 oz. breaded fish sticks	295
4 oz. group C vegetables	100
1 baked potato, salt and pepper	100
	495

2

2 slices Italian bread	110
1 tbsp. butter	100
2 oz. cheddar cheese	220
8 oz. beer or 4 oz. dry white wine	100
	530

1 slice lean roast beef	200
1 small dinner roll	70
8 oz. plain yogurt	130
1 small banana	85
	485

1 cup soup	100
bacon (2 strips), lettuce, tomato sandwich with 1 tsp. mayonnaise	300
½ cantaloupe, wedge of lime	60
	460

3

1 cup soup	100
4 oz. roast beef, lean	300
1 small boiled potato with parsley, salt and pepper	50
Wedge lettuce with 1 tbsp. salad dressing	50
	500

½ grapefruit	40
5 oz. grilled sirloin steak, lean	320
4 oz. group A vegetables	20
3 oz. group C vegetables	75
4 oz. group A or B fresh fruit	40
	495

6 oz. grilled chicken	210
4 oz. group A vegetables	20
2 oz. group B vegetables	20
1 small roll with 1 tsp. butter	120
1 cup fresh strawberries lightly dusted with 1 tsp. sugar	75
	445

MAXI-MEALS

LUNCHES OR DINNERS	CALORIES

1

1 cup soup	100
4 strips bacon	200
4 oz. grilled liver with onions and mushrooms	200
4 oz. group B vegetables	40
1 medium banana	125
½ cup ice cream	140
	805

Spaghetti casserole:	
4 oz. hamburger	225
2 small tomatoes	40
4 oz. mushrooms	10
2 oz. spaghetti	210
4 oz. apple pie (1/12th of 9″ pie)	205
⅓ cup ice cream	90
	780

5 oz. breaded fish sticks	245
4 oz. French fries	300
3 oz. group C vegetables	75
½ cup ice cream	140
1 small apple	60
	820

2

2 oz. smoked salmon	70
1 slice brown bread, lightly buttered	100
6 oz. roast chicken	210
4 oz. group B vegetables	40
¾ cup boiled rice	105
6 oz. group A or B fruit	60
2 tbsp. light cream	100
4 oz. dry white wine	100
	785

1 cup consommé	50
1 roll	100
6 oz. lamb chop, grilled	240
4 oz. group B vegetables	40
1 baked potato, no butter	100
4 oz. caramel custard	300
	830

¼ cantaloupe	30
1 baked potato, no butter	100
8 oz. grilled sole	320
4 oz. group B vegetables	40
1 small piece apple pie (1/12th of 9″ pie)	205
½ cup ice cream	140
	835

3

Cheese and tuna-fish sandwiches:	
4 slices lightly buttered bread	400
½ cup water-packed tuna, low-calorie salad dressing	125
2 oz. cheddar cheese	220
2 small tomatoes, lettuce	50
4 oz. grapes	40
	835

¼ lb. (4 oz.) lean hamburger cooked in 1 tsp. butter	225
1 sliced tomato, lettuce	30
1 slice cheesecake	400
4 oz. group A or B fruit	40
4 oz. dry white wine	100
	795

2 oz. white-meat turkey, 2 strips bacon, 1 tsp. mayonnaise, 3 slices white bread	550
15 potato chips	150
1 small apple	60
	760

THE THINKING WOMAN'S DIET

By Judith Stern, Sc.D.

		SUNDAY		MONDAY		TUESDAY	
BREAKFAST	LOSE	1 cup bran flakes	150	¾ cup orange juice	90	½ fresh grapefruit	55
		½ small banana	41	1 poached egg on	88	1 cup oatmeal	147
		¾ cup skim milk*	66	1 slice whole grain toast	65	¾ cup skim milk	66
		Coffee or tea	0	Coffee or tea	0	Coffee or tea	0
		TOTAL CALORIES: 257		**TOTAL CALORIES: 243**		**TOTAL CALORIES: 268**	
	MAINTAIN	● 1 small banana	81	● 1 cup orange juice	120	● 1 cup oatmeal	147
		1 cup low-fat milk*	120	½ tablespoon butter		1 cup low-fat milk	120
		TOTAL CALORIES: 351		or margarine on toast	50	1 tablespoon raisins	29
				TOTAL CALORIES: 323		**TOTAL CALORIES: 351**	
	GAIN	● 1 medium banana	101	● 2 slices whole grain toast	130	● 1 cup regular milk	159
		1 cup regular milk*	159	1 tablespoon butter		**TOTAL CALORIES: 427**	
COFFEE BREAK		**TOTAL CALORIES: 410**		or margarine on toast	100		
		* milk may be used in coffee or tea		**TOTAL CALORIES: 438**			
	GAIN / LOSE	1 glazed doughnut	170	1 English muffin, toasted, buttered	215	1 Danish, 4¼-inch diameter	274
LUNCH		Garden Vegetable Sandwich	280	1 carrot and 1 stalk celery, cut into strips	30	Ham and cream cheese sandwich	338
		1 piece pita bread, 5-6 inches diameter, filled with		8 ounces plain, low-fat yogurt with ¾ cup fresh pineapple,	130	1 slice pumpernickel bread	
		1 ounce Monterey Jack cheese		diced, or ½ cup canned crushed		1 tablespoon low-fat cream cheese	
		½ tomato, sliced		pineapple, packed in juice	65	3 ounces lean ham (trim off fat)	
		½ cucumber, sliced		iced tea/mineral water	0	½ medium tomato, sliced	
		⅓ cup alfalfa sprouts		¼ cup raisins	116	⅓ cup alfalfa sprouts	
		fresh spinach leaves		**TOTAL CALORIES: 341**		½ cucumber, sliced	
		iced tea/mineral water with lime	0			Iced tea/mineral water	0
		1 small apple	59			**TOTAL CALORIES: 338**	
		TOTAL CALORIES: 339					
	MAINTAIN	● Garden Vegetable Sandwich with 1½ ounces Monterey Jack cheese	280	● 1 tablespoon chopped walnuts with raisins	50	● Ham and cream cheese sandwich with 2 tablespoons cream cheese	417
		TOTAL CALORIES: 392		**TOTAL CALORIES: 391**		**TOTAL CALORIES: 417**	
	GAIN	● 1 large apple	93	● 2 tablespoons chopped walnuts with raisins	100	● Ham and cream cheese sandwich with 2 tablespoons cream cheese	477
		TOTAL CALORIES: 426		**TOTAL CALORIES: 441**		**TOTAL CALORIES: 477**	
DINNER	LOSE	1 cup Manhattan clam chowder	70	¾ cup tomato juice with wedge of lemon	35	5 ounces sea bass	138
		4 ounces lean corned beef (remove all fat)	200	½ chicken breast, baked and basted with juice		Baked at 350° with:	
		1 cup cabbage, boiled	29	and pulp of one orange,		2 tablespoons lemon juice	
		2 carrots, boiled	40	4 drops of Tabasco sauce,		1 tablespoon lime juice	
		¾ cup small boiled potatoes, with minced parsley and		¼ teaspoon ginger, salt	200	½ clove minced garlic tarragon, parsley,	
		1 teaspoon butter/margarine	123	⅔ cup green peas with		salt, pepper to taste	
		2 tablespoons spicy mustard	24	¼ cup mushrooms	76	1 cup spinach with nutmeg	53
		1½ cups mixed green salad dressed with garlic wine vinegar	30	½ cup rice garnished with ½ tablespoon raisins and		Salad: 1 small green pepper 1 medium tomato, chopped,	
		Coffee or tea	0	½ tablespoon chopped cashew nuts	125	thin slices bermuda onion	49
		TOTAL CALORIES: 516		1 wedge lettuce dressed with 1½ tablespoons low-calorie		marinated in 1½ tablespoons low-calorie Italian dressing	23
				salad dressing	33	1 small roll	90
				Coffee or tea	0	1 teaspoon butter or margarine	34
				TOTAL CALORIES: 469		Coffee or tea	0
						½ cup orange or lemon sherbet	115
						TOTAL CALORIES: 502	
	MAINTAIN	● 1½ tablespoons French dressing on mixed green salad	80	● lettuce wedge with 1½ tablespoons Italian or French dressing	115	● 6 ounces sea bass	165
		TOTAL CALORIES: 566		¾ cup fresh pineapple or 1 large sliced, canned, packed in juice	55	⅓ cup white or brown rice, cooked with chicken bouillon and chopped onions	63
				TOTAL CALORIES: 606		**TOTAL CALORIES: 592**	
	GAIN	● 12 ounces beer	155	● 4 ounces dry white wine	95	● ½ cup rice	95
		TOTAL CALORIES: 721		¾ cup pineapple with 1 small orange peeled and cut into wedges	104	1½ tablespoons regular Italian dressing on salad	105
				TOTAL CALORIES: 750		¾ cup sherbet	173
						TOTAL CALORIES: 764	
EVENING SNACKS	MAINTAIN	¾ cup low-fat milk	90	⅔ cup sherbert	152	Blend: ¼ cup frozen blueberries	24
		1 chocolate chip cookie	50	**TOTAL CALORIES: 152**		½ small banana	40
		TOTAL CALORIES: 140				¾ cup low-fat milk	90
						TOTAL CALORIES: 154	
	GAIN	● 1 cup regular milk	159	● 1 cup ice cream	250	● Banana blueberry treat made with	
		2 chocolate chip cookies	100	**TOTAL CALORIES: 250**		1 cup regular milk	159
		TOTAL CALORIES: 259				2 teaspoons brown sugar	34
						TOTAL CALORIES: 257	

● ADD OR SUBSTITUTE

WEDNESDAY	THURSDAY	FRIDAY	SATURDAY
¾ cup tomato juice 35 1 English muffin, toasted (2 halves) 140 2 tablespoons low-fat cream cheese (Neufschatel) on muffin 80 Coffee or tea 0 **TOTAL CALORIES: 255**	1 small orange, sliced 49 Omelette: 88 1 egg, 1 teaspoon water, tarragon, chives, parsley cooked in nonstick pan with Pam 1 slice whole grain toast 65 1 teaspoon butter/margarine 34 Coffee or tea 0 **TOTAL CALORIES: 236**	¼ of 5-inch cantaloupe 30 ¼ cup granola, mixed with ¾ cup plain low-fat yogurt 196 Coffee or tea 0 **TOTAL CALORIES: 226**	1 cup Special K cereal 105 1 cup skim milk 88 ¾ cup fresh strawberries, sliced 41 Coffee or tea 0 **TOTAL CALORIES: 234**
● ¾ cup orange juice 90 2 tablespoons cream cheese on muffin 100 **TOTAL CALORIES: 330**	● Omelette: 2 eggs 176 2 teaspoons water, herbs ½ tablespoon butter/margarine 50 **TOTAL CALORIES: 340**	● ½ cup granola 290 **TOTAL CALORIES: 320**	● 1½ cups Special K 158 1 cup low-fat milk 120 1 teaspoon sugar 15 **TOTAL CALORIES: 334**
● 1½ tablespoons jam 76 **TOTAL CALORIES: 406**	● 1 medium orange, sliced 73 **TOTAL CALORIES: 364**	● 2 tablespoons chopped almonds 86 **TOTAL CALORIES: 406**	● 1 cup regular milk 159 1 cup fresh strawberries, sliced 54 2 teaspoons sugar 30 **TOTAL CALORIES: 401**
1 piece coffee cake, ⅛ of 8-inch diam. cake ring, 2-inch hole 179	2 slices whole grain toast, buttered 205	1½ ounces Swiss cheese with 2 slices French bread 246	1 bagel, toasted, with 3 tablespoons cream cheese 300
¾ cup vegetarian vegetable soup 57 1½ ounces Camembert or Brie cheese 128 2 pieces French bread, 2½-x 2-x ½-inches 88 1 pear (2½-x 3½-inches) 81 Coffee or tea 0 **TOTAL CALORIES: 354**	Cheeseburger 347 Coffee or tea 0 **TOTAL CALORIES: 347**	Tuna plate: lettuce, 3½ ounces tuna, water-packed, tomato, cucumber, 3 radishes, sliced; lemon wedges 165 1 slice whole grain bread 65 1 teaspoon butter or margarine 34 1 medium orange 73 Coffee or tea 0 **TOTAL CALORIES: 337**	Bacon, lettuce and tomato sandwich 297 2 slices toast 1 medium tomato, sliced 2 slices bacon lettuce 1 teaspoon mayonnaise 1 dill pickle 10 1 large tangerine 46 Iced tea 0 **TOTAL CALORIES: 353**
● 2 ounces cheese 170 **TOTAL CALORIES: 396**	● Hamburger, no mayonnaise 319 ½ regular order of French fries 105 **TOTAL CALORIES: 424**	● 1 tablespoon Thousand Island dressing on tuna salad 75 **TOTAL CALORIES: 412**	● Bacon, lettuce, and tomato sandwich 347 3 slices bacon **TOTAL CALORIES: 403**
● 1 cup vegetarian vegetable soup 76 with 1 tablespoon Parmesan cheese 21 **TOTAL CALORIES: 436**	● 1 order of French fries 209 **TOTAL CALORIES: 528**	● 1½ tablespoons Thousand Island dressing on salad 113 **TOTAL CALORIES: 450**	● Bacon, lettuce, and tomato sandwich 413 1 tablespoon mayonnaise **TOTAL CALORIES: 469**
4-ounce sirloin steak, broiled (lean only) 247 1 small baked potato 106 with 1 tablespoon sour cream 25 1 cup string beans 40 1½ cups mixed salad greens, dressed with wine vinegar or lemon juice 30 ½ grapefruit 55 Coffee or tea 0 **TOTAL CALORIES: 503**	¾ cup minestrone soup 66 1½ cups cooked spaghetti 237 ½ cup marinara sauce and 1 teaspoon Parmesan cheese 80 / 7 1 piece (2-x 2-x ½-inch) garlic bread with 44 ½ teaspoon butter or margarine, and minced garlic 17 1½ cups mixed salad greens dressed with wine vinegar or lemon 30 Coffee or tea 0 **TOTAL CALORIES: 481**	1 cup beef consommé with 1 tablespoon scallions, shredded 33 Lemon Veal: 275 4 ounces veal scallops browned, in 2 teaspoons butter or margarine, 2 tablespoons minced onions Sauce: 2 tablespoons lemon juice, capers, parsley ⅓ cup rice, cooked in chicken bouillon 60 6 asparagus spears 26 Salad: 1 medium tomato, 56 marinated in 1½ tablespoons low-calorie Italian dressing and 1 teaspoon basil ¼ cantaloupe with lemon or lime 30 Coffee or tea 0 **TOTAL CALORIES: 480**	1 cup tomato soup prepared with water and a dash of curry powder 84 Shrimp Louis Salad: 176 2 cups mixed salad greens 3 ounces shrimp, peeled, deveined, boiled 1 small cucumber, sliced 1 medium tomato cut in wedges ¼ cup alfalfa sprouts 4 medium radishes with 3 tablespoons low-calorie Thousand Island dressing 45 2 sesame bread sticks 76 1 scoop frozen yogurt 96 Coffee or tea 0 **TOTAL CALORIES: 477**
● 4 ounces dry red wine 95 **TOTAL CALORIES: 598**	● 1 tablespoon Italian dressing on salad 70 ½ cup fresh grapes 53 **TOTAL CALORIES: 604**	● 1 small roll with 1 teaspoon butter/margarine 124 **TOTAL CALORIES: 604**	● 4 ounces shrimp, boiled 202 ½ tablespoon butter or margarine with bread sticks 50 **TOTAL CALORIES: 252**
● 6-ounce sirloin steak 308 2 tablespoons sour cream 50 1 tablespoon Italian dressing 70 1 slice French bread with ½ teaspoon butter/margarine 17 **TOTAL CALORIES: 785**	● 1 cup minestrone soup 88 2 cups cooked spaghetti 316 ⅔ cup marinara sauce 107 2 teaspoons Parmesan cheese 14 **TOTAL CALORIES: 739**	● 5 ounces veal 344 tomato sliced and marinated in 1½ tablespoons regular Italian dressing and 1 teaspoon basil 138 **TOTAL CALORIES: 755**	● 2 tablespoons regular Thousand Island salad dressing 210 1 tablespoon butter or margarine with bread sticks 100 **TOTAL CALORIES: 768**
Trail mix: ¼ cup raisins 116 1 tablespoon almonds 43 **TOTAL CALORIES: 159**	Strawberry treat blend: ¾ cup low-fat milk 90 ¾ cup frozen strawberries 41 1 teaspoon brown sugar 17 dash of lemon juice **TOTAL CALORIES: 148**	½ cup low-fat milk 60 1 piece angel food cake (1/16 of 9¾-inch cake) 104 **TOTAL CALORIES: 164**	¾ cup low-fat milk 90 1 Oreo cookie (chocolate cookie with cream filling) 50 **TOTAL CALORIES: 140**
● Trail mix: 3 tablespoons almonds 129 **TOTAL CALORIES: 245**	● Strawberry treat made with 1 cup regular milk 159 ½ small banana 40 **TOTAL CALORIES: 257**	● 1 cup whole milk 159 **TOTAL CALORIES: 263**	● 1 cup regular milk 159 1¾-x ⅓-x ⅞-inch brownie 100 **TOTAL CALORIES: 259**

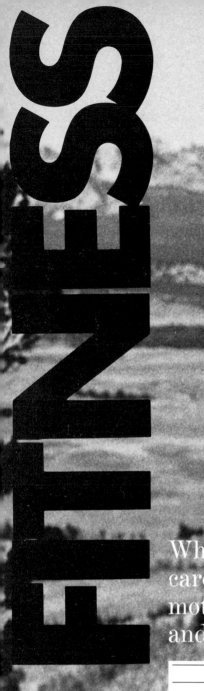

FITNESS

When you talk about long-range physical care, you're talking about a different kind of motivation—that is, valuing your own self and your own body for your own sake

MARIEL'S TRAINING SCHEDULE			
	MONDAY WEDNESDAY FRIDAY	**TUESDAY THURSDAY**	**SATURDAY SUNDAY**
7–9 A.M.	at the training hill—running	at the training hill—climbing	races, bike tour, tennis, racquetball, horseback riding
9–10 A.M.	quick cool-off swim	sprints, agility drills	
10–12 A.M.	weight lifting		
	lunch		
2–4 P.M.	swimming		
4–5 P.M.	stretching	biking	

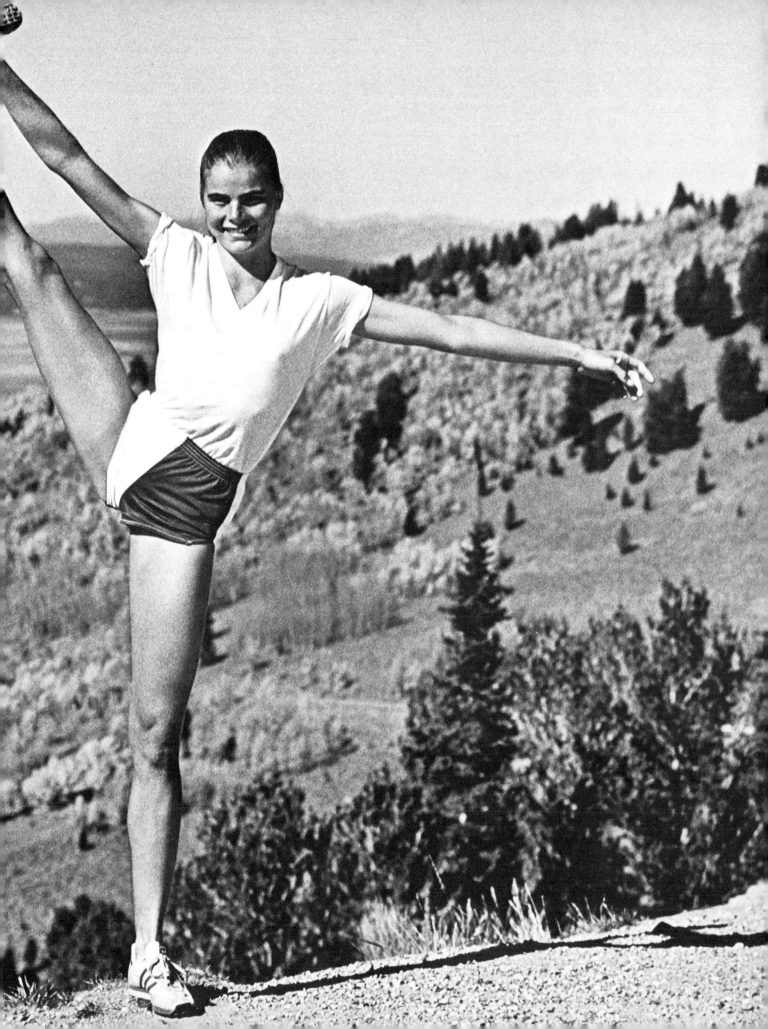

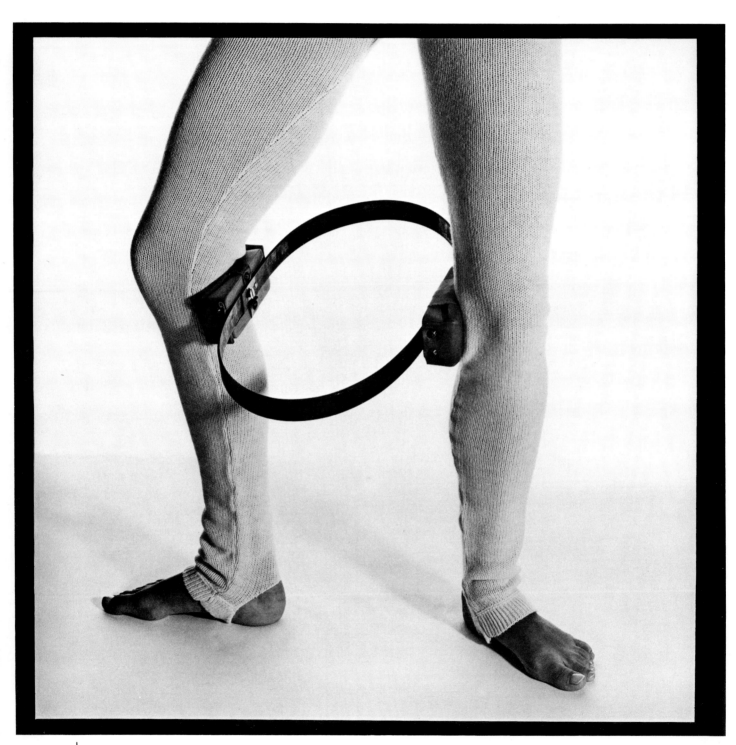

FITNESS: EVERYTHING YOU NEED TO KNOW

Chapter edited
by Alexandra Penney

by Edith Loew Gross

When we talk about self-maintenance—about keeping in shape—we are talking about a concept that couldn't have come on the agenda until our own time. It would have had no meaning for past generations, when the average life span simply didn't warrant a long-term view of one's health and looks and overall physical well-being. Today, as a result of medical advances in the fields of childbirth, infectious diseases, kidney disease, cardiovascular disease and cancer, the life-expectancy figure for women is into the eighties—and a woman in her early forties could safely be having her first child, while the woman of 54 might be entering the job market for the first time or starting on a college degree.

The point is, we are dealing with a different reality for women: It isn't only that we're living longer but that we have, as well, something to say about how we're going to live. A great deal to say, in fact, since in terms of health and fitness we are probably better informed than any group of people at any time in history, and therefore better able to control the quality of our lives. Moderation is the key, and excess the spoiler.

To help you reach strength goals, there are several small "machines" you can work out with. To strengthen thigh muscles, the Pilates Studio uses Pilates Magic Circle.

We know, for example, that to eat properly —meaning nutritionally balanced foods in moderate amounts—is to provide the body with the most basic climate of good health and that the "crash" in crash diet stands for the damage it can do to muscle tone, skin tone . . . the entire system. We know that to take precautions in the sun at age 15 is to avoid wrinkles at age 30 and possible skin cancer; that to avoid smoking is to avoid courting lung cancer, emphysema, heart disease or lines on the upper lip; that to do some form of exercise 10 minutes a day every day is ultimately more effective—and easier on the heart—than a fast set of tennis now and then. It will build stamina, keep muscles toned, spine supple, circulation flowing, energy high—all those qualities that we associate with youth, and that we know may be absent in a teenager and present at any age . . . provided the motivation is there.

In other words, you have options: You can just hang in there or you can—if you choose —live very, very well. Curiously, this is not, says psychoanalyst Jean Baker Miller, quite so simple a choice as it may seem. According to Dr. Miller, who is also associate professor of psychiatry at the Boston University School of Medicine and author of *Toward a New Psychology of Women* (Beacon Press), "Women have been geared for so long to being the

93

server, the helpmate, the person who is there to be supportive of others. And along with that, the person who defined her own appearance by how pleasing—how attractive—other people found her to be. So when you move to talking about long-range physical care, you have to move to a different kind of motivation—that is, valuing your own self and your own body for their own sake. Even now, that's very hard for women to encompass, because to really be moved by that sort of motivation you have to have had some sense of pleasure that you've generated from yourself and for yourself. And for all the talk, I don't think women allow themselves pleasure too easily. They find it difficult to say, 'I'm doing this for myself,' or, 'I think I'd like that, I'd like to try it.' Usually, there's some other motivation; either they're doing it for how they will appear to someone else, or it's 'I'd better do this exercise routine now so I will still be attractive at 40,' which is true, incidentally, but it isn't the same as doing it just because it brings you pleasure. To find this inner motivation is a process we're just beginning on—that hasn't been there for us. And since it is an almost unknown experience, one major step would be to make a little bit of experience for yourself—to do some form of exercise, or whatever—that will be important only for you, and see how good it feels, and how good it would feel to do more. Not because it will prevent you from looking older, but for the direct pleasure involved.

''I think that what has been made of age for women is absolutely criminal. Middle age has hung over us—even over the very young —as the dread ahead. It goes back to the time when a woman's only role was to have babies (except for a short period when her role was to look pretty), and middle age, which was signaled by the menopause, meant an end to that and therefore an end to her real value as a woman.

''We know now that there are very few things, either physical or mental, that actually correlate with the decline of menstrua-

tion; hot flashes do, and a certain diminution of vaginal secretion, which is easily taken care of. But the rest—the depression, the headaches, the dizzy spells, the nervousness—they don't correlate at all. And many of us are coming to believe that they are part of this whole psychological thing—this myth— we've been sold. So well sold that even 20-year-olds are pressured into doing exercises on the grounds that in 20 years it will help them to look younger. That kind of program gets dropped in a week; the motivation is too distant to sustain.

''The obvious reality is that one does get to be 40 and 50—even 80 these days. And as one gets older, one will look older. But it's equally obvious that if you're fit and in good health —if you've taken care of yourself—you will look and feel quite different from someone who hasn't. Younger, if you like. Because being fit presumes certain characteristics that we tend to think of as young and that can, to a great extent, be maintained: muscle tone, circulation, strength, endurance, vitality—no age has a monopoly on them.

''I know of one woman who, at 62, took up squash and flying—clearly, just for her own pleasure and fun and exhilaration. This is a conception of oneself, and an attitude about age, that is very special: To do new things that are going to give an excitement to your life, to say 'I have the right to start this new venture, just for me'; to do what feels good because it feels good, and no one else is necessarily going to know—to me, that is the key.''

FITNESS FACTS

Today, how you look and how you feel are up to you. Throughout your life, there are going to be changes. At 40, the kind of exercises you should do differ significantly from the kind you do—or did—in your teens. At 30, you are a different person with different needs than you were at 20. At 50, you have a whole set of other problems—and adjustments to make. And so on. These changes don't take place automatically; they happen gradually. You become aware of differences—of changes in your body shape, your capabilities—at every decade.

At the heart of good health is: exercise. It's the bottom line, the base to everything—to your looks, your vitality, your mood. It gives you more than your fitness . . . it gives you freedom, too—to be able to run, to work unfatigued, to wear what you want because all clothes fit. When you see a woman in shape, her vitality, her energy is unmistakable. Behind it: good sense, good health, regular exercise and a larger goal—long-term self-maintenance . . . re-evaluated at every decade. What those changes are, how you make them, and most importantly how you reach your goal (your options) are what this chapter is all about.

Today we have more knowledge about our bodies and what it takes to keep them going . . . including the facts that follow . . .

THE FIRST FACT: What takes longer, lasts longer. An investment of time and effort is the kind of investment that pays off and keeps paying off. Good example—that of a woman who, from the age of 20, has watched her diet, kept everything in moderation, and has made it a rule to *walk* everywhere. Same woman, age 60—her shape, her level of fitness are very much like those of an in-shape 20-year-old!

FACT: All the experts, all the doctors in the world, cannot do for you what you can do for yourself. The words that count today are words like "preventive" and "self-maintenance" which tells a whole story in itself. What the experts can do is show you how to take the responsibility for your own well-being and how to make the most of it.

FACT: Habit is a very powerful tool. Use it as an ally. Good habits, once established, form a pattern—one that lasts and works over a lifetime. The habits of everyday exercise and skin care; the habit of consistently choosing the right foods and letting the wrong "temptations" go by; of balancing activity and rest. Basically simple things. Simple, but very effective. The only real way to prove it is to prove it yourself: by taking three months, better still by taking six months, during which time you start to exchange some of the bad habits (and you know what they are—smoking, overeating, lack of exercise, to name three) for some of the good ones. At the end you will have convinced yourself!

FACT: Today, age is no longer important. How old you are is not a valid reason to do—or not do—anything. And age is no longer a barrier to change. There is no point—from the teens to the seventies to past the seventies—at which you cannot stop, make changes, and have those changes count. Granted, the earlier you do it the better—if it's a matter of starting to exercise or cutting out cigarettes. But don't think you reach a point beyond which it doesn't make a difference. It always makes a difference.

Naturally, there are certain age-dependent changes—you may need a different kind of spot exercise, a different kind of treatment mask, a different medical checkup. Those changes and how to deal with them are documented in the pages ahead. What you won't see anywhere is advice on "looking younger" —something that has become totally irrelevant. What counts—as you should be aware by now—is looking better, living better, living up to your potential at every age.

FACT: "Glamour" isn't what it used to be. There was—not too long ago—a certain image of a glamorous woman: a woman who did nothing but pamper herself, who rested all day to "save" her energy for evening, a woman who wouldn't dream of being caught without makeup—or being caught in the rain because of what it would do to her hair. She was a woman who "cared" about the way she looked. And then, there was the type of woman who didn't care at all. She was classified as being "athletic" or "intellectual," depending. . . . If she "did" anything, it was in terms of physical activity; but makeup, time at a hairdresser—all out of the question.

Today—and it's an enormous change—

there is a different reality . . . and a very different woman. A woman who not only runs or swims, but trains with weights to give her the stamina it takes to get through a busy day and an evening of disco-dancing; a woman who knows that to have energy you have to spend it; a woman who has the kind of haircut that looks as good on a tennis court as it does at the theater. You wouldn't use the word ''glamorous'' to describe this woman; although she looks very, very good. The words instead: attractive, vital, modern.

FACT: An active woman represents more than a new ''type''; she represents the way we live today. Which brings us back to the woman—and the vitality—we started with: a woman who's active, in the sense of being out in the world and on the move, because of what's true across the board: Women are doing more, traveling more, demanding more. And what's important now to a woman like this is the way she presents herself and the way she feels. The first concern is with herself; not in a narcissistic way, but in a way that comes from a healthy (the operative word) self-awareness. When you start with that, all the facts make sense . . . and all things are possible, as you will see on these next pages. . . .

But the most important ''fact'' has to do with *exercise and age*. And the rule is: It's never too late to begin. Exercise, says Willibald Nagler, M.D., of the New York Hospital-Cornell Medical Center, can be done—even by a beginner—at any time of life, any level of fitness . . . and the least taxing, most total exercise is walking (about which you'll be reading more later in this chapter).

Exercise is an antidote for age, the best ''medicine'' you can take to prevent aging. ''As we get older, our bones become thinner and softer. They lose substance,'' says Dr. Nagler, ''especially after menopause. Our shoulders become stooped and hang forward. The discs in our spines change, and the muscular/skeletal fluids in our cartilage begin to dry up and drain out. We all develop some form of osteoarthritis, because as we grow older the surface of our bones, which is smooth when we are younger, becomes uneven and rougher. All of which could lead to a decreased range of motion. Exercise prevents this, and it helps us all deal better with osteoarthritis. Doing regular exercise keeps us flexible and strengthens our bones.''

Exercise is the key, says Dr. Nagler, and the most important kind is weight-bearing exercise, such as walking—very briskly three or four times a week. This will keep your bones strong.

If you're older and you want to start exercising, says Dr. Nagler, you can do as much as a younger woman can . . . but, you must exercise gradually; your increase in activity must be slower, which also means your improvement will be slower (have patience!). Use longer warm-up periods, says Dr. Nagler. Then, exercise for brief stints; start out doing only five or 10 minutes of exercise; work up slowly to 20 (it may take you a few weeks or a few months).

What about racquet sports? You can play any of them, even if you never tried before, says Dr. Nagler. There's no reason you can't start at any age. But he suggests seeing a good pro first to learn the game and the strokes properly. If you want to run, you can do that, too. The best way: by alternating running with walking. Walk fast, then run, then walk fast again. At the beginning, do this for 10–15 minutes, doing more fast walking than running. Gradually shift the balance to more running, less walking and work up to a half-hour of walk/run time.

One caution, says Dr. Nagler: gymnastics. Don't attempt them if you're not in shape; it's too difficult. So is yoga, if you haven't been exercising, because if you're not careful, you can slip a disc or pinch a blood vessel in your neck if you snap your head around too suddenly.

A GOOD ALL-AROUND EXERCISE PLAN

You need three kinds of exercise for real fitness—stretching, strengthening and endurance. "Work gradually up to 15 minutes of stretching and strengthening daily for good posture and a good figure. And up to 20 minutes of endurance exercise, at least three times a week," says Willibald Nagler, M.D., chairman of the department of rehabilitation medicine at the New York Hospital-Cornell Medical Center. Here is how Dr. Nagler's plan works.

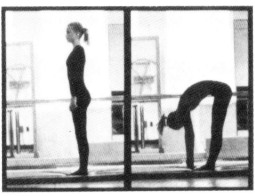

1

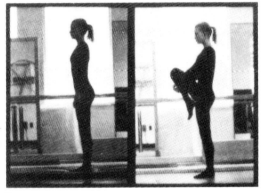

2

1/_Front Bend: Standing, feet 12 inches apart, knees slightly bent, bend from the waist, touch fingers to floor. Rise and stretch._
2/_Knee Kiss: Standing, feet together, bring right knee to chest and hug it, using both arms, lower. Repeat with left knee._

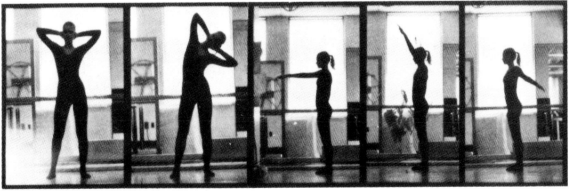

3   **4**   **5**

3/_Side Bend: Feet apart, hands behind neck, bend from waist to right side and back to center. Then left side._
4/_Arm Circles: Windmill right arm, making large circles, in both directions (toward front, then back). Windmill left arm._
5/_Neck: Hand against right side of face, press head against resistance. Hold 5 seconds. Then left._

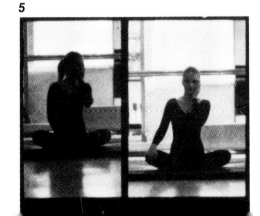

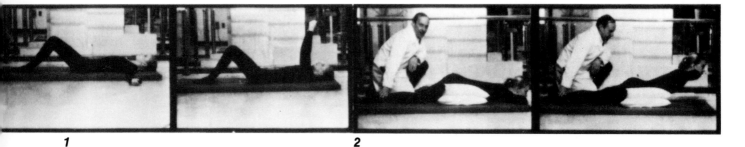

1 **2**

1/Chest Muscles: *Lie on back, on mat, arms out at side, barbells in hand. Bring arms up and together. Lower.*
2/Upper Back: *Lie on stomach,* pillow underneath you, and close hands behind neck. Arch head and trunk up, without raising feet. Hold 5 seconds.

STRETCHING

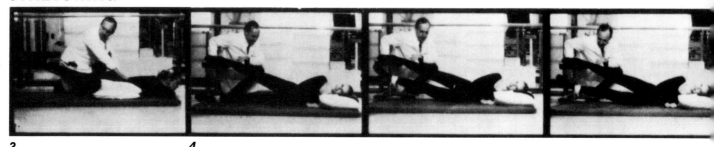

3 **4**

3/Lower Back: *Keep trunk down, raise legs instead. (Not for those with a back problem.)*
4/Inner Thigh: *Lie on left side, legs straight. Place right* foot on chair seat. Raise left leg to meet right one, then down—best with weight around ankle of moving leg. Switch sides, repeat.

STRENGTHENING

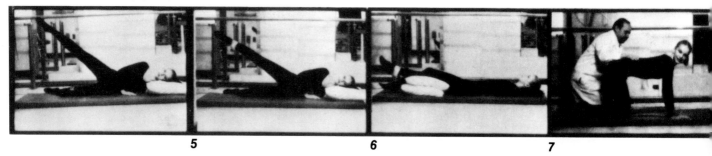

5 **6** **7**

5/Outer Thigh: *Lie on left side, left leg slightly bent, upper leg straight. Raise right leg up, then lower (best if weighted). Repeat on other side.*
6/Knees: *Lie on back, pillow under knees. Straighten* right leg. Down. Then left. Weight adds resistance.
7/Cat Back: *Get on hands and knees, back straight. Arch back, pulling in abdominal muscles, breathing out. Hold 5 seconds, return to straight back position.*

9/Feet: *Walking on heels, then toes, helps to strengthen, but will not prevent or cure flat feet.*
10/Ankles: *Sit in chair. Put weight on foot. Raise toes. Hold 5 seconds, then lower. Repeat with other foot.*

9 **10**

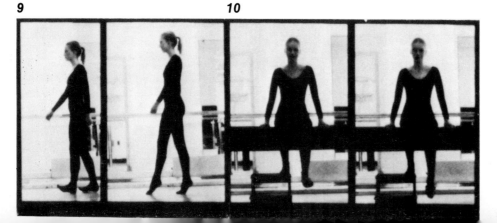

STRETCHING AND STRENGTHENING BASICS

Build up gradually to 15 to 20 times for each exercise. Left-right counts as one. Don't force or bounce—you can sprain a muscle or tear a tendon.

Never exhaust yourself. Don't exercise to the point of hurting or shaking. Ease into your routine over a period of weeks. Check with your doctor before plunging into an exercise program—especially if you are out of condition.

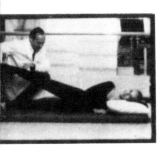

ENDURANCE BASICS

To build endurance, you must bring your heart beat up to 130–140 (or more, if you are very young) by using major muscles over a period of time —running, biking, swimming, dancing, playing tennis or fast walking are all good ways to do this.

Before each stint, warm up at least five minutes to limber muscles and joints, raise pulse. Never stop cold: cool down slowly to avoid faintness, nausea. Do stretching exercises as part of warm-up and cooldown.

Exercise has to be progressive. Run further at the same speed, for example, or the same distance but a touch faster.

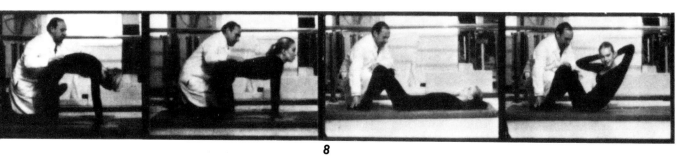

8

8/*Sit Ups: Lie on back, knees bent, hands clasped behind head. (Someone can hold feet down, or place feet under* *piece of furniture). Curl up slowly, breathing out. Bring right elbow to left knee. Down. Repeat to other side.*

ENDURANCE

11/*Jogging in Place: Good shoes are a must. Do leg stretches before and after. Build up to 20 minutes.*
12/*Rope Jumping: Work up to doing it fast, with a* *twirling flick of the wrist, upper arms close to the body. Three minutes, a minute's rest, then another three. Good for calves, ankles, too.*

11   12

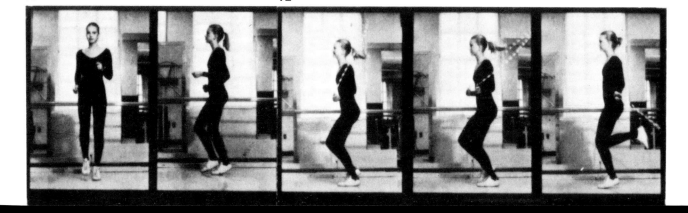

WHAT YOU SHOULD KNOW ABOUT: POSTURE

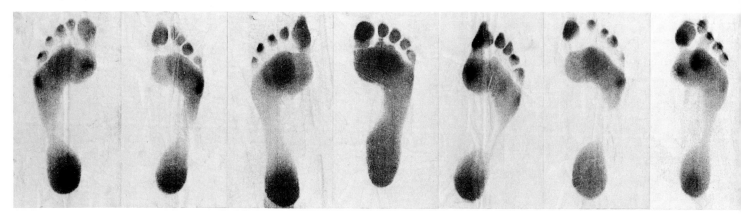

Alexander Hersh, M.D., attending orthopedic surgeon at the Hospital for Special Surgery in New York, uses footprints in diagnosis and "read" these for us. 1. As close to an "average" foot as possible: normal arch, even weight distribution on heel, ball of foot, toes. 2. A corn may be causing the fifth toe to turn in. 3. Slight tendency to flatness. 4. Mild flat foot; a good, broad foot to stand on. 5. Very high arch; foot rolls out a bit. 6. Toe-tips indicate curling of toes—not uncommon in high-arched foot—painful if toe tops rub shoe. 7. Dark spot on ball of foot may be a callus caused by, and painful when wearing, high heels.

Nothing is more aging than incorrect posture, says Naja Cori, a body alignment/conditioning specialist, and the older you get, the more exaggerated your posture faults become. The best way to prevent its happening: to learn correct posture (under supervision) and retrain your body. The good news: Age is not an obstacle to retraining; you can still make improvements when you're 70, though you may have to work harder.

The key—at any age—is a flexible spine. You should be able to attain the correct postural position by pressing your spine against the edge of an open door—it should be straight (the curves "eased out") from tailbone to shoulder blades.

Posture exercises should be a counter-balance. Analyse your lifestyle and daily body actions. If you bend over a desk all day, you need exercises that "work" the body in the opposite direction.

Half of your battle is learning correct posture. There's less of a strain on your body; you have more energy. When your body is not in the proper alignment, it's having a tug of war with itself!

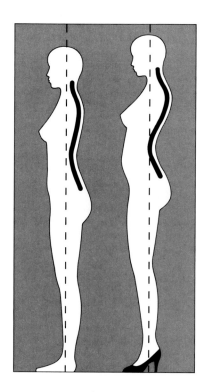

How feet influence posture: the "before" and "after" of high heels. High heels push body weight forward and shift the plumb line of good posture, thrusting out bosom, derrière—and throwing the spine a curve. Most spines are resilient, but doctors encourage women to change to low heels frequently.

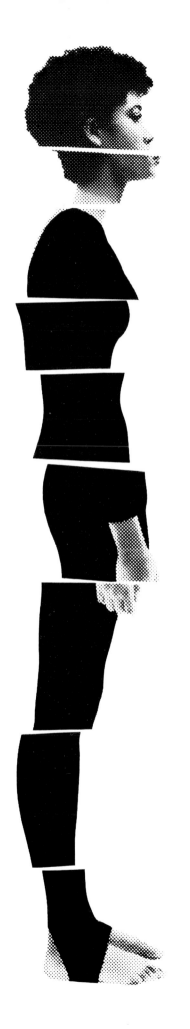 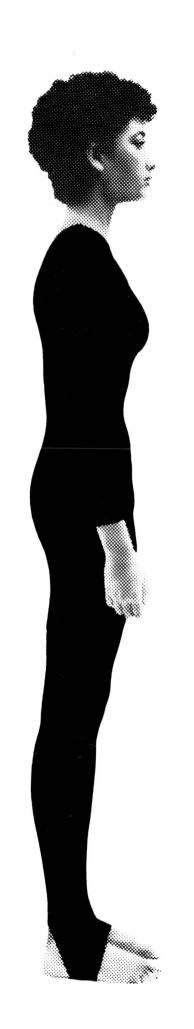

When your body is properly aligned, every movement you make helps to tone the muscles. You get a benefit simply by using your body

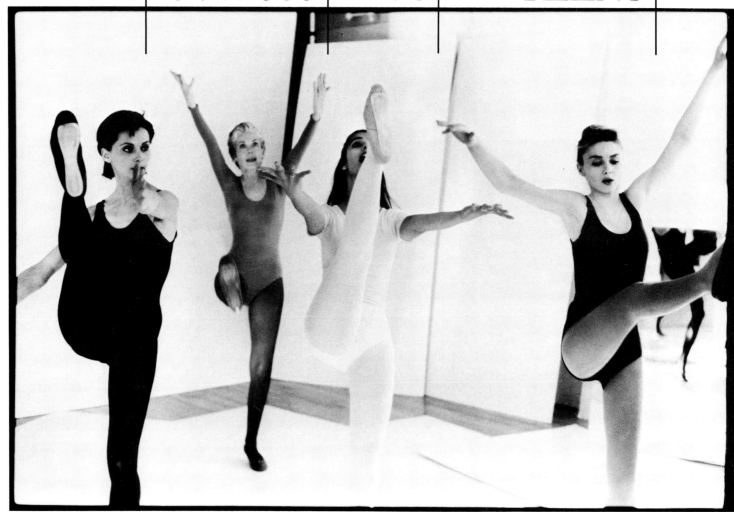

EXERCISE

by Diana Lea

How to find the right exercise program for you at any age: a what-to-expect guide to five basic exercise methods, from five different exercise experts.

Barbells? Handstands? Ballet stretches? They all work. The hitch is finding out which exercise system is going to be the right one, at what age, for you—meaning not just which one you're likely to stick with, but which one

The "no-age" age. It all starts here.... Dressing do's and don'ts based on age no longer exist. What counts most is the shape your body is in. Everything begins with that.

you'll enjoy, which makes the sticking-with no sweat. The crucial difference lies in the approach : Some people prefer working with a trainer, some on their own at home, others with a group. Some prefer stretching on the floor, some pushing against resistance, others balancing on rings.

Whichever you wind up with, from gymnastics to weights, the results will be surprisingly similar : A good exercise system will give you better circulation, and aerobic conditioning, and a body that shows what fitness is. Results start showing in less than a month if you start off by going 3 times a week and eventually level off to twice a week. (As always, check with a doctor before beginning any exercise program. And if you're a beginner, go *slower*.)

GYMNASTICS

According to the gymnastic experts at New York's Gala Fitness, women who are grossly overweight or who have suffered mastectomies (apparatus work relies on pectoral muscles) will have difficulty learning gymnastics. Most women are held back by the fear of hanging upside down from trapeze or rings —a natural fear, but not unconquerable for almost anyone who sticks to a gymnastic class. A typical hour-long beginner's class of four to six women begins with calisthenics—body stretches, jogging in place, leg kicks, sit-ups —to pick up the circulation, loosen up the body and work on a few trouble spots. Next comes mat tumbling—easy somersaults, handstands—good for all of you. The last 20 minutes involve apparatus work—swinging and balancing on low rings (still possible to touch the floor), working on a stationary five-foot-high trapeze. Instructors never allow competition to push a woman onto the high apparatus before she is ready.

A big plus of gymnastic exercise is the carry-over effect : because gymnastics concentrates on strengthening upper torso muscles, tennis and golf swings take on a new look ;

skiers find the emphasis on balance and coordination equals added slope agility.

ONE IMPORTANT NOTE: Gymnastics is *not* for older women who have not kept up with an exercise program throughout their lives. If you're just starting, stretching or calisthenics (more about them follows) will be better. Gymnastics, if you're not in shape for them, can injure you.

SPRING-RESISTANCE

Based in movements from yoga, Zen and rehabilitation therapy, spring-resistance exercises involve controlled, rhythmic stretches done against strong springs (found hidden under cubes, at the ends of straps). This method probably works best for the woman who hears her own drummer, who doesn't require constant supervision or a competitive stimulus. For the first few sessions, an instructor should give you undivided attention ; then it's like graduating to the honor system (though monitoring is always necessary).

The goal of spring-resistance exercise, says Romana Kryzanowska, director of the Pilates spring-resistance exercise program in New York, "is to stretch tight, stubby muscles away from the joint so that each limb can move freely." At Pilates, which limbers up some of the great bodies of the ballet world, one-third of the time is spent on floor mats, the other two-thirds on springs. Each program is worked out on an individual basis so that each exercise evolves from the one before, with new ones frequently being added so that boredom doesn't creep in. What might an hour-long routine involve ? For someone who spends the day at a desk, jackknifes, spring push-ups and scissor kicks on a mat ; for a ballet dancer, backbends and leg "spring" stretches. It all depends on what shape you're in. "No matter which exercises are done," says Romana, "deep breathing and body alignment should always be stressed . . . shoulders relaxed, back flat against the floor or wall, abdomen pulled tightly up and in."

PILATES' SYSTEM OF BODY CONTROL TO LAST YOU A LIFETIME

Romana Kryzanowska, director of Pilates Studio, New York, teaches you how to take charge of your body through a system of controlled movements against the resistance of springs that show you where your muscles are, how they work. It is advisable to have your doctor's consent before starting.

On exercise mat:

1,2/*The Saw (good for homework), reaching beyond toes to stretch, strengthen legs, loosen shoulders, stretch back and waist.*

3/*The Teaser, sit-ups with legs extended in air; stomach and lower-back strengthener.*

4–7/*The Corkscrew (also good at home): swinging legs up, over, down and around (while holding onto handles) to strengthen stomach, lower back, firm hips.*

On the Universal Reformer:

8/*The Down Stretch for shoulders, entire body.*

9/*The Long Stretch—stomach firmer, fanny lift.*

10–12/*Tight back muscle massage: with legs in straps, rolling spine back onto table to stretch it out.*

13–14/*Pulling straps forward and back to firm biceps, triceps.*

Relaxing fun and games on the "Cadillac":

15/*Relaxing into lower back.*

16/*Stretching legs on bar.*

17/*Reaching for top bar.*

18/*Full back stretch.*

19/*Pull-up to strengthen arms, shoulders.*

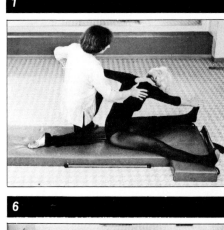
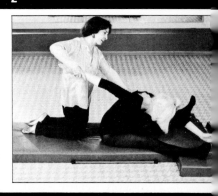
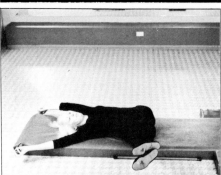
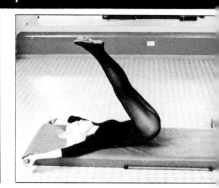
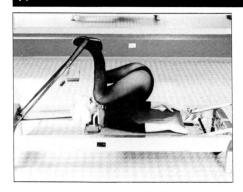
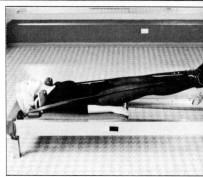
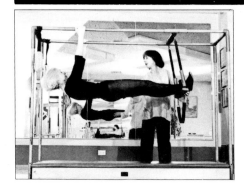
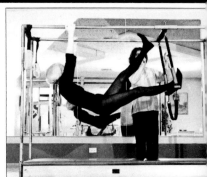

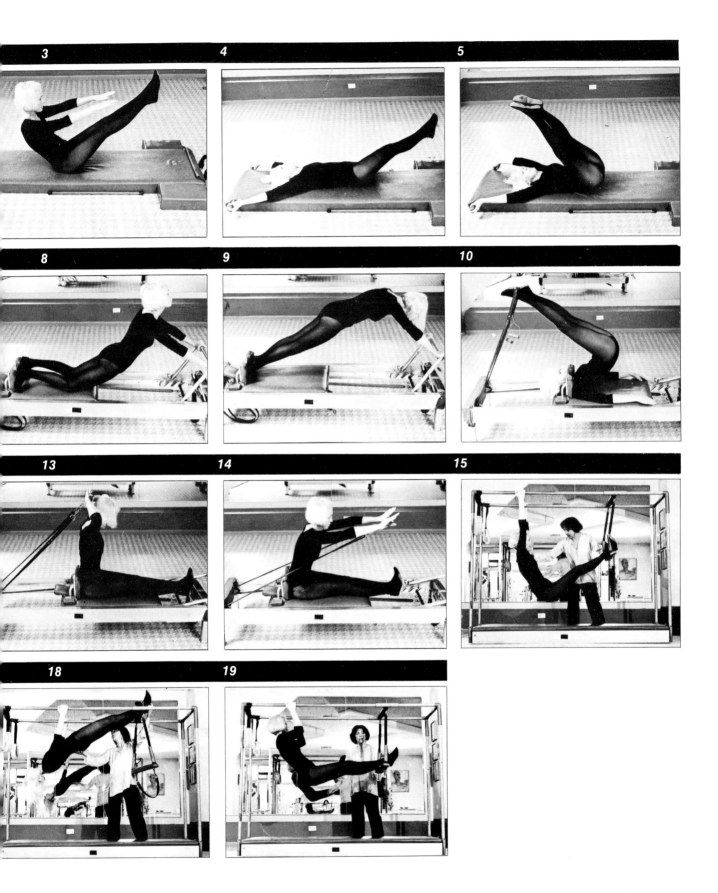

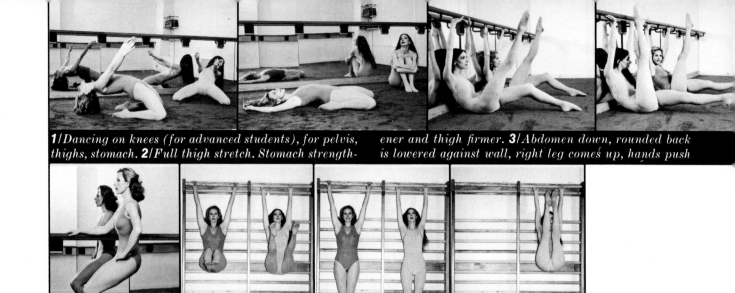

1/Dancing on knees (for advanced students), for pelvis, thighs, stomach. 2/Full thigh stretch. Stomach strength-ener and thigh firmer. 3/Abdomen down, rounded back is lowered against wall, right leg comes up, hands push

stretch. 8/Balanced stretch to tone legs, stomach; reach-ing for ankles while keeping back straight. 9/Thigh strengthener and toner. 10/Testing abdominal strength. 11/Spine stretcher. 12/Ultimate test of stomach muscles.

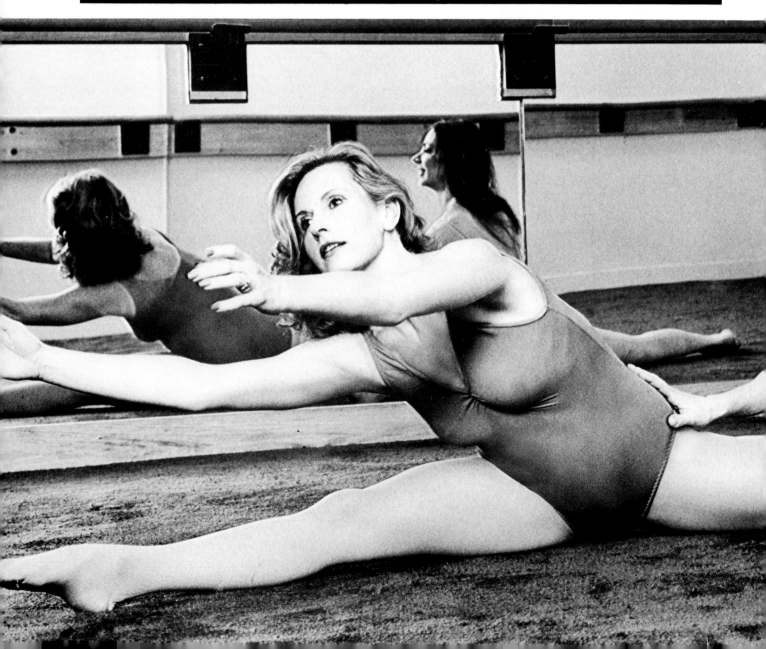

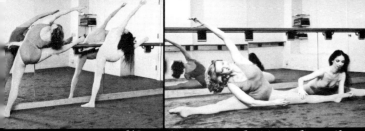
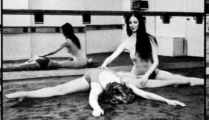
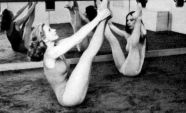

against barre. **4/**Legs alternate, one flattens to floor, other lifts up. **5/**Stretching for waist, inner thighs, backs of legs. **6/**Stretching to side, while someone keeps other knee straight. **7/**Chest to floor, with legs in second position

CALISTHENICS

"Exercise" exercises—twists, lifts, bends, stretches—have been energizing the energetic for years. They are demanding, "but they should be," says Lydia Bach, of the Lotte Berk Method in New York. "After all, they're one way to compensate for all the activity that modern conveniences deny us." Frequently adapted from modern ballet, Hatha yoga, pelvic movements and orthopedic exercises, these exercises (described by one fan as "a shot of zest") are designed to build stamina, increase flexibility, create leaner muscles, and improve circulation—and to teach you to use your muscles properly, as a smoothly functioning whole. "For instance," explains Lydia, "because we don't use the abdominal muscles regularly, we force the back muscles to carry most of our weight. The result is backache, tension, fatigue. When abdominals are strengthened, they help support the back."

Lotte Berk classes begin with a warm-up (all exercise classes should) and typically include all-over stretches (the key, according to Lydia, to a graceful, limber body) plus groups of exercises concentrating on every area of the body. They can be especially effective for "hanging bottoms" and thighs. Surprise: "The front thighs are the easiest part of the body to firm," says Lydia.

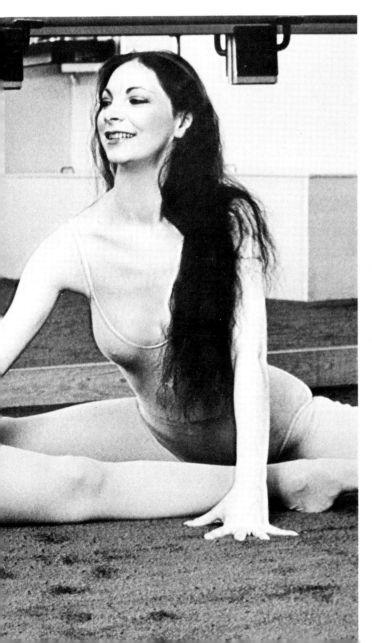

STRETCHING, STRENGTHENING AND STAMINA

You can't possibly work on one without involving the other two. You will develop long, stretched-out muscles that are also strong—not strong bunched ones (the bunchy kind are geared toward explosive, quick movement, not toward endurance). Pia Lindstrom (far left), anchorwoman on New York's NBC-TV NewsCenter 4, in her late thirties, works out with Marjorie Thompson (near left), director of the Lotte Berk Method, N.Y.

ALIGNMENT

The body must have a strong center. Strengthening your stomach muscles strengthens and straightens the back.

107

WEIGHT RESISTANCE

To Billie Jean King, Diana Nyad, and other all-out athletes, a workout on Nautilus weight-resistant machines—found in well-equipped gyms all over the country—is a workout of champions. Unlike barbells, pulleys and other weight-lifting equipment, weight machines (which, at first glance, look like instruments of torture) do not apply straight-line resistance against just one or two muscles. Instead, a system of rotating resistance, which allows the limb full range of movement, exercises both the specific muscle and its entire body part. The machines also apply resistance at the beginning and end of each movement, when the muscles are contracted. "This is the secret to building muscle tone," explains Michael O'Shea, director of The Sports Training Center in New York.

Because weight-resistance-machine workouts aim at keeping pulse and breathing rates high, this method is definitely not for the exercise dabbler. Rather it is for the woman who doesn't mind sweating side by side with men, who thrives on being pushed and prodded by a professional trainer. It is, as one advocate put it, "impossible to cheat. You either move that weight—or you don't!"

"AT HOME" EXERCISES

Any woman disdainful of sweat has come to her spot on this page. Exercise expert Barbara Pearlman believes women shouldn't feel "as if they're panting through laps." A dancer for 20 years, she sees exercise as a form of aesthetics, "graceful stretches to the Beatles or Bach." For maximum results, Barbara offers the following tips: First, set aside 15 minutes a day so you can work slowly, meticulously; second, don't try to attain your final position at first start—work up to it, don't strain; third, inhale when you stretch, exhale when you release; fourth, switch to a relatively high-protein diet "with breakfast and lunch like a princess, dinner like a pauper"; fifth, concentrate on the movement—not the evening ahead; sixth, stick to sequences—exercises are designed to lead into each other.

SHAPING UP FOR SPORTS AT ANY AGE

by Charles T. Kuntzleman, Ed. D.

It's a popular notion that sports are a good way to become fit. But it usually doesn't work out that way. You rarely see athletes getting in shape by playing their sport. They do extra exercises to put them in top form.

In the tennis world, Billie Jean King runs, bicycles, stretches, and lifts weights to stay on top of her game. Her bicycling and running keep her game from falling apart. She has the staying power to defeat a less fit opponent. Weight training increases her strength and helps drive the ball across the court with more power and speed. Calisthenics and yoga stretches improve her flexibility, reduce her chances of injury, and give her a smoother swing and serve.

You should take a tip from the pros: Get fit to play your sport, rather than playing your sport for fitness. When fit, you'll enjoy your game more, do better, and be less prone to aches and pains.

Getting in shape to play your sport becomes more vital as you grow older. When you're 18, being fit for your sport is, of course, important. But by the time you are 30, it's mandatory. Athletes who continue to excel when they are in their thirties and forties are fit athletes.

To get into top shape for your favorite sport, you must condition your heart and lungs, strengthen your muscles, and stretch your tendons and ligaments.

CONDITIONING YOUR HEART AND LUNGS

Without a satisfactory level of heart–lung endurance, performance falls off rapidly in almost all sports. Running is the best activity to condition your heart and lungs. To do this, you'll want to run hard enough to get your pulse rate up to your target heart-rate level, the one that is best for building your heart and lung stamina.

How long you should stay at your target heart-rate depends upon your sport. The Length of Time Chart shows you how long you must run to get into good shape. Start at Level #1 and work up to the highest level recommended for your sport. The first number tells you how many minutes you should run. The second number tells you the number of days per week. For example, at Level #1, 10/3x means you are to run 10 minutes three times a week. If you want, you can walk-jog instead. After a period of time, move to Level #2 and run 13 minutes three times a week.

LENGTH OF TIME AT TARGET HEART-RATE LEVEL										
Activity*	Levels**									
	1	2	3	4	5	6	7	8	9	10
Basketball	10/3x	13/3x	16/3x	18/3x	20/3x	22/3x	24/3x	26/3x	28/3x	30/3x
Bowling	10/3x	13/3x	16/3x	Maintain						
Golf	10/3x	13/3x	16/3x	18/3x	20/3x	Maintain				
Squash	10/3x	13/3x	16/3x	18/3x	20/3x	22/3x	24/3x	26/3x	28/3x	30/3x
Tennis	10/3x	13/3x	16/3x	18/3x	20/3x	Maintain				
Skating (Ice & Roller)	10/3x	13/3x	16/3x	18/3x	20/3x	22/3x	24/3x	26/3x	28/3x	30/3x
Skiing	10/3x	13/3x	16/3x	18/3x	20/3x	22/3x	24/3x	26/3x	28/3x	30/3x
Softball	10/3x	13/3x	16/3x	18/3x	20/3x	Maintain				

* For walking, running, swimming and bicycling, simply walk, run, swim or bicycle for fitness. Use your target heart-rate level as a guide.

** The length of time you spend at each level depends on your feelings and fitness level. When you feel you are ready to move to the next level, do so. If you're under 30 years of age, you may spend one week at each level; if you are between 30 and 40, two weeks; and if you are over 40, three weeks or more.

AT-HOME AEROBICS— A BASIC STATIONARY RUNNING PROGRAM	
WEEKS 1 & 2	**WEEKS 7 & 8**
• Run 2 min. (at least 70 percent max. H.R.) • Walk in place 1 minute • Run 2 min. (at 70 percent) • Walk in place 1 min. **6 MINUTES TOTAL**	• Run 2 min. (at 70 percent) • Run 1 min. (at 85 percent) • Run 1 min. (at 70 percent) • Walk in place 1 min. • Run 3 min. (at 70 percent) • Walk in place 1 min. **9 MINUTES TOTAL**
WEEKS 3–6	**WEEKS 9 AND BEYOND**
• Run 3 min. (at 70 percent) • Walk in place 1 minute • Run 3 min. (at 70 percent) • Walk in place 1 min. **8 MINUTES TOTAL**	• Run 2 min. (at 70 percent) • Run 1 min. (at 85 percent) • Run 1 min. (at 70 percent) • Walk in place 1 min. • Repeat this entire cycle 3 times **15 MINUTES TOTAL**

STRENGTHENING YOUR MUSCLES

To do well in sports, you need strength. The best way to get it is with weights. Unfortunately, many women think that exercising with weights will build unsightly muscles. Research disproves this; weight training will build strength and a better figure.

In weight training, the set system is used. This means you do eight repetitions of each exercise. And you do these three times. For example, you do eight repetitions of barbell curls, rest for one or two minutes, do a second set of eight, rest for one or two minutes, then do a third set of eight. After the third set, you go on to the next exercise. It is best to lift weights every other day, not every day.

There are thousands of weight-training exercises. Here are eight. You need only do those marked for your sport. (For exercises done on your back, lie on an exercise pad, thick carpet, or bed.)

SPORTS

EXERCISE	Swimming	Softball	Skiing	Skating	Running	Squash & Tennis	Golf	Bowling	Bicycling	Basketball
Arm press	●			●	●	●	●	●	●	●
Upright rowing				●	●				●	●
Supine pull-over	●				●	●	●			●
Barbell curls	●	●			●					
Supinator-pronator				●	●	●			●	
One-half squat	●	●	●	●	●	●	●	●		●
Toe raise	●	●					●	●	●	
Sit-ups	●	●	●	●	●	●	●	●	●	●

ARM PRESS
Stand with a barbell in front of the chest, palms forward. Extend the barbell over the head with your arms straight. Repeat.

UPRIGHT ROWING
Stand with your feet spread apart, holding your body upright. Knees and back are straight. Grasp a barbell in the middle with hands touching, the palms down. Raise the bar up to the chest, by bending the elbows and bringing the bar up. Return. Repeat.

SUPINE PULL-OVER
Lie on your back. Extend your arms above the head, palms facing up. Raise your arms to a 90-degree angle, and then return to the original position. Keep the arms straight through the entire movement. Return. Repeat.

BARBELL CURLS
Stand with arms extended downward, the barbell against your thighs and your palms facing up. Flex your forearms and bring the bar to the shoulders. Return. Repeat.

SUPINATOR-PRONATOR
Sit on a bench with your forearm on the table. Extend your wrist and hand over the table. Grasp a dumbbell bar with a weight on one end. Hold in an upright position. Lower the weight to the one side so that the palm is facing downward. Return. Repeat.

ONE-HALF SQUAT
Stand with feet comfortably spread. Hold a barbell on your shoulders behind the neck. Bend your knees to perform a one-half squat (90 degrees). Return to a standing position. Repeat.

TOE RAISE
Assume a standing position, barbell resting on your neck and shoulders. Place balls of your feet on a 1- to 2-inch block of wood. Heels on the floor. Rise up on your toes. Return. Repeat.

SIT-UPS
Lie on your back, knees bent, and arms across your chest. A weight may be placed on your chest. Curl your body up into a sitting position by first drawing your chin toward your chest and then lifting your upper body off the floor. Keep your back rounded throughout the movement. Sit up as far as possible. Return to the starting position. Repeat.

Body Shaping: Stretch, strengthen, make the body you want. Arnold Schwarzenegger has developed a fitness plan using dumbbells. Each exercise zeroes in on a body trouble spot. Final Stretch: Each move done slowly, one after another to make a whole. Head up, lunge to side and touch floor. Head lowers, leg straightens, torso arches, then turn forward, hands reach feet. Other-side arch; final knee bend.

110

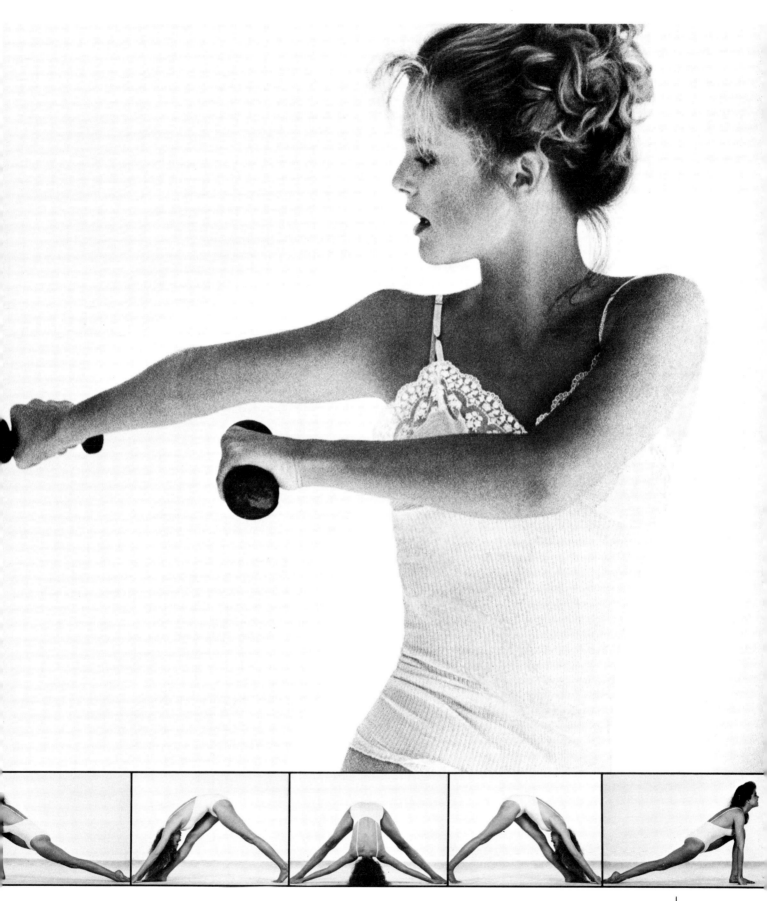

STRETCHING YOUR LIGAMENTS, TENDONS AND MUSCLES

Flexibility is important to prevent injuries. If you lack flexibility, you will be prone to strains or tears of muscles or tendons. The result may be weeks of disability, pain or dull aches. To improve flexibility, do yoga-type exercises or positions. These positions and movements focus on stretching selected muscles and ligaments.

Muscle flexibility is the range of motion possible at the joints (or bending places) of your body. If you can't touch your toes without bending your knees, for example, you lack flexibility in your lower back and legs.

Do flexibility exercises like these before and after all sports—and do them slowly. For example, when doing the sitting toe touches, move very gradually. Go to the point where you feel your muscles being stretched. Hold. Now concentrate on relaxing those muscles. Soon you'll be able to slip down just a bit further. For some people, it may be a quarter of an inch at a time, for others, it may be several. This pattern is to be followed on all the exercises described.

SITTING TOE TOUCHES

Sit on the floor with your legs extended in front of you, feet together. Reach for your toes with both hands, and bring your forehead as close to your knees as possible. Return to the sitting position.

CALF/TENDON STRETCH

Stand about two to three feet away from the wall. Lean forward, with your body straight. Place your palms against the wall at eye level. Step backward. Continue to support yourself against the wall. Remain flat on your feet until you feel your calf muscles stretching.

SPRINTER

Assume a squatting position on the floor. Extend one leg back as far as possible. Your hands should be braced on the floor. Hold. Repeat with the other leg.

STANDING LEG STRETCH

Use a table approximately three feet in height. Place one foot on the table so that the knee is straight and the leg is parallel to the floor. Slowly extend your fingertips toward the outstretched leg on the table. Repeat with the other leg.

STANDING LEG STRETCH TOWARD THE FLOOR

Stand sideways to the same table used in the preceding exercise. Raise the leg nearest the table and rest foot on table, keeping knee straight. Slowly bend at your waist and extend your fingertips toward the foot on the floor. Hold. Return to the upright position. Repeat with the other leg.

BACK STRETCH

Stand erect with your feet shoulder-width apart. Bend forward slowly at the waist. Let your arms, shoulders, and neck relax. Stretch until you feel a slight pull in the muscles on the backs of your legs. That will give you support. Hold. When you come back up, bend your knees to take the pressure off your lower back. Return to an upright position.

SIDE STRETCH

Stand with your feet about shoulder-width apart, legs straight. Place one hand on your hip and extend your other arm up and over your head. Bend to the side on which your hand is placed on the hip. Move slowly. Hold. Repeat on the other side.

SHOULDER STRETCH

Stand with feet about shoulder-width apart. With both arms over your head, hold the elbow of one arm with the hand of the other arm. Slowly pull the elbow behind your head. Do not force. Hold. Repeat on the other side.

EXERCISE TIPS:

An interview with John L. Marshall, M.D., of New York Hospital-Cornell Medical Center

To be effective, an exercise program has to be done regularly. And the basic rule is that you must do it at least three times a week. If you are trying to make significant improvements, then something like five times a week is better; but if you are just starting out, if you are older, go *slowly*. A lot depends on how much you are putting into it. If you are exercising every day but it is not stressing you effectively, you may find you are better off doing it less often and more intensely.

I like to have people work on cardiopulmonary endurance three times a week and have them also do stretching and strengthening exercises for the musculoskeletal system three times a week. This can be worked out on an alternate-day schedule or combined on the same three days. I prefer alternate days; the change back and forth keeps things more interesting. But if time is a problem, then combine everything into one session and do it at least three times a week.

What about specific guidelines? Well, stretching should take you about 10 minutes. If you are doing endurance exercise like running in the same session, do five minutes of stretching before your cardiopulmonary workout and five minutes after. That way, the flexibility exercises serve as a warm-up period and a cool-down period. Easy does it for stretching—go slowly, don't force yourself, and don't bounce.

Strengthening next. This can take you 20–30 minutes if you want to be reasonably complete. But shorter periods are worthwhile, too. Certain exercises are especially important because you are not likely to·get their effect from sports or endurance activities. For instance, you do not get upper-body strength from most sports. You can remedy this by doing push-ups, arm-hangs (if you have a bar to hang from in a doorway), arm curls, and squeezing a tennis ball for your forearm. If you can't do a real push-up, do a modified push-up, using your knees instead of your toes as the fulcrum.

Abdominal-strength exercises are essential. The sit-up is a basic one. Do it slowly, with knees bent, bringing your chest and shoulders off the ground slowly, and then unwinding and coming down to a resting position. If you do it that way, it takes only eight or 10 before you get fatigued. And, incidentally, strengthening exercises should be done only to the point of muscle fatigue—not to the point of pain.

There are several things you should always be careful about in doing these exercises.

> **❝ To be effective, an exercise program has to be done regularly . . . A lot depends on how much you are putting into it. The basic rule is that you must do it at least three times a week ❞**

Avoid full squats or deep knee-bends, with or without weights, or duck walks—anything that puts pressure on the knee. Straight-leg exercises, like lying on your back, lifting your legs up and doing scissors, or raising your legs together—are not good if you have had any kind of back trouble. You should do back exercises with your knees bent. And butterfly exercises—where you lie on your belly and move your arms and legs like a butterfly—are not good. Many doctors recommend this kind of exercise, but I am against it. Anything that causes the back to go into extension, or into any stress, may cause difficulty.

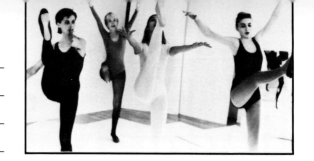

DEALING WITH
TROUBLE SPOTS
AT EVERY AGE

a. *For upper arms, push-ups (below, first two photos): Keep knees bent— it's easier for women (who don't have the arm power of men). Lower your-self slowly to floor. Do sets of five.* *Work up to 25 times (it takes months!).*
b. *For "baby fat" leg-slimming (a common teen problem spot), squat thrusts: Crouch down, hands on floor* *(below, center). For more support, move hands forward (below, right). Thrust legs out behind you (below, far right). Return to squat position. Stand; repeat. Work up to 10–25.*

AT FIFTEEN

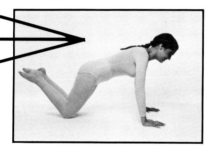
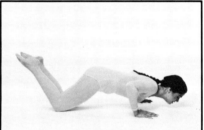
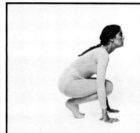

a. *Sit-ups (below) for the abdomen, the best way: with legs bent, feet free (less strain), and hands behind but not touching neck (prevents pressure on spinal column). Alternate, com-ing up to sitting position, to right, to left, then to middle. Do sets of five; work up to 25.*
b. *Toe touching for legs, for flexibil-ity: Do with feet apart, feet together, right-leg crossover, then left-leg crossover (three photos, below, cen-ter). Touch toes four times in each position.*
c. *Spot work to do in addition to (and before) aerobic exercise, such as* *running in place. Knee bends to strengthen thighs (two photos, below, far right): Standing, bend knees, slowly lower body. Stop when your upper leg is parallel to the floor— damage to your knees may result if you go lower than that. Do this exer-cise eight to ten times.*

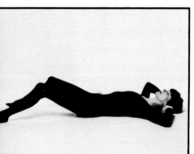
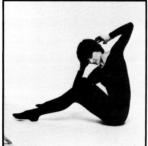
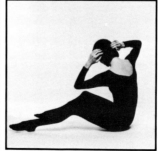
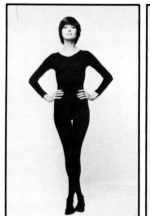
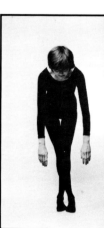

IN YOUR THIRTIES

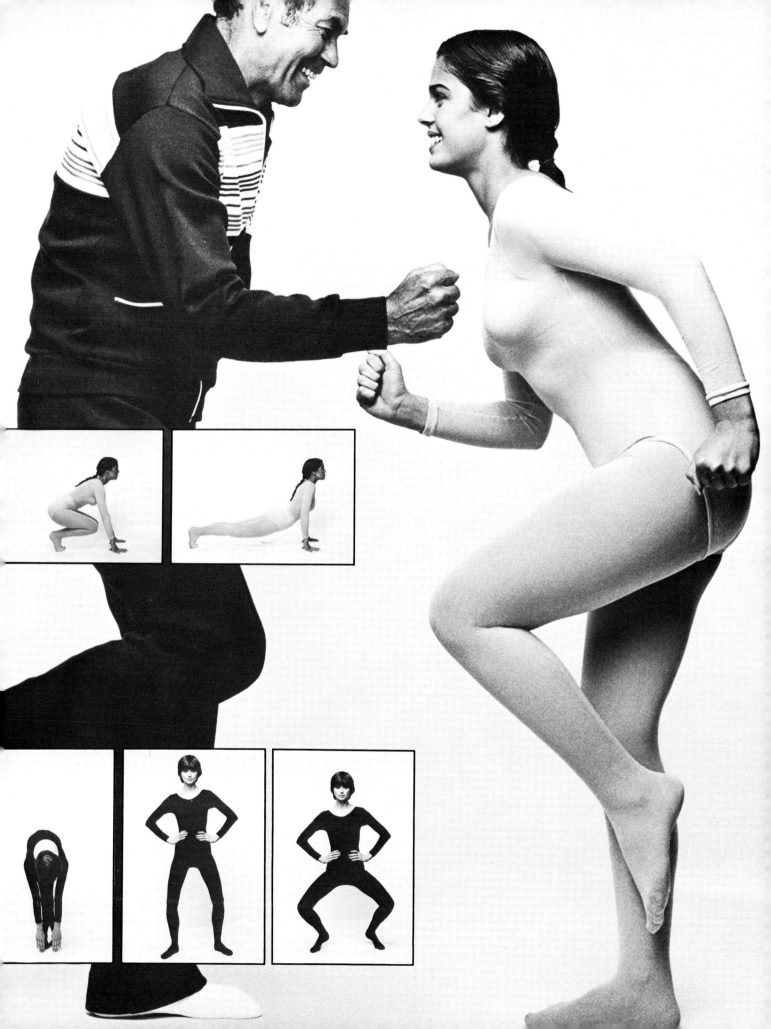

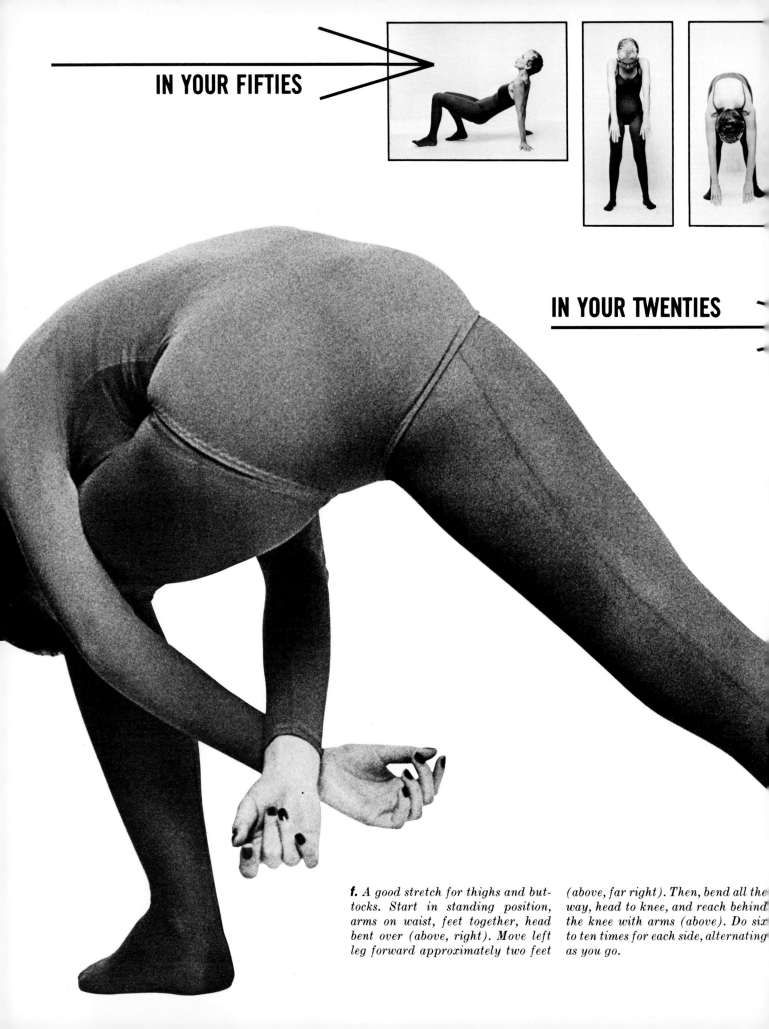

IN YOUR FIFTIES

IN YOUR TWENTIES

f. *A good stretch for thighs and buttocks. Start in standing position, arms on waist, feet together, head bent over (above, right). Move left leg forward approximately two feet* *(above, far right). Then, bend all the way, head to knee, and reach behind the knee with arms (above). Do six to ten times for each side, alternating as you go.*

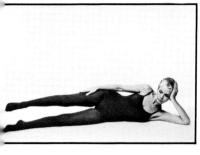
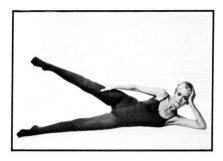
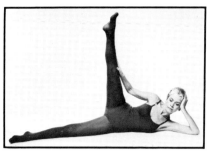

a. *The "crabwalk" (above, far left) prevents flabby upper arms, tightens legs: In position shown, with hands, feet on floor, buttocks raised, "walk" forward (10 seconds) and back (10 seconds). Repeat four times.*
b. *For breathing (two photos above, left): inhale; touch toes. Exhale and stretch arms overhead. Do this in continuous motion only four times; otherwise you may feel lightheaded.*
c. *Leg lifts: On floor as shown (three photos above), raise top leg—gently —as high as you can; lower. Work up to 10 times. Repeat with other leg.*

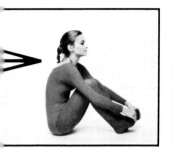
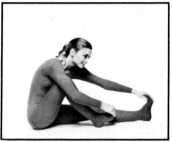
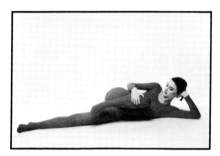
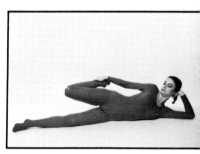

d. *A good exercise for stretching the hamstring and toning legs: Start by sitting on the floor with knees bent, hands on toes (above, far left). "Walk" left leg down till it's stretched out—straight—on the floor (above, left). Do six times for each leg; work up to 10 for each.*
e. *To promote hip flexibility. Lie on left side, bend right knee and bring up to chest (above, right). Holding onto the ankle and keeping knee bent, gently pull leg back (above, far right). Do five to six times for each side.*

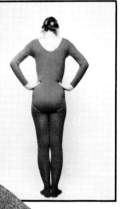
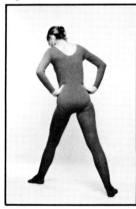
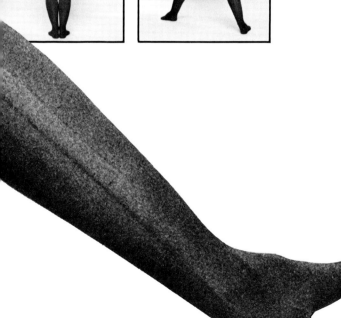

WALKING
by Carol Kahn

If jogging is a bore and running is too painful, how about walking? If you want to lose weight, tone muscles, build endurance, why not try a low-risk, high-yield exercise that involves simply putting one foot in front of the other?

"Too many people have the idea that walking means dragging along for a little bit," says Irving M. Levitas, M.D., director of the cardiac-stress laboratory in New Jersey's Hackensack Hospital. "Ask yourself honestly, how much walking have you done this week? Moving at a brisk pace. Not just from the house to the car or from the parking lot to the nearest building."

Walking is nature's way of assisting the blood in its journey back to the heart, Dr. Levitas points out. With each step you take, the muscles of the legs squeeze against the veins, helping to pump the blood upward against gravity—that is why the leg muscles

117

have been called a "second heart."

Walking, if vigorous, is an excellent aerobic exercise. It makes the heart and lungs work harder and take in more oxygen to fuel the working muscles. And the greater the abiility of the body to absorb oxygen, the more fit it becomes.

There are certain advantages that walking has over other aerobic exertions. For one thing, it is free and instantly available. And it can be done just about anywhere. It doesn't involve a lot of expensive gear—comfortable shoes with low or medium heels are the main thing. It is also an ideal activity for anyone who is overweight or out of shape. And because you are earthbound—rather than airborne for successive instants, as with jogging —it spares your joints and tendons that traumatic thump that comes every time you land.

To put walking back into your daily life, try relying on foot power more, horsepower less. The body, Dr. Levitas explains, has internal regulators called "biostats," and, like thermostats, they have built-in settings that determine such matters as when we feel hungry and what level of energy we need to expend. "As we turn up the biostat for physical activity," he says, "we feel a biological call to exercise."

But short spurts of activity are not enough for endurance and fitness. You really need a regular exercise plan. Try the "rubberband method" for building endurance recommended by Lenore Zohman, M.D., director of the cardiopulmonary unit at New York's Montefiore Hospital and Medical Center, and Albert A. Kattus, M.D., adjunct professor of cardiology at the University of California, Los Angeles. In this plan, "you increase the distance before you upgrade the intensity," Dr. Zohman explains. "Work up gradually to a goal of four miles an hour." Dr. Zohman rates three miles an hour as adequate dynamic exercise if your capacity is low, three-and-a-half miles an hour as usually good dynamic aerobic exercise, four miles as definitely dynamic and aerobic. Once you get much above

that speed, you are likely to break into a jog.

In addition to conditioning the heart, there are other benefits to walking. Dr. Zohman's patients report that it aids digestion and elimination, ups their energy level, combats insomnia, and makes them feel better. When they get in shape, they seem to require less sleep. In fact, she says, 30 minutes spent walking may be paid back in that much less sleep being needed.

And walking is an excellent way to slim down. Grant Gwinup, M.D., professor of medicine in the division of endocrinology and metabolism at the University of California, Irvine, had overweight women walk for one to three hours a day, eating everything they wanted, for one year. The women lost an average of 30 pounds, even though they had repeatedly failed to keep their weight off with diets. "You should combine a dietary program with a sensible exercise program that uses aerobic activities like walking, jogging or cycling in order to prevent excessive loss of muscle tissue," says Frank Katch, Ph.D., chairman of the department of exercise science at the University of Massachusetts.

And a diet-exercise combination makes sense for another reason, he adds: You neither have to walk yourself into the ground nor have to be hungry all the time. Since it takes an expenditure of 3500 calories to lose one pound of body fat, cutting back five hundred calories a day will result in one pound less every week. But you can lose that pound by eating only 250 calories less and walking an hour at a comfortable pace.

Remember that the number of calories burned by physical activity will vary according to body size—a heavier person has to use more energy than a slimmer one for the same activity. In one hour of walking, that difference becomes really significant, with the larger woman expending 414 calories to the 252 calories used by the lighter person.

Both a teenager and an over-50, in narrow-legged pants and boots, tweed jackets and sweaters. The same kinds of clothes—and the same freewheeling spirit.

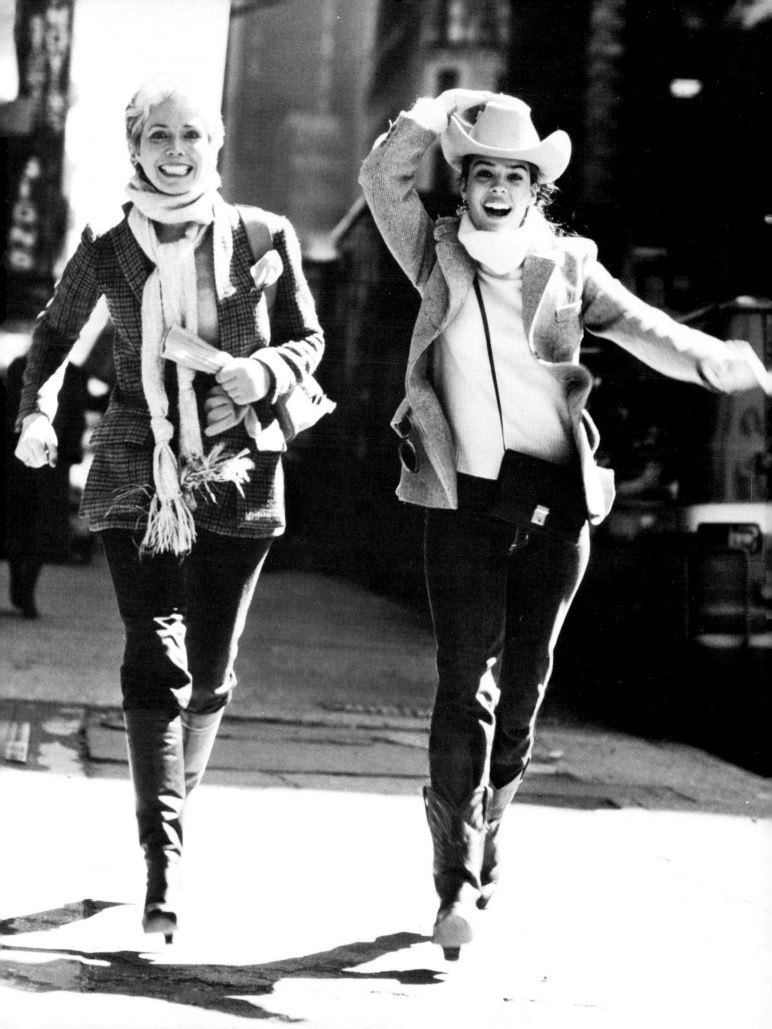

FITNESS
FONDA STYLE

"I don't think it's important to look young or to look thin. The most important thing is to be healthy."

Jane Fonda has never looked better, never felt better than she does right now. Mother, wife, actress—Jane Fonda has come into her own, taken charge of her life, approaching everything she believes in—from acting to politics to women's rights—with force and enthusiasm. She attributes her confidence, radiance, energy for living to her other great passion: exercising . . . which she's been doing every day for the past 25 years. "I found early on that exercise has a tremendous effect on my morale. And when I'm working hard, I have a tendency to let everything good go. But I always hang on to my exercise. It gives me energy, staves off depression—it makes all the difference in the world."

Glimpses of Jane Fonda, right and below, during her daily workout. Fonda's new belief in interdisciplinary exercise—an hour and a half of aerobics, calisthenics, dance (ballet, jazz, or disco), with an emphasis on leg- and thigh-firming—is the basis of her workout.

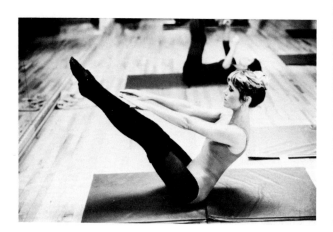

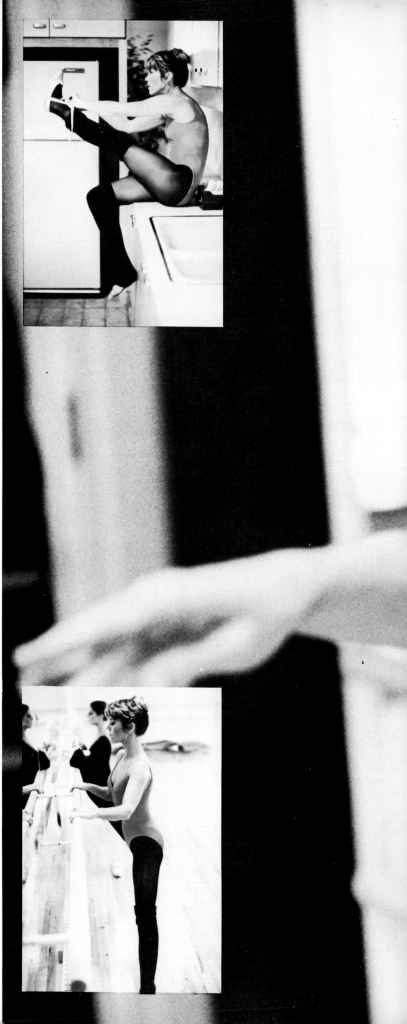

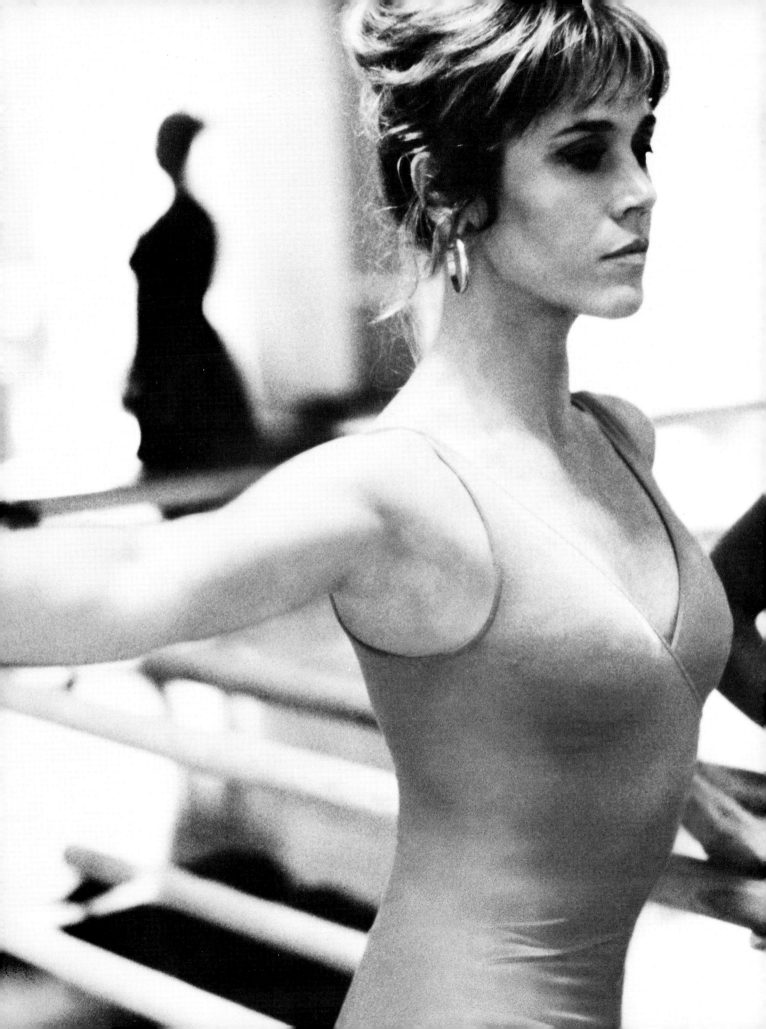

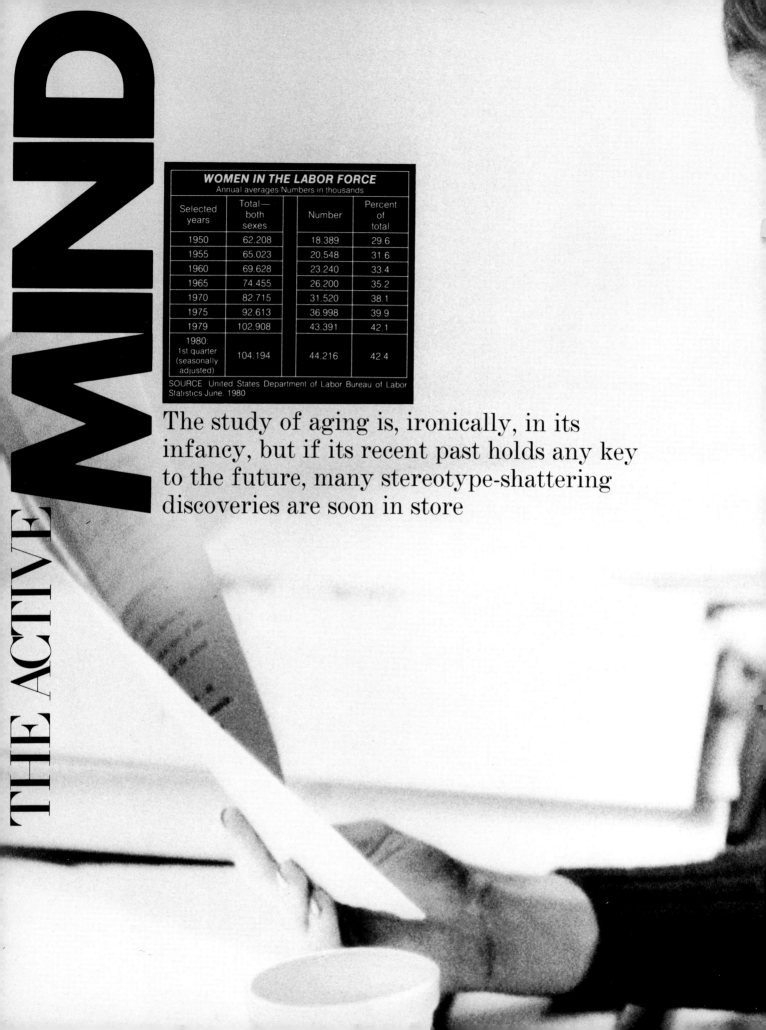

THE ACTIVE MIND

WOMEN IN THE LABOR FORCE
Annual averages Numbers in thousands

Selected years	Total—both sexes	Number	Percent of total
1950	62.208	18.389	29.6
1955	65.023	20.548	31.6
1960	69.628	23.240	33.4
1965	74.455	26.200	35.2
1970	82.715	31.520	38.1
1975	92.613	36.998	39.9
1979	102.908	43.391	42.1
1980: 1st quarter (seasonally adjusted)	104.194	44.216	42.4

SOURCE United States Department of Labor Bureau of Labor Statistics June. 1980

The study of aging is, ironically, in its infancy, but if its recent past holds any key to the future, many stereotype-shattering discoveries are soon in store

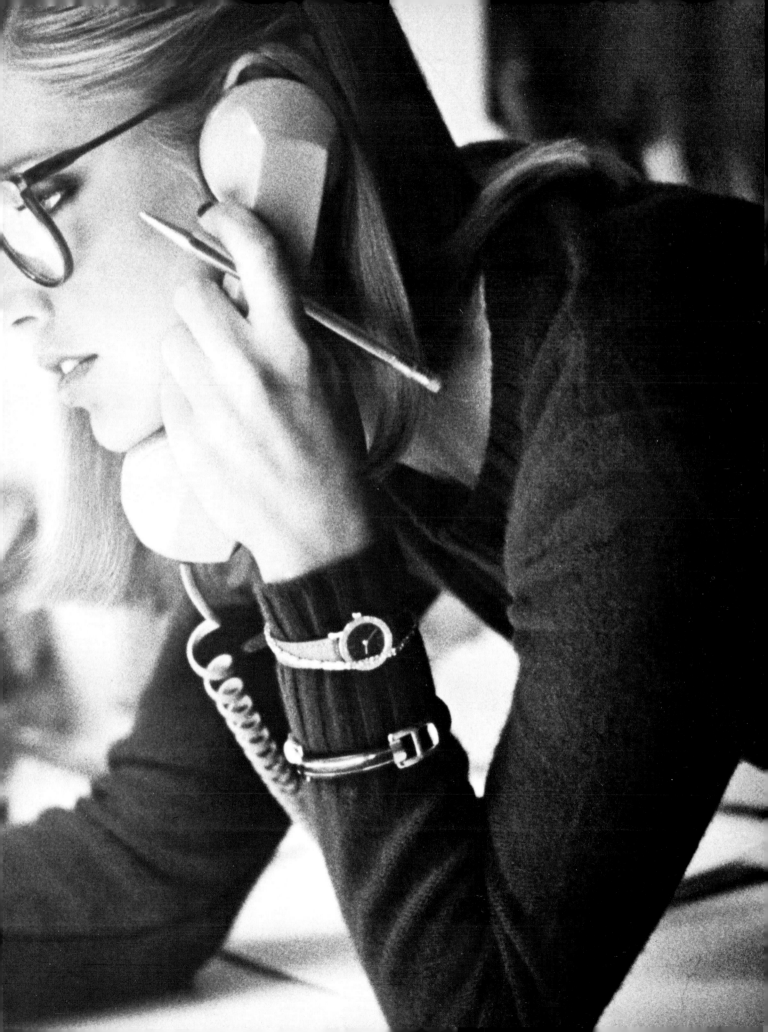

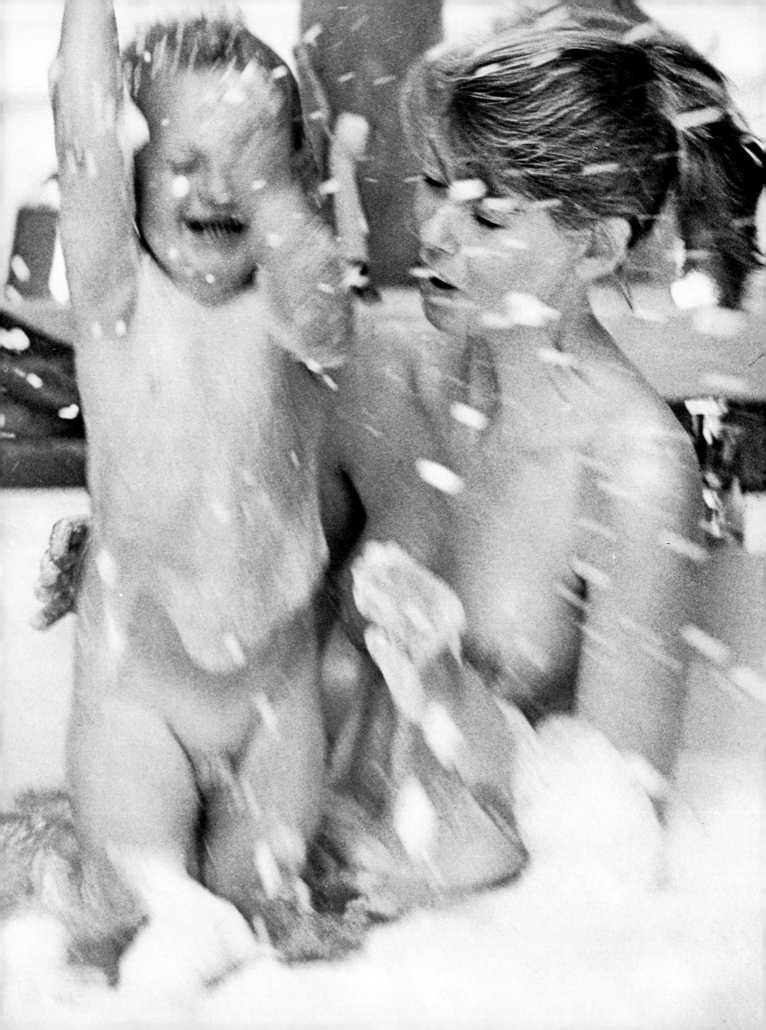

THE ACTIVE MIND

by Blythe Holbrooke

Just as aging affects the body, so it affects the mind. As with the body, the effects of aging on the mind differ radically from part to part, function to function, and individual to individual, depending on environment, diet, exercise and general health, personal adjustment, heredity, body chemistry and other factors as yet unknown. The systematic study of aging is still quite young, and the great debates are many, but the bottom line is that changes—both simple and complex—occur as the body passes through the decades. The key question is what these changes mean, for better or for worse, and if for worse, what you can do right now to help.

MEMORY AND AGING

Will I lose my mind? There are different kinds of memory. Some kinds of recall are greatly diminished by age, while others remain largely unaffected. Happily, substantial memory losses, if they do occur, happen much later than is popularly thought, generally not until the mid-seventies. While nonverbal recall drops markedly as we age, there is small (if any) decrease in vocabulary or short-term memory (the ability to do things like repeat a

The systematic study of aging is still quite young. The great debates are many, but the bottom line is that changes—both simple and complex—occur as the body passes through the decades.

string of unrelated digits). Dr. David Arenberg, an expert on memory and learning in the old, thinks this may be because with short-term (immediate) memory, the desired response is already the focus of attention. Dr. Arenberg suspects that much of what is considered memory failure in the old is really failure of concentration. It is not that the memories are no longer there, or even that the old are unable to retrieve stored information, but rather that increased distractability prevents their focusing on recall tasks long enough to pull the stored information.

This theory seems to be borne out by the fact that mid-range memory (what happened a few months or years ago) is most affected by age, while long-term memory (what happened 20, 40 or 60 years ago) seems more stable. (The results of tests of long-term memory in older people have been mixed. It is hard to tell whether one seems to remember what happened decades ago because one actually remembers the incident, or because one recalls all the stories told about it in the interim.) But while saying that the old remember best what happened to them when they were very young may or may not be true, the converse is certainly false. Short-term memory is relatively unaffected by age.

The ability to retrieve stored information quickly, however, can be affected as the years go by. Older people do best on memory tests that are self-pacing. If allowed a little additional time, the name that's slipped from memory will probably be recalled. As we age, we tend to underachieve on I.Q. and memory tests because we are less motivated than younger subjects. While "less motivated" sounds quite serious at first, it simply means that older subjects tend to put things in a larger perspective, and not strain themselves trying to repeat "nonsense" syllables on memory tests. Motivation is naturally high when it comes to remembering the names of clients, grandchildren or favorite butterflies.

Actual practical memory is very hard to test, but it seems that unless you are an architect, mathematician or engineer who needs to remember highly abstract formulas or de-

❝ *Does I.Q. decline with age? As with memory, the answer is not a simple yes or no* **❞**

signs, the "no loss" of vocabulary is more relevant to the practical effect of aging on your memory than is the significant drop on the nonverbal side. Even in the generally high-loss abstract memory, 11–20 percent of the older subjects tested showed no loss of memory at all and performed better than some of the 20-year-olds in the control sample!

INTELLIGENCE

Does I.Q. decline with age? As with memory, the answer is not a simple yes or no.

There are two basic kinds of intelligence. "Fluid," nonverbal intelligence is most directly tied in to the functioning of the nervous system (__is to__ as__is to__, __, __, __ or__? The answer is __.). "Crystallized" intelligence is the ability to use judgment (based on experience) to solve problems. (Crystallized intelligence encompasses vocabulary and knowledge of specific fields like science or history.) Crystallized I.Q. is related

to environment and education as well as a certain fluid intelligence base. Pure fluid I.Q. declines more with age than crystallized intelligence. In fact, there are many management and planning decisions we do best with more experience; that is, with greater age.

"Depending on how we define I.Q. and cognition, there is very little decline in physically healthy older people until the mid-seventies," explains Dr. Carl Eisdorfer, University of Michigan, one of the foremost authorities on the aging brain. And even very late in life, some theorize, the I.Q. decline may result from lack of stimulation or post-retirement depression, not an aging brain. Dr. Gisela Labouvie-Vief thinks that at least part of the decline could be a function of the way we educate people, lumping all their learning into the early years, often giving them scant reinforcement for speculative thought for the next 40 years. She has had some success with her work on making intellectual receptivity a more lifelong trait. Nevertheless, aging causes undeniable and, at times, critical physiological changes in the brain.

IRREPLACEABLE BRAIN CELLS

We are born with a brain weighing 350 grams, which grows to a maximum of about 1400 grams when we are around 20. From then on, there is a continuous decrease in brain weight until by our ninth decade there has been a decrease of around 10 percent. What causes the loss is not, as yet, understood, but it results in a shrinkage of the brain's convolutions, and in a widening of the grooves between them. The brain covering also thickens. Again, the reasons and significance of this are not yet known.

What *is* known is that the brain is composed of billions of non-regenerative cells. We have our maximum number of brain cells at age one-and-one-half or two, then it's downhill all the way. It was once thought that we each lost as many as 100,000 nerve cells a day after 20, but the loss is no longer thought to be so steady, so high—or even calculable, for that matter.

We lose nerve cells at different rates throughout the nervous system. According to physiologist Dr. Harold Brody, a pioneer in mapping out the processing going on in different sections of the aging brain, in certain areas like the cerebral cortex and all but one part of the

" We have our maximum number of brain cells at age one-and-one-half or two, then it's downhill all the way "

brain stem, the number of cells does not decrease with age at all. We do not yet understand why there is cell loss in certain parts of the brain and not others. Dr. Brody notes that heredity, blood supply, misuse or internal biological clock may be factors. Blood pressure (too high or low), environmental factors, drinking, smoking or drug habits and basic body health probably have a hand in it too. Curiously enough, those cells which are the last developed are also the first to go. These "associational" cells are the most highly developed, performing integrating activities within the brain. Synaptic contacts (the telegraph by which nerve impulses travel) can also deteriorate with age.

The questions, "but do these losses really matter?" and, if so, "how much?" remain. Happily, the answer is, in the normal older or even elderly person, no; let alone in the normal 55-year-old! We have from 20 to 40 *billion* neurons in our brains. Each neuron has about 1000 connections, giving our neurons more possible connections than there are molecules on earth! With that kind of reserve capacity we can afford to lose quite a few million neurons before it shows, according to Dr. Eisdorfer. Of course, he points out that no two brains are the same. Original endowments

and disease history have a lot to do with how well your brain ages. Until recently, for example, it was thought that the trembling and nervous disorders of Parkinson's disease might just be an unfortunate side-effect of age. Then the incidence of Parkinson's disease began dropping off. Why? Scientists looked back and saw that between 1917 and 1921 there was a terrible epidemic of a particularly deadly flu that killed many and, scientists now believe, destroyed millions of brain cells in those who fell ill, but apparently recovered. When the survivors were 25, or even 40, the loss of brain capacity didn't affect them much, but as their remaining brain cells dwindled with age, they developed the symptoms of Parkinson's disease, which was previously though to be simply a part of normal aging!

IS SENILITY PART OF "NORMAL AGING"?

One of the great fears associated with old age is that we will "lose" our minds and memories, become senile. Many seem to believe that senility is just a normal part and parcel of growing old. This is not true. While it cannot be overemphasized that the health of the body is mirrored in the health of the mind (even a "terminal drop" in tested I.Q. slightly prior to death has been found), the odds are pretty good against your becoming senile, even in your eighties. Only five percent of those over 65 are senile, and still only 20 percent of them will ever become senile, no matter how long they live. Even among those people thought senile, about 30 percent are really suffering from some other, reversible disorder, like depression or chronic drug overdose.

While senility is a disease of old age, it is not a part of normal aging. (There is a world of difference between minor concentration and memory lapses of old age and the massive disorders of senile dementia.) While all people, even 16-year-olds, die with some senile plaque on their brains, very few normal people are found at the high or low end of the plaque density spectrum. Not that scientists are quite sure yet what this really means or what actually causes senile dementia. Heredity? Early illnesses? A virus? Long-lamented, senile dementia is only now coming under intensive study.

STRESS AND COPING

The problem is most often not stress, but coping—coping with a diminished set of friends, responsibilities, stimulation, position, love, even less money. Much depression is "reactive," that is, the older person's understandable response to his diminished role or the death of a spouse. The vast preponderance of white male suicides may indicate the greater disappointment of their higher expectations, and the greater changes in a more outward-oriented and, prior to old age, more other-reinforced style of life. Dr. Robert N. Butler of the National Institute on Aging notes that our society's work roles are so structured that "people are either burned-out or bored to death" by the time they reach retirement.

While we often experience more losses as the decades pass, there may also be physiological factors contributing to depression in later life. According to Dr. Monica Blumenthal, a psychologist, an increased biological vulnerability to depression, due to changes in the brain's chemical messengers, can occur. Fewer of the natural uppers, norepinephrine and dopamine, are produced, while at the same time the body manufactures more of the enzyme that destroys them. If the brain is already doing things marginally, the chemical balance (so very important to maintaining normal mood) can be upset, and depression can result. Fortunately, depression is the most treatable mental illness. Old as well as young respond well to a combination of drugs and psychotherapy. And today, many more therapists are concentrating specifically on post-retirement problems in both males and females.

But what about special abilities in the nor-mal older person? Doesn't creativity decline with age? Are older people more rigid than the young? Conventional wisdom certainly says they are, but some gerontologists don't buy the stereotype of the closed, uncreative older person. Historical studies have shown that while certain types of creativity, notably highly theoretical mathematical abilities and genius in certain physical sciences, seem to flourish, then diminish as early as the twenties (though he lived 85 years, Sir Isaac Newton had discovered gravity and differential calculus by the time he was 24), other types of creativity involving less fluid and more crystallized intelligence—like literature, philosophy and diplomacy—show no change. In fact, peak creative work in these disciplines often takes place in the forties, fifties and sixties, or even in the late eighties. Goethe was in his eighties when he gave us *Faust*, Verdi wrote grand opera *(Falstaff)* into his eighties, and Thomas Mann gave us *The Confessions of Felix Krull* in his final, 80th year.

The bottom line on aging and creativity is simply that, with the exception of math and certain physical sciences, the correlation between age and creativity is not clear at all. As with intelligence, the link is more between creativity and good health. Again, as with intelligence, barring major trauma or illness the creative person will, in all likelihood, continue to be creative. How creative? It all depends. . . .

THE CHANGING SENSES

Gourmets, wine tasters and all those who savor the many perfumes of life will be happy to learn that smell and taste barely change with age, if they change at all. Some studies report a slight loss of taste and smell after 60, others do not. In those studies finding a difference, the ability to detect sweet was an issue and a number of men had trouble picking up salty tastes, but older women did not. Smell sensitivity seems to remain constant in either sex, while sensitivity to touch seems unchanged until about 55, at which point it begins to decline, as does sensitivity to pain.

We commonly believe that we see less well as we age, and this is generally true. The ability to see far away differs as we age, but until the fifties the change is slight and comes from loss of elasticity in the lenses. The ability to see well close up is a different matter. This deterioration starts in childhood, with the greatest changes coming between 40 and 55.

As we grow older our lenses also become progressively thicker, letting in less light, so that in general a 65-year-old will need twice as much illumination as a 20-year-old to receive the same amount of light. Not surprisingly, night vision is also affected, as is depth perception under low illumination.

Color vision undergoes changes, too. As we grow older, the lenses of the eye yellow, filtering out the shorter wave lengths (blues, greens and violets), while leaving our ability to see the longer ones (reds and yellows) almost unchanged. Perhaps this explains the otherwise tasteful grandmother's penchant for blue-white hair; she simply doesn't perceive the shadings of blue. Some older people should avoid relying only on their own perceptions with subtle blues and greens, especially when taking different pills in the blue-green spectrum. Of course, with color perceptions as with all aspects of aging, individual differences can be immense. Some vital 90-year-old artists are still painting the truest blues!

General hearing ability also changes with age, in men more than in women, and in the higher, much more than the lower, frequency range. Thus, at 80, your interest in Joan Sutherland's art may diminish as you start collecting the records of a favorite basso. As with many of the faculties affected by aging, the rate accelerates with greater age. Thus, hearing loss between 25 and 50 will be slight, that between 75 and 85 proportionately greater. Studies show that a higher percentage of those exposed to ''noise pollution'' are poorer hearers in later life.

AGE, ADJUSTMENTS AND PERSONALITY

But aren't older people supposedly less open and more rigid? The answer, according to Dr. Paul Costa of the National Institute on Aging (who has made a study of openness and age), is ''no. We don't find any effects on openness from age. If a person is open, age doesn't seem to diminish that.'' At any age, an individual's openness or flexibility is tied into his culture's (and parents') child-rearing approach.

On the basis of early cross-sectional studies, psychologists had originally thought rigidity was linked to age. But then they noticed a curious phenomenon: Those over 66 tested as relatively closed to experience, but so did those 30–40; while the 56- to 60-year-olds appeared as open as those 20 and under. What was going on? Checking back, psychologists found that the 56- to 60-year-olds had grown up stimulated by the open Roaring Twenties, while those then 51–55 grew up during the Great Depression.

Not that none of us changes for better or worse as we get older. One's own personal psychohistory hurts or helps. If a person's adult life has been an unending string of putdowns and disappointments, he will become more rigid and closed. But that can happen at 30 as well as 60, and is not by any means a part of the aging process per se. On some tests a number of older people do test as more rigid in their approach to certain problems, but as aging-specialist Dr. Jack Botwinick points out, that could simply be because the problem was solved in one way in the past, so that the habit is more strongly reinforced.

SUCCESSFUL AGING: MORE OF THE SAME?

While some analysts, like Erik H. Erikson, talk about age as a time for staged withdrawal, recent studies show that the best-adjusted older people don't radically change their personalities or lives, but rather take a little off the pace of the kind of life they've always lived. "Age is just another background variable, affecting, but by no means determining, personality," says Dr. Costa. Thus, the extrovert will do best by continuing to be active and outgoing, while the lifelong scholar would make a dangerous mistake by pushing himself into a flurry of other-oriented activity. *Continuity.* Successful aging comes from being able to maintain one's lifestyle in the fullest sense of the word, acknowledging which activities you can no longer perform and finding adequate substitutes. If you used to go out and play touch football every Saturday, get out and golf, swim, play croquet or garden. If you have difficulty hearing, don't withdraw, get a hearing aid. If you feel you can no longer see as well, change your glasses and turn up the lights. Older people are much more affected than younger ones by the same amount of medication. If you feel dopey and overmedicated, see your doctor right away. If you're tense and anxious, opt for exercise instead of drugs. (Exercise helps burn up anxiety drugs only mask. Be sure to check with your doctor before beginning any program of physical exercise.) If you're feeling dull and sluggish, don't write it off as age. Have a thorough physical as you would were you younger.

Find a lover. There is no age limit to the sexual function, or the need for tenderness and companionship. (Tests show we seem to function better longer if we have a confidant.) If you're depressed, remember it's never too late to seek counseling. If you take a little longer to do things, give yourself more time. If you don't remember names as well as you used to, write them down!

Realize that with age some of your priorities may change, and that this is just fine! Don't worry if you're not half so eager about "making it" at 71 as you were at 29. Keep in mind that there are pluses to growing old. We can have a better sense of what's really important. Consequently, we are often better able to organize our days in a less manic fash-

ion, taking time for both the practical and the transcendent, like really noticing that tree. While we often don't make decisions as quickly as we did when young, we have more confidence in our decisions once we have made them.

Retirement certainly can kill you if you spent your life always chasing after the next deal. While more gerontologists are against mandatory retirement for 65-year-olds, don't put off some kind of taking it easier indefinitely. Enrich your life now! Start preparing for leisure in later years by taking up interests you can pursue later on. And while you're planning ahead, don't forget about providing for your retirement. One of the best predictors of successful adjustment to retirement is income! (Can it be that living well *is* truly the best revenge?) Don't shy away from

" *Find a lover. There is no age limit to the sexual function or the need for tenderness and companionship* **"**

continued education just because it may take you a little longer to pick things up. Remember, even the healthy 80-year-old shows only a marginal loss of I.Q.; in tests conducted by Dr. David Arenberg at seven-year intervals, anywhere from 10 to nearly 20 percent of those tested show no change in any kind of tested mental ability! Sometimes even a slight improvement!

What is the secret of these special individuals? Dr. Arenberg found that those who maintained their performance level had good general health and were, on the average, more active, energetic, friendly, responsible, productive and emotionally stable than those who didn't. But this is just a start. Clearly, as we age, we have far greater potential for functioning "young" than has been recognized.

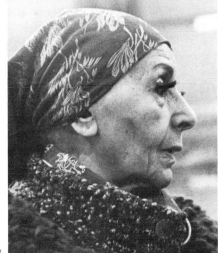

Nevelson

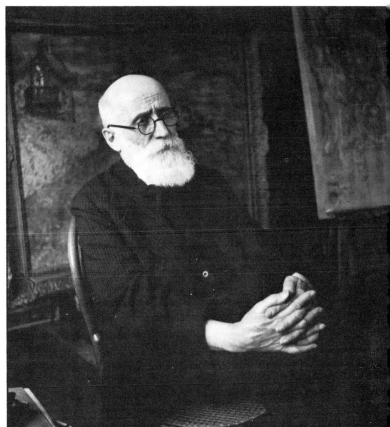

Vuillard

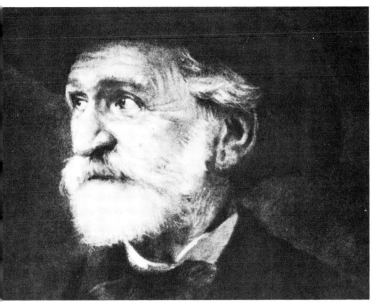

Verdi

Dr. Arenberg is now turning his attention to those happy few who seem to lose none of their mental abilities. This seems a more promising route to a ''fountain of youth'' than any contemplated by the early explorers. Dr. Eisdorfer and Dr. Brody's trailblazing work on the importance of brain cell loss and the effects of aging on different parts of the brain also continues. The study of aging is, ironically, a science still in its infancy, but if its recent past holds any key to the future, many important stereotype-shattering discoveries are soon in store.

"Crystallized intelligence," involving creativity in the arts, flourishes in later years, as evidenced by the masterpieces of Louise Nevelson, Giuseppe Verdi, Edouard Vuillard and Thomas Mann.

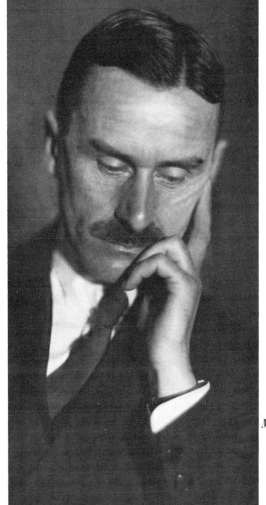

Mann

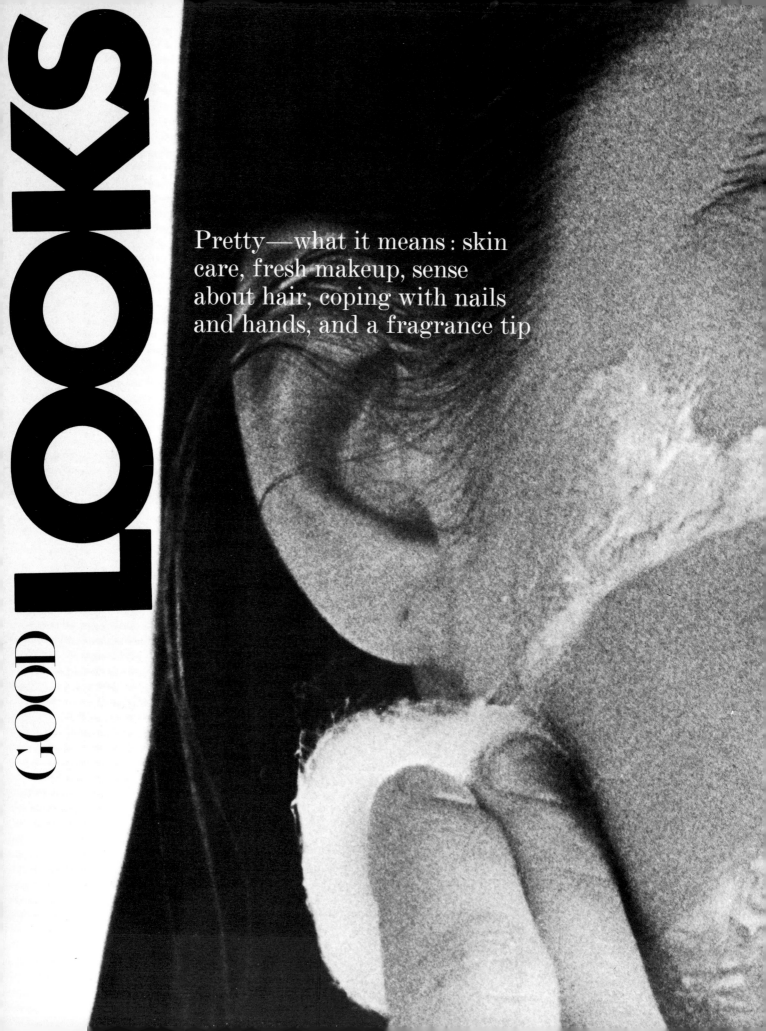

GOOD LOOKS

Pretty—what it means: skin
care, fresh makeup, sense
about hair, coping with nails
and hands, and a fragrance tip

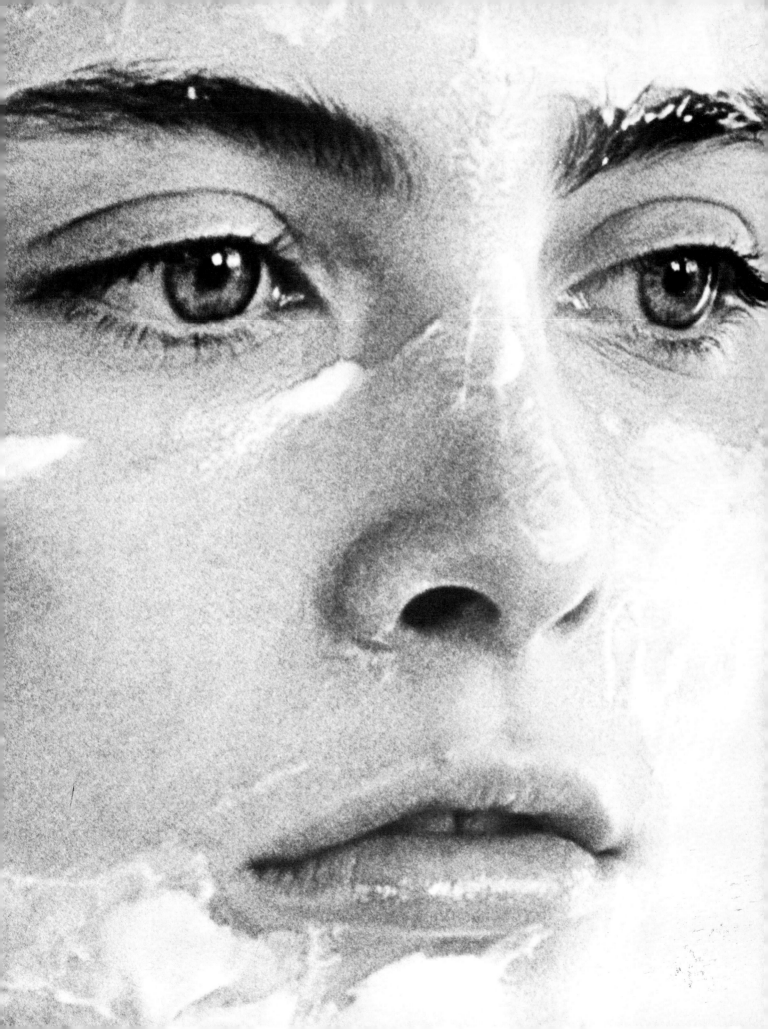

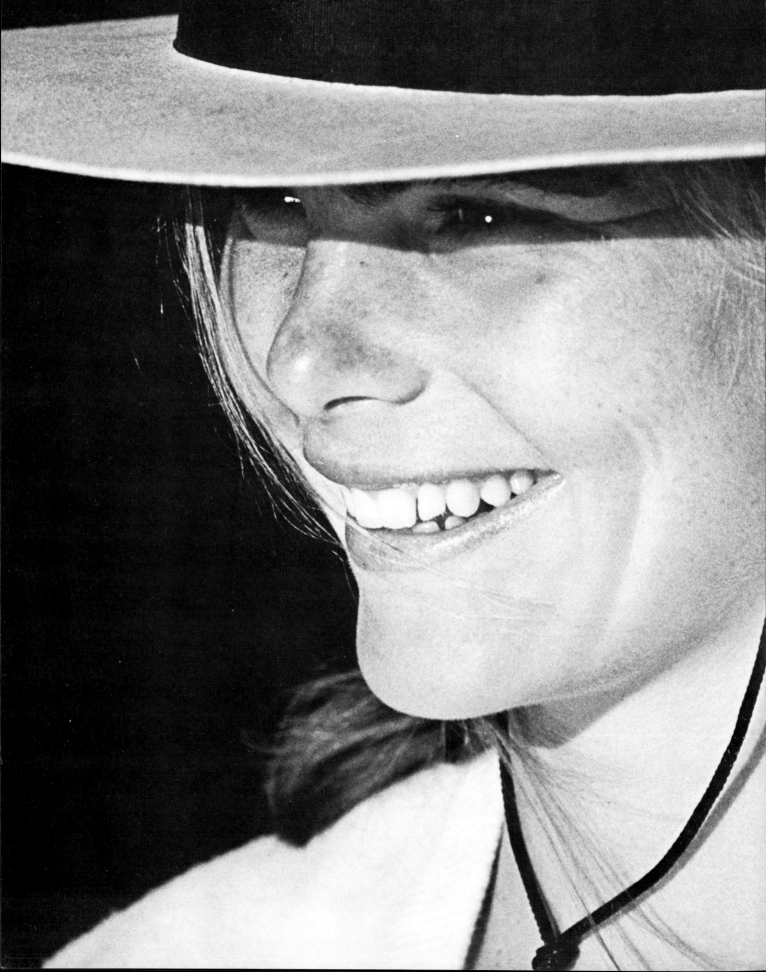

PRETTY: WHAT IT MEANS IN THE 80's

Chapter edited
by Alexandra Penney

by Jill Robinson

You can't buy the latest thing in beauty. You have to change how you think.

Better news: You probably already have.

Beauty has always started behind the eye, always been a matter of semantics, the private idea of the beholder.

To me, Beauty was always passive. I saw Beauty leaning backward and away, in bias-cut satin (she looked like the great model Dovima). She was flawless, adored, always given masses of flowers and precious jewels in leather cases that opened and closed with an expensive snap I'd recognize a mile away. When I was 14, I bought Violets-in-the-Snow lipstick. Late one night, with my lipstick on and my head swathed in emerald-green veiling, I stared into the mirror, convinced that if I could just climb out my window and make my way to the nightclub Ciro's, I would be applauded as a new Beauty. Clark Gable and Errol Flynn would duel to dance with me. Then, at 16, standing in a powder room after a premiere, between Elizabeth Taylor and Lana Turner, I realized Beauty was magic. I made the discovery women made then that Beauties were born of different stuff than people.

Mariel Hemingway's beauty regimen: the most basic skin care, frequent shampoos, minimal makeup, sunbathing never—she gets enough healthy color exercising outdoors.

Beauty's definition, happily, has changed. My own perception, and yours, has grown up, opened up. It is not romantic. It is not magic. You can't tell the stars from the people. What we want now is a kind of mental Gorgeousness that goes beyond beauty or prettiness.

Gorgeousness is Beauty in motion: moving from the inside out with a plan. Gorgeous, to me, implies an active creature, taking charge and growing, unfolding, enveloping. You can't apply Gorgeousness for a big evening or pick it up anywhere under the sun in a quick 10-day course and expect it to stay there. You don't have to shoot it in the right light, from the right angle. Gorgeousness catches women moving, working, slouching, thinking and lusting. Gorgeousness is Beauty Liberated.

Gorgeousness is an attitude, a frame of mind and a way of life. It is a new kind of inner beauty that is not to be confused with serenity or complacency. An expression occasionally caught is inquisitive. This new Beauty is involved with the right to know. She asks the hard questions and expects precise, expert answers.

Gorgeousness is energy. The tough secret way to get it and keep it is intelligent, planned maintenance. The thought of that makes me want to take a nap. To call it beauty-sleep is a cop-out. We all know 10 minutes of yoga exercises will do more.

For with all the freedom from the rigid,

135

captive standard of beauty defined by eye alone, comes this terrible sense of responsibility for knowing and doing what is really good for us. We know as much about exercise and nutrition as some doctors (sometimes, we suspect, we know more).

This enlightenment involves consistent follow-through. I'm the only person I know who still orders dessert. When people go on vacation now, it's often to a tennis camp or a spa. No one expects miracles there: One goes to a spa now to learn a program to be carried through every day, a schedule of fitness that will teach us an appropriate individual rhythm to maintain the essential equilibrium between relaxation and the tension we need to get through our days.

This is the new priority in beauty: We don't want our bodies to get in the way of what we do. And this Gorgeousness is the side effect. In fact, aesthetic consideration is the side effect now of all our Beautywork—or things which used to be thought of as Beautywork. We are interested not in quick cover-up effects but in long-range feeling better. It is this aspect of women's liberation that has, by the way, most successfully caught on with men. The information we've demanded and received has enlightened them, given them treatment products they do use, sent them to spas, made them notice what they eat, quite literally stood them on their heads.

Gorgeousness has less to do with the youth myth than with feeling better. Life is longer, we want the quality of that life to be better. It has little to do with wrinkles or gray hair —fairly inevitable badges of honor and wisdom—more to do with productivity and ongoing sexuality. We finally got the message there, too: Sex is feeling better, moving better. You have to be older really to know, really to understand your way out of inhibition and into the commitment that makes it worth all that adolescent angst. You have to be older to understand just how much youth got in the way.

Anyway, youth has added at least two decades lately. Think of prematurity this way: before we were mature enough to understand that self-indulgence in drinking, overeating and inactivity (sitting around and worrying about what we could not accomplish) is the great aging process. Or limiting process. There is nothing wrong with age. Gorgeousness begins with energy enlightenment. That can begin any time. This is my 40th year. I could not cross the monkey bars when I was 10, but I've finally (starting at 37) gotten myself into good enough shape to take up tennis now. Well, next week. (It is one thing to observe all this, to write about it, quite another to instill that consistency.)

Major point here: Gorgeousness is at once starting from the self and moving *away* from self-involvement. We start with our own self-awareness, an intelligence about what our bodies, skins, teeth, hair need—we develop the routine that works, and then we can move out of self-consciousness. No more boring Beauties drifting away their days, drowning

" Beauty's definition has changed . . . It is not magic . . . What we want now is a kind of mental gorgeousness that goes beyond beauty or prettiness "

in mirrors of despair over each line, each eyebrow that won't lie down. You can have a day when you think your hair looks like a rat on alert, when you've been working triple time (house or office or, most likely, both), when your personal sky is, indeed, falling in pieces, and someone will say, "You look gorgeous." Probably true. It's energy galvanized. If you've kept to your maintenance plan, you can afford days, even a week or two, of chaos. The body releases the adrenaline it has been saving. It will ask for some quiet time later on to store it up again—that quiet time may even resemble a terrible low. But you can get through that time, too, without alarm, because you have all this information. You know the mechanics. You know the tuning process.

Rhythm—this is part of the work we've learned to do, understanding the personal rhythm we need to keep fit, knowing what to use and when. Knowing it finally almost by instinct. You can't be gorgeous by nattering on and on about how you're going to do this and that, musing it over and over, driving friends crazy with repeated (and inevitably lengthy) resolutions you do not keep. A true resolution is one you simply do. You start. You don't discuss it. That's why we're not having resolutions here. You know by now what kind of maintenance rhythm will work for you. What should be involved in the program. If you don't, you know where to find the information (or you haven't been reading the best-seller lists in the last decade).

Beauty is the amazing aftereffect of a lot of intelligent work. Part of Gorgeousness is also the intelligence to design your individual standard and stay with it; it may involve several pieces of many different fitness techniques, cleaning-up rituals. Creativity in beauty involves more than knowing just how to wear three shades of eye shadow (although that's fun, and we'll come to that—it also belongs). Beauty is science now, a kind of preventive medicine, and the people who work in that know we cannot be lured by mystery, by magical promises or packaging. The talk is more technician to student; often, chemist to technician. Nutrients, pH factors, anti-pollutants, proteins, vitamins—these are part of the language we expect. We want to know how it works and what's in it. Skepticism has started rewarding us with answers. This new discipline extends into our relationship with doctors and dentists. Whoever used to ask how to brush teeth? Now we not only know how but precisely why. Responsibility—our own—is the essential now.

Perhaps the reason we never used to ask questions was that we suspected there weren't answers. But the questions actually did begin to force the answers. Feminist writers such as Betty Friedan and Barbara Seaman began to ask the questions. Susan Brownmiller, in the devastating *Against Our Will*, questions the entire culture. And it is up to us to follow through. It's responsibility, again, that is the watchword, the key to the active spirit we call Beauty now.

❝ This new beauty is involved with the right to know. Women ask hard questions and expect precise, expert answers ❞

Self-respect, not dependency; selection, not sexual plumage: passivity is non-beautiful. I think art always prefigures what will happen in social attitudes, and as art moved out of academic ideals, beyond anthropomorphic figuring, as it freed its own definitions, so ideas about human beauty have opened and changed. Art moved into abstraction, into structure, into consideration of things the eye does not necessarily see, and so beauty has moved into action, the mind, the basic nature of our media: the condition of cells, bones and blood. Beauty, then, like our art, is beyond ornament. It is a broader statement, rough and perplexing, even as some of us appear to others. The standard, however, is concerned with an intrinsic sense of beauty and form and balance. It is our great good fortune that, in human beings, this new standard takes our well-being as its point of departure. This new sensibility is what sophistication should be all about.

So much for sheer black stockings, which, in the time I was playing around with green veiling, represented the Sophisticated Lady.

Except (here's what I promised about fun): Gorgeousness must also involve wit and whimsy. This is essential to humanity, and the new Beauty is a human person. Lapses (the occasional croissant, I say hopefully, having just finished one), burrs, quirks make us really gorgeous. We must permit movement of approach. Steps back and forth in the day's dance. Guilt is not gorgeous. Rigidity is as boring as plodding immersion in constant self-discovery—a contemporary affliction to be avoided rather more than the empty calorie or lunchtime spent trying on blushers because the names of the colors are so terrific. . . .

You can't include this in a maintenance plan because it defeats the purpose : the occasional spunk of letting yourself just be. I think when they planned the Declaration of Independence and they put in the part about the pursuit of happiness, they meant times like this, when one isn't thinking or planning, when one is avoiding all the seriousness which life is really spent pursuing. One can't pursue happiness, of course, but one can permit it, the occasional nonpolitical playing around. As Joseph Heller, the smartest of the man writers, says, ''Where did we get the idea people are supposed to be happy?'' We don't get much of the new Gorgeousness by utterly happy means, for instance. Maintenance is work ; this is why we have to shore each other up with encouragement, suggestions, and articles like this that remind us what the point of it all might be.

I mean, if someone came up with an eye shadow called Lilacs Caught in Prism, which promised to fragment itself about the eyelid in slippy, gleaming myriads of little rainbows, I would leap from my lotus position and run right out, certain to see, in my mind's eye only perhaps, such a vision of Beauty. And the mind's eye is still where Beauty dwells, napping though she may be while Gorgeousness does the work of the world and makes us strong. Rejection of Gorgeousness, her regimen, her great good sense, is not to be implied by an occasional dreaming tryst with Beauty.

SKIN CARE FOR A LIFETIME

An interview with Norman Orentreich, M.D.

Good skin care begins on day one—with proper sun protection. This is probably the single most important aspect of skin care there is.

We have known for quite a while that all ultraviolet radiation is cumulative and that every hour of sunlight a person gets—whether at age one, two, five, or 50—adds up. But we did not realize until fairly recently that an hour of radiation is far more damaging to a child than to an adult. This finding is new. Studies in which a record is kept of the carcinogenic effects of sunlight on laboratory animals for a period of time in the early part of their lives, in the middle, and in the latter part show that the earlier damage—the same unit of damage—is worse. This is likely to be true for man, too. Our cells' genetic material is probably much more susceptible to damage when we are very young.

Of course, if you can stay out of the sun for several years, your skin will recuperate to some extent. But the harm caused by any period of exposure can never be completely reversed. So children should be taught to use sunscreens while they are still quite small and not get a deep tan. It may look healthy, but the look is deceptive.

ADOLESCENCE

Your skin needs scrupulous care during adolescence because the hormonal changes that take place in your body at and after puberty

Editor's note: Dr. Orentreich is a clinical associate professor of dermatology at New York University School of Medicine.

frequently lead to oily skin and acne. The basis of treatment for this teenage condition is exfoliation—which involves a certain amount of controlled irritation, with soap and water and a washcloth, scrub brush or abrasive sponge, or with chemical preparations like salicylic acid, resorcinol or benzoyl peroxide.

The important thing is to minimize comedo formation by regular mechanical or chemical exfoliation, because the longer an open comedo (blackhead) lasts, the bigger it gets, and the more damage it will do. Open and closed comedones go through the same stages—once they reach a certain level of maturity, they inflame and then "cure" themselves. When you use controlled irritation to treat a comedo, you bring everything into sync and force the inflammation to occur early. If you just let it go its course and get bigger and bigger, then when it finally explodes, you get a significant pustule—which can enlarge the pore and leave a scar.

I don't think that every case of acne or oily skin calls for a dermatologist. Mild acne, such as an occasional premenstrual pimple, does not usually leave scars. The family doctor can advise you about treatment and prescribe medication. But if there is a regular crop—large or small—of comedones and pustules, you should see a dermatologist. He can give you an individual program of therapy along with gentle "acne surgery"—to express the contents of comedones and drain pustules and cysts.

TWENTY TO THIRTY-FIVE

Between 20 and 35, you peak endocrinologically—that is, you have reached your maximum hormone levels. Your oil glands and sweat glands (eccrine for moisture, apocrine for scent) are most active. Your sense of smell and taste are most acute. You are at your peak sexually.

Oily skin is an ongoing problem for a great many young women during the twenties and thirties. And as long as it persists, frequent washing with soap and water can be helpful, along with a daily shampoo.

Acne, like oily skin, is a manifestation of this peak period of hormonal activity. But it may indicate a slight hormonal imbalance when it goes on so long—and hormonal tests are useful in helping to pinpoint the exact cause. If the tests do show an imbalance, medication can be prescribed to correct this.

Large pores are another problem you are apt to see more of during those years because oily skin and acne both contribute to the condition—a large pore is nothing more than the skin surface outlet of a large (and more active) oil gland.

Exposure to sunlight is something else you have to think about. Remember, this is a time when you probably spend more hours out of doors—jogging, biking, skating, skiing and such—than you are likely to at any later period. So the amount of sun you get is bound to be considerable, and you really have to zero in on protection. You are, after all, still in a very susceptible phase, a young phase. Use sunscreens and sun blocks regularly—and generously.

Wrinkles first appear during this period. And in order to forestall them, there are four things you can do. Reduce continually repeated facial expressions. Cut out cigarettes (smoking causes lots of little lines on your upper lip and may even be linked to crow's feet, although we do not have strong evidence on this yet). Have your eyes checked; poor accommodation leads to squint lines, and this is something most women do not pay enough attention to. (If you wear glasses, be sure to get them fitted properly.)

And use a good sun block whenever you are in the sun for any length of time, even in winter; this, more than anything else, helps ward off wrinkles.

Following pages: How you cleanse your skin is far more important than how often—and a doctor is usually the best authority on the right cleansing and treatment methods for you. The goal: to help you understand your skin so you can adapt your care to changes in your environment, in your lifestyle.

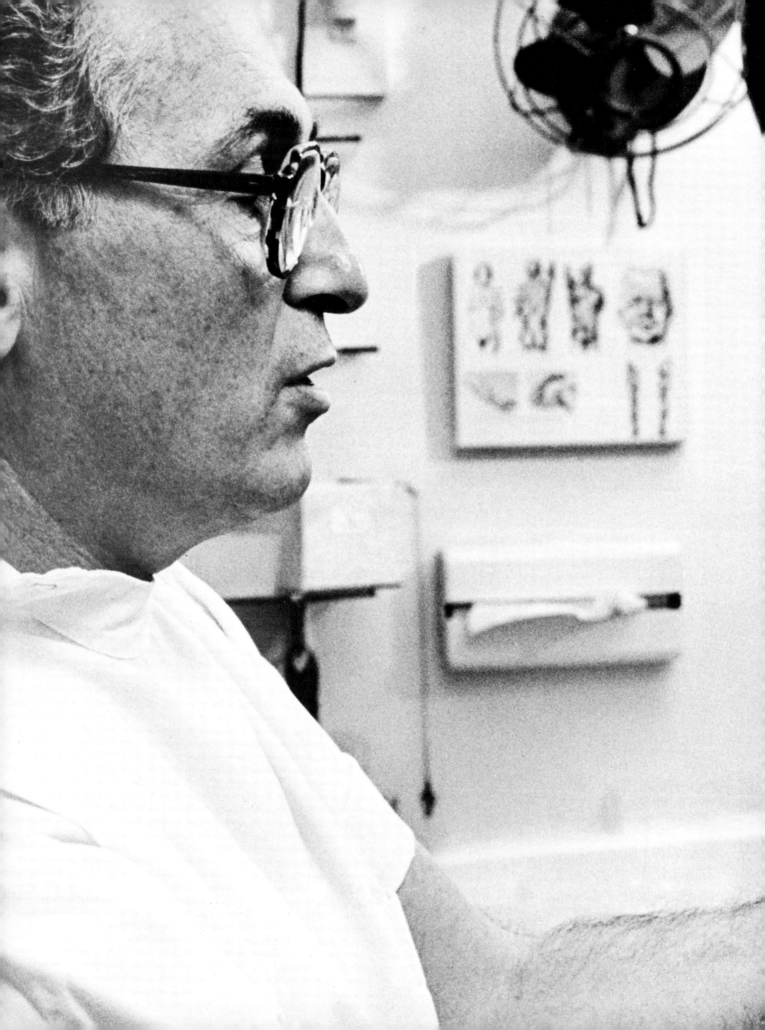

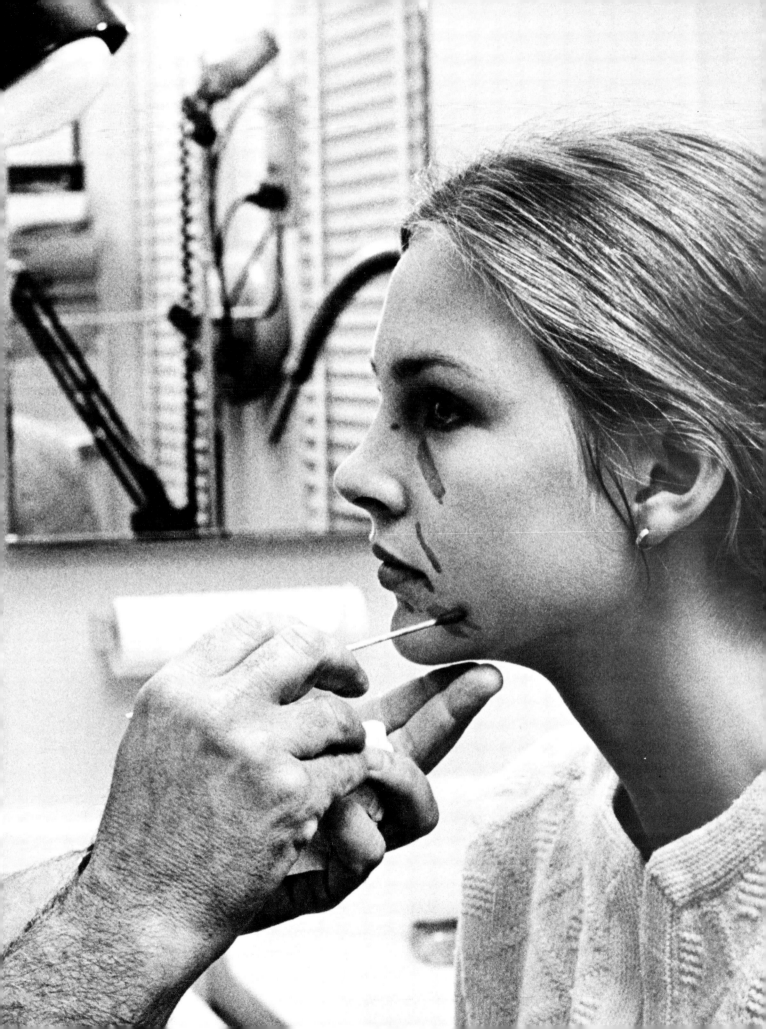

THIRTY-FIVE TO FIFTY

It is after 35 that you have to come to grips with the fact that change is inevitable—and start zeroing in on the situation. Fast! For one thing, your skin is getting thinner, less elastic—more noticeably so if you have not been using sun blocks. For another, it is beginning to show changes in pigment—the color is no longer uniform. And if you are still smoking, squinting and frowning, you have little set grooves on your upper lip, around your eyes, and on your forehead. But more than that, there is a gradual increase in skin surface area—it is rather like wearing a skin that is several sizes too big for your face. Women frequently start to feel it's time to pick up the slack a bit.

As a matter of fact, I rarely can look at a woman over 35 without feeling that some replacement, resurfacing or redraping therapy would help. It is a time when you are not so young that doing something is premature and not so old that doing something is not going to be worthwhile.

Take plastic surgery (redraping).... The right time is, simply, when you need it and want it. Obviously, the risk in operative procedure is less in a healthier and younger individual, and the healing is quicker. However, one thing about plastic surgery that you do have to bear in mind is that, in about five to 10 years, you are usually back where you started from—and ready for a second operation. I do think you have to be realistic about this.

With dermabrasion (resurfacing), I find that the improvement holds up well through the years, provided you avoid too much sun. I can usually tell a patient that in 10 years' time her skin will look better—I've seen people 20 and 30 years later, and even then their skin shows persistent benefit. There is still aging, but it is aging of an inherently more youthful skin, and the person looks naturally younger.

Collagen augmentation (replacement) of lost tissue—with minute amounts of expertly injected pure medical-grade silicone or other materials—is another procedure that can help, but you do have to keep up the "maintenance" augmentation.

I think that, of the three kinds of therapy, dermabrasion gives the most overall improvement and has the most lasting effect. It just makes people look better—as if they had protected their skin all their life.

Chemical peeling is still another resurfacing technique. And it is certainly easier to do than dermabrasion, but I generally do not like

> **"** *Smiling also helps by masking the defects. Not by a smile—more a Mona Lisa smile, a half smile* **"**

the results you get with it. There is no careful way to control the chemical/skin interaction —whereas the mechanical/skin interaction of dermabrasion can be precisely controlled. Also, with chemicals, you get a demarcation line between the treated and untreated areas that you can avoid with dermabrasion. The dermabrasion can be light, moderate or deep, depending on the condition of any given area, and areas can blend perfectly. What's more, dermabrasion can remove skin damaged by ultraviolet rays and so reduce the risk of skin cancer—this, I think, is most important.

FIFTY-PLUS

Your skin gets quite a mottled look as you get older. If you look at a young person's skin, it is a single shade. An older person's has at least three shades, sometimes four—it is an irregular alteration and distortion of pigment. Here and there are brown spots that do not belong—not like a child's uniformly colored freckles, which do belong. Whether you call them liver spots or age spots or actinic keratoses, they are areas of skin damaged by ultraviolet rays. And since these can be pre-cancerous, you should check with a dermatologist. In fact, I firmly believe that after 50, all sun-exposed skin should be examined annually for precancerous changes. While dermabrasion can treat precancerous facial problems, for the rest of the body I use cryotherapy (freezing) or curettage.

There is one very annoying problem that you gradually begin to be aware of—a gully, a groove, in the cheek area between the lower eyelid and the nose. The skin above gets unbelievably thin and the skin near the nose gets thicker. It is very hard to correct this except with replacement therapy—collagen, silicone or the like. Smiling also helps by masking the defect. Not a big smile—more a Mona Lisa smile, a half smile. This is one facial gesture that is really helpful—every woman past 35 should be a Mona Lisa!

You have to be "on," too. You have to have good posture—stand up straight, hold your head up straight, chin slightly up, tongue against the roof of the mouth (it lifts a sagging chin).

Dry skin is more and more of a problem, the older you get. Some of this results from skin cells dividing less frequently—that is, the rate of skin-cell division falls off by about 50 percent between the ages of 30 and 80—a decrease of about 1 percent a year. And there is an increasing tendency for dead skin cells to remain on the skin. Exfoliation really helps: It sloughs off dead skin cells and also steps up cell-division time, making skin cells perform more youthfully. You can get this step-up by slapping the skin or using a washcloth or—my preference—an abrasive sponge. But be sure to follow this with an emollient.

As a woman's skin starts to get seriously dry, she usually tries to solve the problem by using just a standard moisturizer. She does not realize that skin-cell replacement has diminished as well as natural lubricant production. The key thing is getting the skin to be more the way it used to be. To do that, you have to rev up cell-replacement time by chemical exfoliation or mechanical epidermabrasion to reactivate the skin cells. And then apply a moisturizer.

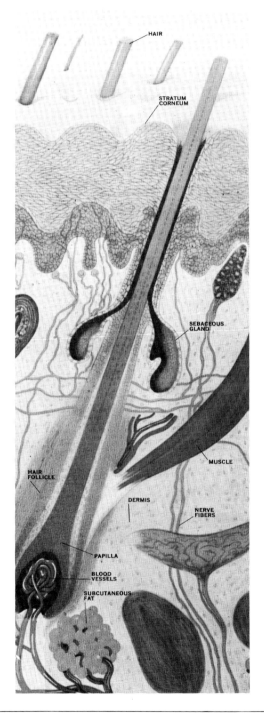

Here is a cross section of skin diagrammed. The skin you see, the stratum corneum, is just the tip of the iceberg ...What really counts—what goes on underneath—depends on the foods you eat.

SKIN SHOCK: TRAVELING FROM ONE CLIMATE TO ANOTHER

Q *If you're living in a winter climate and heading south for some sun, what should you be most aware of in caring for your skin?*

A According to Paul Lazar, M.D., clinical associate professor of dermatology at Northwestern University Medical School: In the natural sequence of events, one goes through a relatively gradual seasonal transition, which allows the body to prepare itself for the differences in temperature and humidity. With the advent of fast transportation, however, winter-adjusted skin can be plummeted into a summer environment. Almost instantly, the skin has to adjust to this sudden change—and may not be able to do so adequately. For example, you may not be able to perspire as much as you need to at first, or shed skin cells fast enough—two physiological changes that are stepped up in hot weather. Dysfunctions in either area could lead to prickly heat or rashes, particularly under the arms or breasts, or around the groin —where skin rubs against itself. One note: Most people think of skin scaling as dry skin, which it usually is not. They make the mistake of applying lots of heavy cream or oil instead of a specific treatment or a lightweight product in an attempt to combat the scaling and lubricate the skin.

Q *Can you spell out exactly what is best when going from cold to hot?*

A I suggest using a lightweight moisturizer rather than a heavy one—and using it more often if you have to. Put it on in the evening, too, when it's cooler and you're not sweating as much as you would during the day. If you play sports outdoors, keep a damp towel around to wipe off perspiration periodically. This will cut down on skin irritation. Remember, however, that as you wipe off perspiration, you're also wiping off sunscreen, so reapply your sunscreen often.

Q *What if you live in a warm climate, such as Houston, and travel north to ski, say, in Vail?*

A In this case, you have to be careful of skin dryness and winter itch, which can be prevented in two ways. One is the frequency with which you shower or bathe. The other is how often you lubricate your skin. Both frequent cleansing and hot water tend to dry out your skin. If you ski (or do any exercise), you may find that you're showering more often—and then jumping into a hot whirlpool right afterward to soothe tired muscles. To help prevent dryness, lubricate your skin every night, after every bath or shower—and always while skin is still damp. Use a good sunscreen outdoors, too, because you need sun protection in cold climates as well as hot ones. If you don't already, start using a lip balm and moisturizer well before you head to a cold climate—so you get into the habit and use both regularly.

Continued on page 153

The New Beauty also asks hard questions and expects precise, expert answers to such diverse questions as smoking, drinking, pill-taking and the possibility of turning time around.

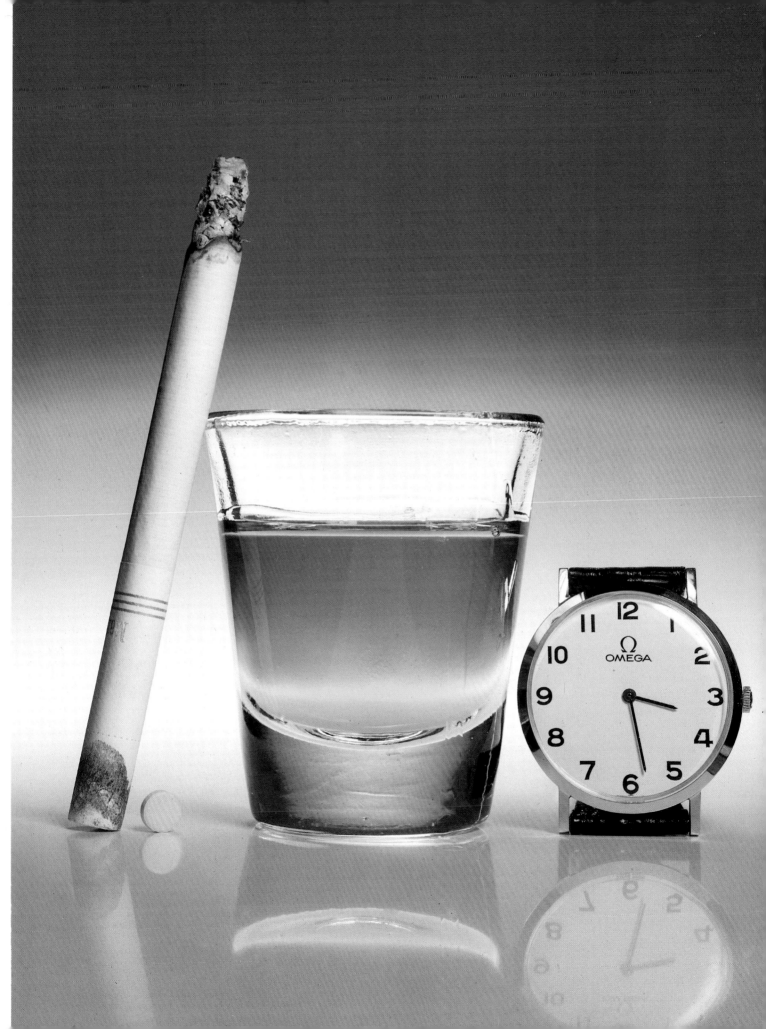

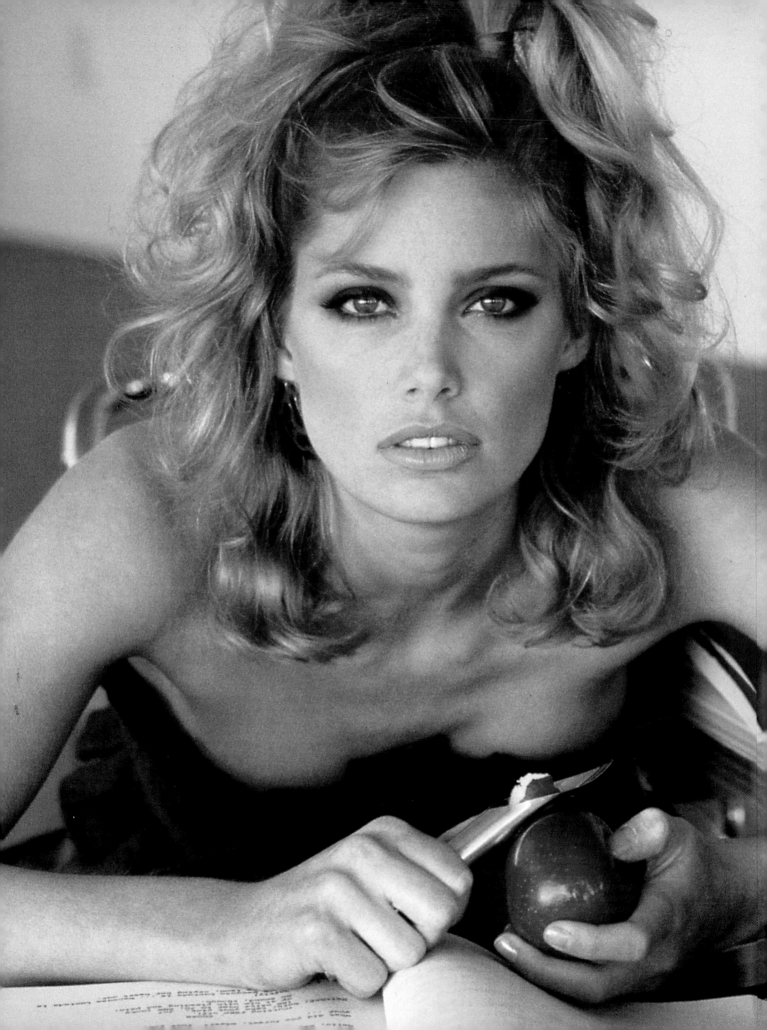

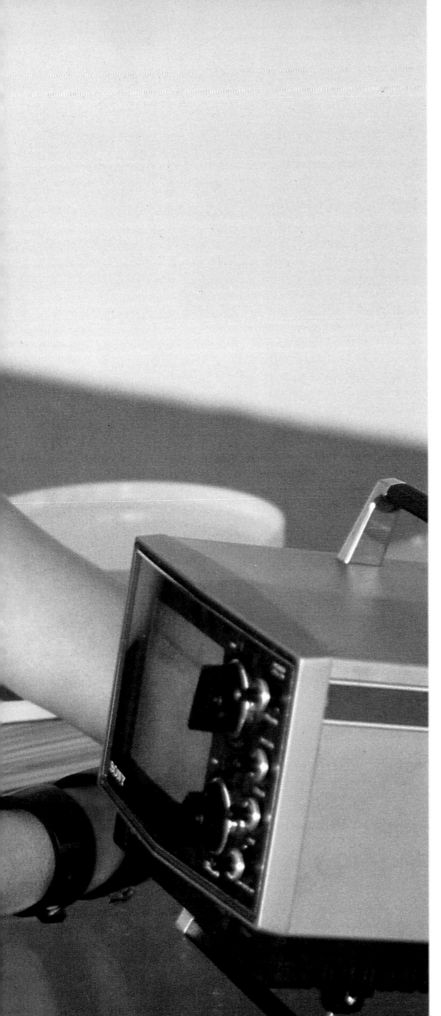

The changes that are happening are happening everywhere. A difference of style, of attitude. You see good looks that are thoroughly uncomplicated, easygoing—modern makeup and fashion at its most relaxed...at its healthiest best ...a great leap away from the sort of stylized, rigid looks that earlier generations succumbed to.

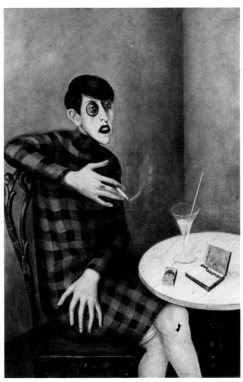

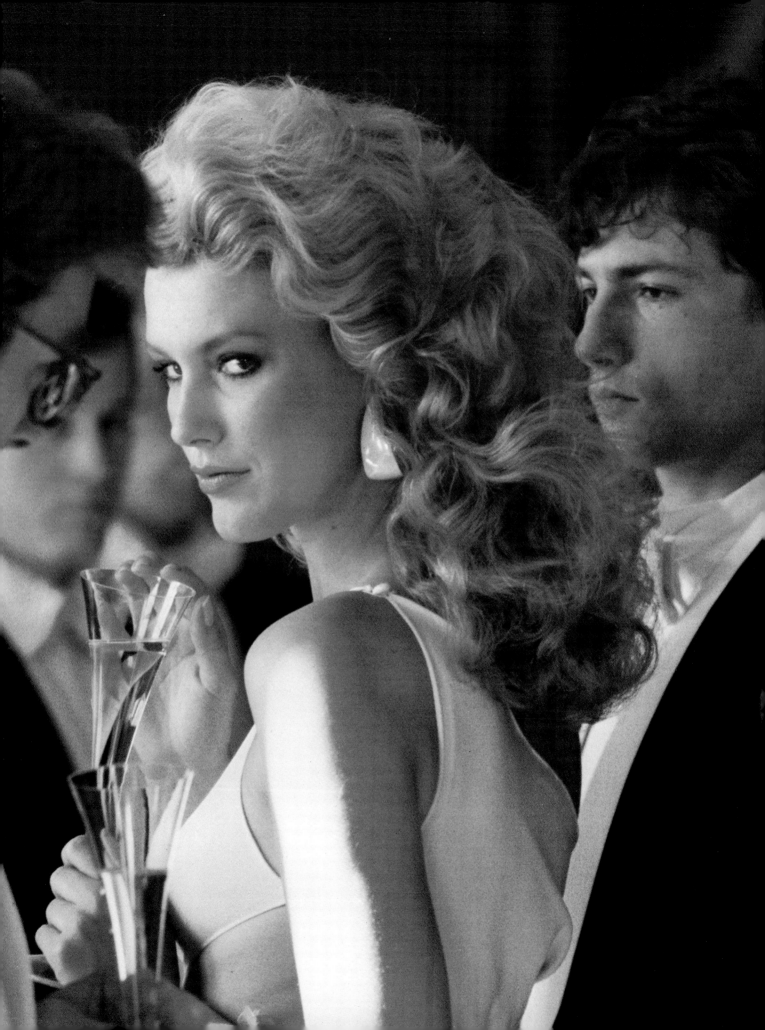

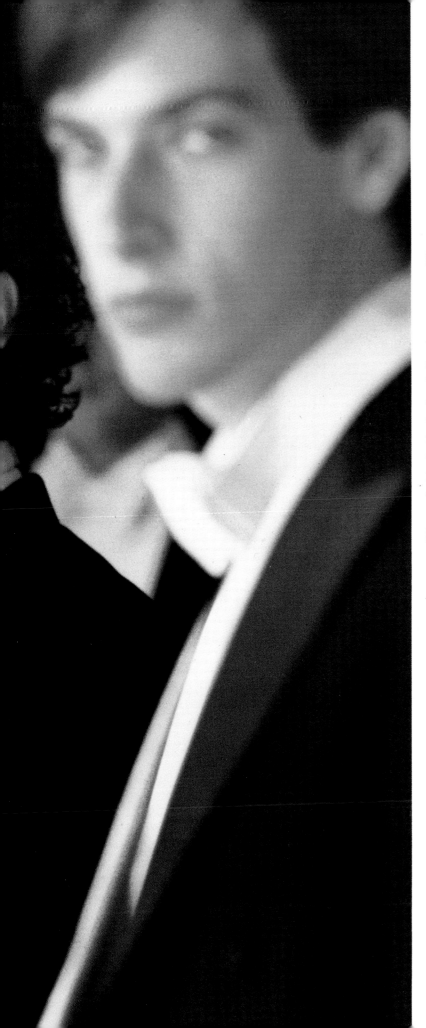

FRAGRANCE

As you get older . . .
Your olfactory senses diminish and it becomes more difficult to distinguish among and smell scents. All of which means: Don't become heavy-handed about fragrance—because other people can still smell, even if you can't. Another time to ease up on fragrance: in the morning, when your senses are just "waking up" and scent is also more difficult to detect.

Hair is your most important beauty accessory. You can subtract (or add) years to your age, depending on your hair's style and color.

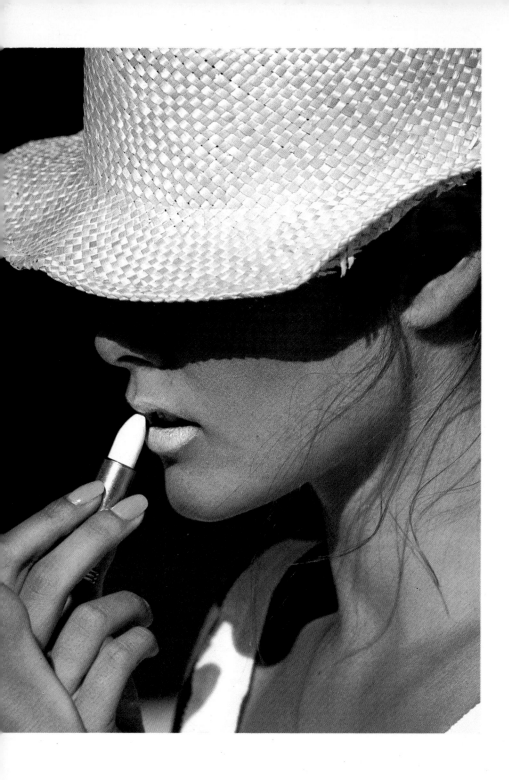

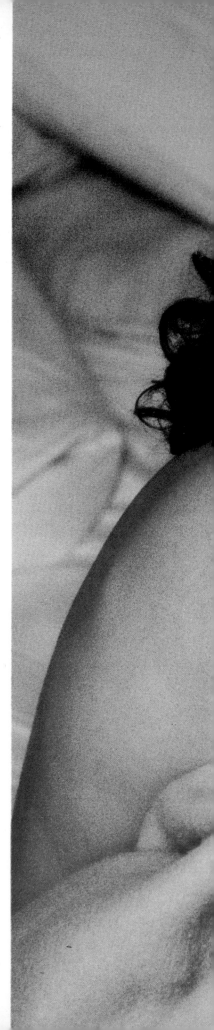

W hat's different today is a cleanness. Above, it's not a sun block but a white lipstick: to pale the mouth, make any lipstick color softer ... To get the look of a tan without the dangers.

Letting go. The pleasure of waking up rested, refreshed is part of good looks. The way to do that— for most of us—is seven or eight hours sleep.

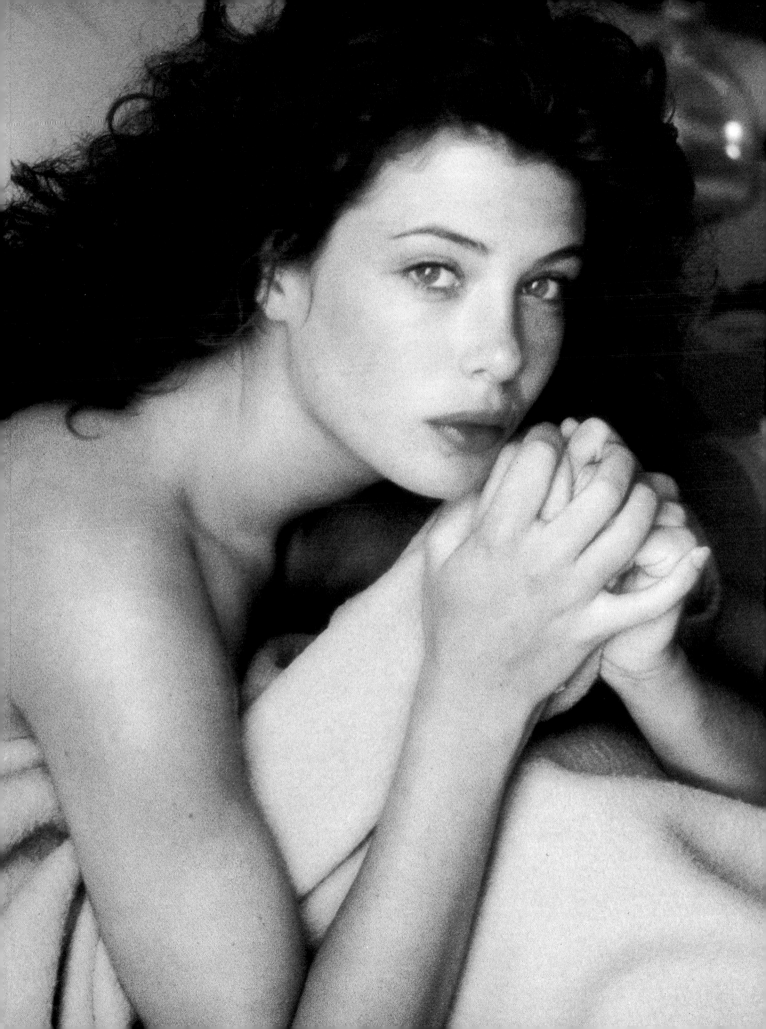

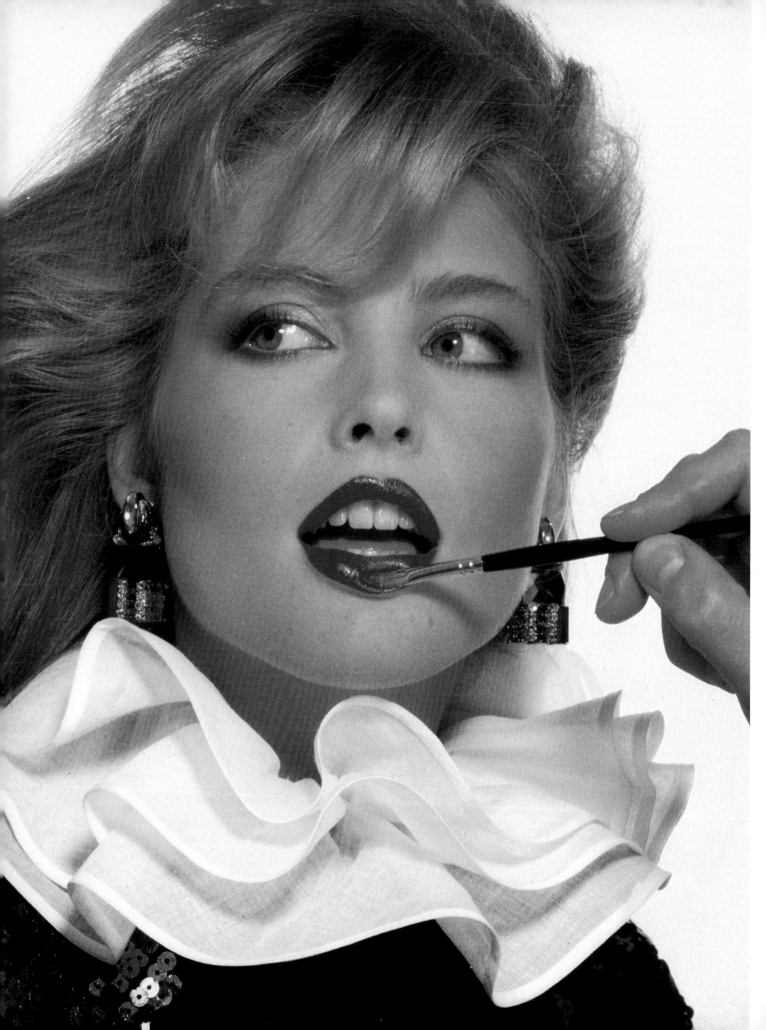

MAKE-UP

The way makeup should look today—at any age—is sheer, natural. Makeup should be used to heighten skin coloring, never to cover it up or change it. The mood you're after is, in a word, attractive. That is what being "pretty" (and "beauty") is all about *now*.

"My key advice to a woman over 40," says makeup expert Pablo Manzoni, "is: Never look ridiculous. In my book, this means: Stop trying to look younger. At 40, a woman is in her glory. After 50, however, there is a major turning point—physically and mentally. At 50, the key word is: adjust. You must learn to rethink your looks. Too many times a woman over 50 will lock herself into certain beauty routines that have become dated: Her looks have been frozen in an earlier decade. You find she is still wearing the makeup of that decade. Another mistake: makeup that is exaggerated—either too shiny or too matte.

"Women should learn to look at themselves from three different points of view. First, from a distance, to get a head-to-toe silhouette, to see a proportion. Second, from the waist up to look at the relationship of shoulders to the width and volume of hair (and, after 50, it should be lighter and shorter). The third view—the face.

"Certain things will always help you look better. As you grow older, a thinner, sheerer makeup. A cream rouge and blush in a burgundy shade—it's the most natural (no one really blushes 'pink' or 'orange'). Place it on

---

"My key advice to a woman over 40," says makeup expert Pablo Manzoni, "is never to look ridiculous. This means: Stop trying to look younger."

top of the cheekbones, as close to the eye as possible. Not on cheeks! Eye shadow should complement eyes, never match. The three most flattering shades for all eyes: gray with a blue in it, brown with green overtones, plum. Never use a frosted; it accentuates puffiness."

Adds Kenneth Battelle: "Use makeup with a light hand. Lines are minimized by less, not more. Use less foundation. Use a moisturizer under your base to give a more transparent look. Powder can be aging. For women who tend to wrinkle, powder brings out every line.

"I find, for a woman over 40, paler lipsticks are more flattering—pinks, corals, lighter reds."

MAKEUP: Q & A

Way Bandy answers the most-often-asked questions—from over-40 women—about putting on makeup

Q. *How do I know my coloring?*
A. Start with your hair, eye and skin colors as a guide—experiment until you find the shades that seem to do the most for them. For example—if you have red lips, gloss them over with more red—a very soft red with a touch of plum in it.

Q. *I love sheer makeup. How can I use it effectively to "contour" my face?*
A. Contouring works well only for very soft evening lighting or photography and is best left to the "pros." However, everyone can have a beautiful cheekbone. Place your color just underneath the bone, blending it back all the way to the ear—as you can see in the day makeup, page 155. Over this, along the underside of the cheekbone, add a narrow band of deeper color. Putting a little wing of soft tan on the outer corner of the eye gives cheeks a real lift also. Use neutral colors and keep everything simple. There should be no straining for a look.

Q. *My eyebrows have always bothered me. What can I do to make them "fit" my face?*

A. Eyebrows should never be noticeable. That is, they should blend into the entire look of the face. If yours are too heavy, use your eye shape to guide you. Tweeze brows carefully.

If the color of your eyebrows seems dark, use a facial hair bleach for one or two minutes to cut the color and lighten it by a shade or two.

If your brows are too sparse or if the shape is too irregular, use soft blond taupe powder or pencil and gently reshape or define the brows. Blend the color by going through brow hairs with a small brush—it softens any pencil lines or powder color you have applied.

"Makeup should be an extension of your natural coloring," says Way. "If, for example, you happen to have pale lips, try heightening that coloration. If your lips are reddish brown, use deep-auburn pencil that's closer to your natural lip tone. Sallow skin? Go with it—use the yellow undertones in your skin. And if your lashes are naturally dark, make something of that. If you have freckles, don't try to hide them—use sheer enough makeup you need to enhance your features and stick to that." Way's basic what-to-own makeup guide is illustrated on this page.

Q. *Should I use eyeliner? Which kind?*

A. One way of "lining" the eyes is to use a pencil or a powder in soft taupe, gray, or tan. The effect is a smudge of shadow all around the upper and lower lids. Another easy way to give definition, shape and intensity to eyes is to apply dark brown or black pencil liner under the upper lid near the lashes. And, incidentally, the older you get, the more this does for you!

Q. *How do I know which type of foundation—and which shade—is best for my skin?*

A. If your skin is oily, use a water-based liquid foundation. If your skin is dry, an emulsified liquid foundation works better —it contains both water and oil; the emulsifier causes the two to mix. To select the right color of liquid foundation, match it to the skin on your neck; this way your face and neck will be the same tone.

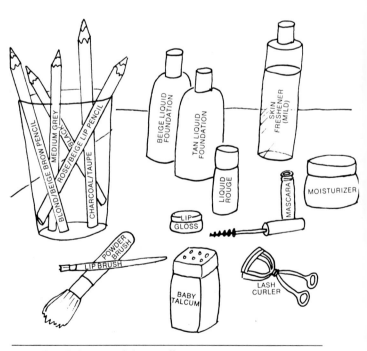

Way Bandy's essential utensils

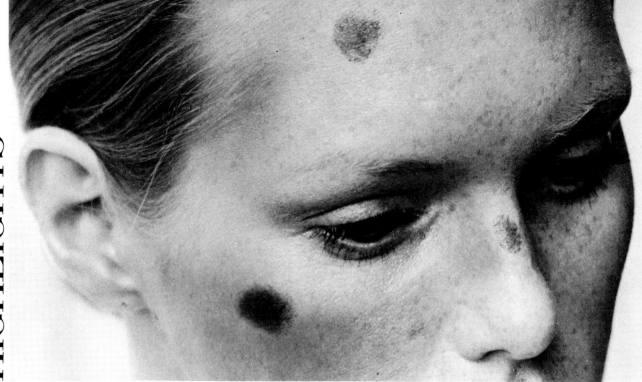

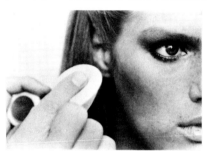

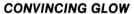

CONVINCING GLOW

The key for a daytime makeup is to look healthy, as if you had been out on a boat. Begin makeup with four dots of moisturizer: one on each cheek, the forehead, the chin (the nose doesn't need any extra grease); blend, then blot it. Choose a foundation to match your neck because otherwise you get a demarcation line. Always apply foundation with a sponge for the smoothest blending; it's the greatest friend of anyone who wants to do a good makeup. Blend foundation up from the jawline to the hairline. Then apply cream rouge, above, in five dots: two high up on the forehead, one way up on each cheekbone, and on the bridge of the nose. Blend with a sponge up to the temples, lower left. Cream rouge, upper left, is a more believable way to blush because it has a gleam to it. Rouge always right on the cheekbones rather than underneath them.

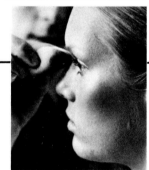

HOT TO CONTOUR

The idea behind highlighting and shading is to balance the face. With a narrow face, you should highlight more than shade. For a round face, shade from about the top of the ear to the center of the cheek to try to achieve a cheekbone, below far left. If your nose is fuller on one side than on the other, slightly shade the full side and slightly highlight the other, below second left. Shading is done with a gray-brown "no-color," applied before your foundation and blended into it, below third left.

POWDER TRICKS

With very finely milled powder for a foundation, you can buff color all over, then do delicate contouring with the same powder in the areas to be shadowed—two possible areas, below right.

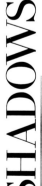

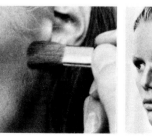

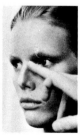

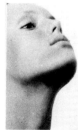

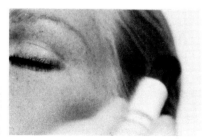

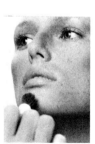

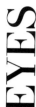

EYES

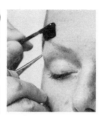
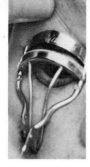

TIPS FOR TWEEZING AND FOR STRIKING EYES

Brush your eyebrows up and down constantly as you tweeze, far left. This shows the natural shape; you can see what should be plucked and what should not.

Curl lashes as much as possible before applying mascara, left. The more lashes are curled, the more open the eye seems to be—lashes will cast a shadow on the lid rather than over the eye itself. Apply mascara and then brush through lashes.

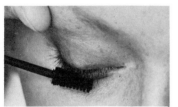
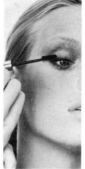

MASCARA AND SHADOW

Always apply mascara on the top of the lashes first, far left, then from underneath. Often the upper surface of the lashes is sunbleached. Even when it's not, coating your lashes with mascara on two sides gives them greater thickness. Your mascara should always be a natural eyelash color—black or brown—rather than an artificial emerald green or whatever, even at night.

By shadowing the whole area from lash to eyebrow, left, you cause the brow bone to recede and the eye itself to look deeper, stronger, more important. But the shadow must look like a natural shadow or the effect can be too heavy.

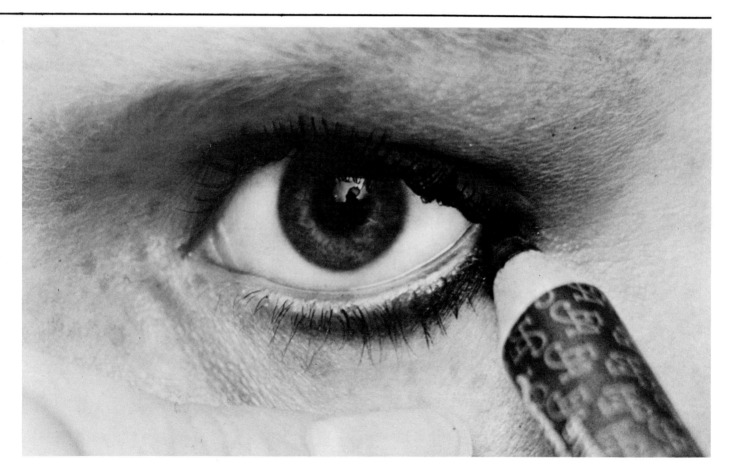

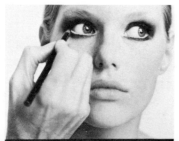

TO BRIGHTEN EYES

A navy-blue pencil, above, inside the lower lid at night. For day: a white pencil.

A flesh-color pencil, left, along the inside of the lower lid takes that red edge off and makes the eyes look larger at the same time.

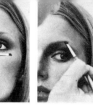

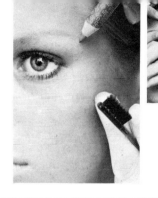

EYEBROWS: SUBTLE, DEFINED
A feathery eyebrow is ideal. Here, near right, it is filled in with a pale-blond pencil. To define and darken the eyebrow, center and far right, use a powder eye shadow in a soft, smoky tone.

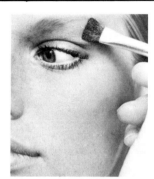 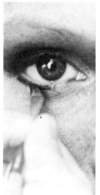 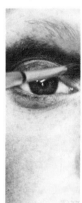 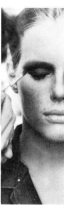 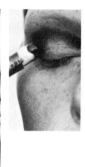

ON THE BROW LINE
Recede the brow bone with a soft cocoa/pecan shadow, near right, all the way to the brow.

TO DEEPEN EYES
Start by shading with dark brown, second right, on the upper lid. Then use very soft black shadow over the brown and blend the two, third right. The entire eye area from base of lashes to brow is shaded, fourth right; for extra depth, a curve of brown pencil is blended into the crease of the eye.

BALANCING LIPS AND EYES
Trace the outline of the lips with the same medium-brown pencil, top near right, used for the eyes. Not a harsh outline: blend, smudge with a cotton swab, second near right. Fill in with a very light brownish lipstick, then add clear lip gloss because it's prettier than a dry lip.

COLOR HARMONY
Using the same color on the mouth and eyes really pulls in the harmony of the face. The brown crayon used to shadow the eyes is used again to accentuate the shape of the mouth, bottom. Then this is blended out so it gives just a suggestion of depth and definition to the mouth, not a hard-edge outline.

SHARP FOCUS/SOFT FOCUS
Line lips with a gray pencil, top far right, then fill in with colored gloss, bottom far right, for a strong, dark mouth. For a natural mouth, just brush on the outline and fill in with the same color blend.

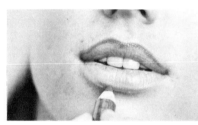

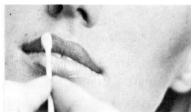

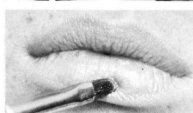

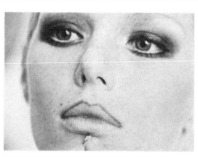

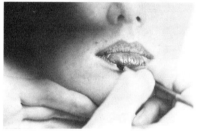

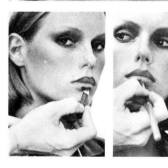

LIPS

157

DEFINITIONS OF SKIN TYPES

- **SKIN TYPE I**
invisible pores
thin, sensitive skin
tendency to flake
easily irritated
tendency to fine lines
often has broken capillaries
flat texture
often has freckles
burns easily
- **SKIN TYPE II**
very shiny
enlarged pores
coarse and rough in texture
tendency to blackheads
   and blemishes
ashy complexion
sallow in color
tans easily
- **SKIN TYPE III**
no shine
pores same size all over,
   barely visible
moist, supple, smooth,
   even texture
no blackheads or blemishes
good elasticity
no real tendency
   toward lines
tans slowly
- **SKIN TYPE IV**
any combination of skin
   types I, II, III—
   anywhere on your face

ENVIRONMENT

	EFFECTS	SKIN TYPE I
SUN	Ages the skin; causes lines, uneven pigmentation.	Sun is particularly bad for you. Use products—sunscreens, foundations, moisturizers—with a high SPF.
POLLUTION	Makes skin dirtier faster.	Frequent washing dehydrates skin. Use moisturizing cleanser; remove dirt, soot, chemical debris.
WIND	Chaps and burns the skin.	Use extra emollient cream for protection. Cover face with a scarf, whenever possible.
COLD	Shocks the skin.	Wash with lukewarm instead of hot water. Apply moisturizer while skin is still damp. Use eye cream during the day.
HEAT	Prevents perspiration from evaporating quickly from skin's surface. Makes skin dirtier, some skins produce more oil.	You're lucky! Heat is good for your skin—it helps keep it moist. Switch to a lighter moisturizer in hot weather.
AIR CONDITIONING	Dries out the skin.	In both cases, energy conservation counts—especially for skin. Areas like eyes, neck, cheeks need more care. use a night cream before bed. In the winter, use a humidifier.
STEAM HEAT	. . . drying, too.	
RAIN	A natural "moisturizer."	Rain is good for your skin—it puts it in best-looking state. The less you cover your skin on a rainy day, the better.
EXERCISE	The more you exercise, the better you'll feel, the younger you'll look.	More exercise means more showering . . . but not necessarily with soap; try loofah-and-bath-oil scrubs.
AGE	Skin regenerates more slowly.	A strict regimen, from cleansing on, that always replenishes skin with moisture.
TROUBLESHOOTERS		Moisturizers, night treatments, eye creams.

SKIN TYPE II	SKIN TYPE III	SKIN TYPE IV
moderation, sun can help your skin. But ways use an SPF sunscreen, even if it is a low number. You can choose from e range—it depends on how much tan u want. Use water-based foundation.	You can take sun in very small doses but always use a sun product with a moderate SPF. Chances are you don't need a foundation at all, use a light moisturizer.	
se astringent; wash several times a day th soap—clean skin is especially important to you (reduces oiliness).	Wash with a superfatted soap or a cleansing bar twice a day.	
se protection only where you need it! In ur case, around the eye area, on mouth, bove upper lip. Your skin tends to be ss moist now.	Use a moisturizer—switch to a slightly heavier formula.	
nce you cleanse often, use products at don't strip all your natural oils.	Be sure your toner has no alcohol. Use an eye cream and lip protector.	
his makes your skin produce more oil. kin gets dirtier faster. Wash more frequently. Use an astringent—gently—roughout the day. Wear no makeup if ossible.	Use a light astringent to clean, moisturize around eyes only.	"Combination" skin types should consult directions from columns I, II, III, depending on your skin's condition.
is is a good condition for your skin. It elps normalize your skin, improve summer rashes . . . the less you put on your kin the better.	Use at low setting if conditioner is extremely drying. Use moisturizer when needed.	
ter cleansing, leave your skin bare. en use a spot treatment at night—when u need it, where you need it.	Use a humidifier in the winter. In the summer, keep your air conditioner at a low setting.	
this kind of humidity, your skin will feel reasy. Cleanse thoroughly. Use an astringent.	Do nothing different.	
ake lukewarm showers. Never wear akeup or treatment while exercising. eep your hair tied back off your face.	While showering, use a damp washcloth without soap on face, follow with a clarifier before makeup.	
ou're the luckiest of all the categories. hile your skin will need less frequent eansing as you get older, it will also how fewer signs of aging.	As you get older, your skin will lose moisture—when you see fine lines begin to appear, step up your moisturizing program.	
il-control stick, powder, astringent, exliators.	A steady regime of good care. All you need are the basics—cleansing, toning, moisturizing.	

● CROSSING THE LINES   Whatever your skin-treatment regimen, whichever plan you've opted for, you don't have to stick to it day in and day out; in fact, you shouldn't stick to it, because your skin changes—from season to season, from year to year, even from day to day. For example: If you have been out in the cold a lot and you have been using a soap cleanser, switch to one that's more emollient, one that will put something back. When you travel, your skin changes, too. You have to take along more than just your daily cleanser/toner/moisturizer. Your skin may be "shocked" if you suddenly go from a cold climate into a hot one. If you go from a cold climate to an even colder one (if you go skiing, for instance), your skin-care regimen should change, too. The point: Know your skin, its needs, what changes—guidelines in the chart, above.

HAIR

Your hair is your most important beauty "accessory"—you can subtract (or add) years to your age, depending on your hair's style and color. Here's what you should know about keeping your hair looking its best.

Women should examine their looks every five years to see what mistakes they may be making, according to hair expert Kenneth

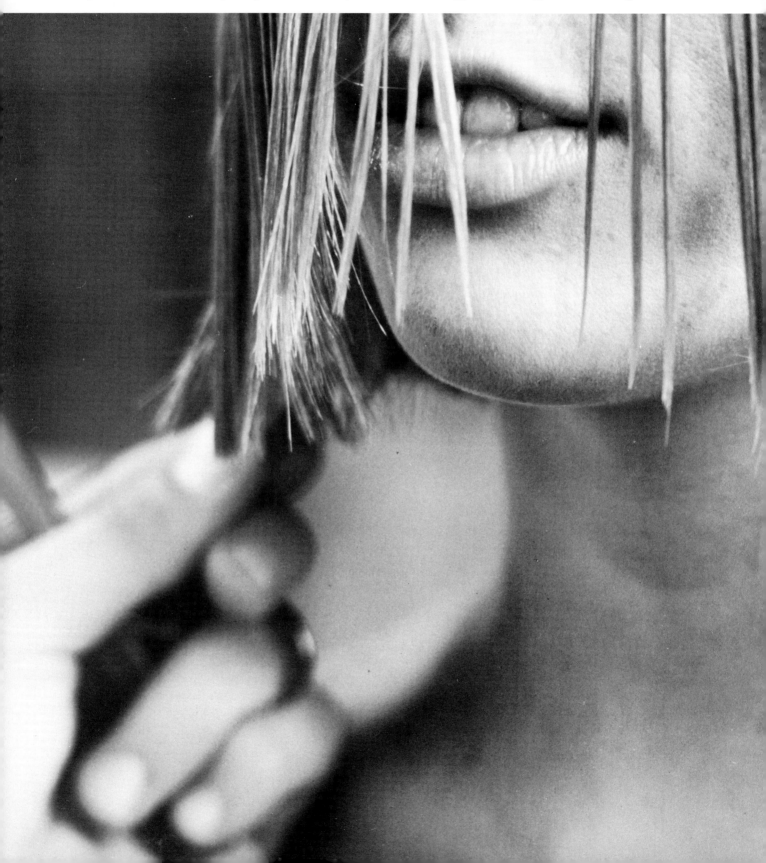

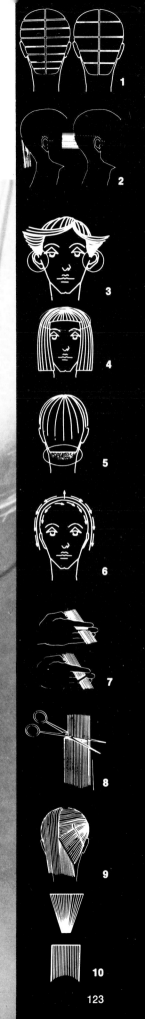

1 / For fluffy results, cutter should take many partings, left. If you want it chunky at the back, he should take fewer partings, right. 2 / Lifting and lowering the hair will produce different effects. 3 / If a woman has big ears, hair can cover them. 4 / Short bangs suit few people. 5 / For tailored necklines, make a crisp haircut. 6 / If you have awkward growth directions, then leave hair long. 7 / Each piece to be cut must be between cutter's fingers. 8 / First parts cut serve as a guide for the rest. 9 / Ends will ultimately create the look. 10 / In preparing hair for scissors, use fine comb.

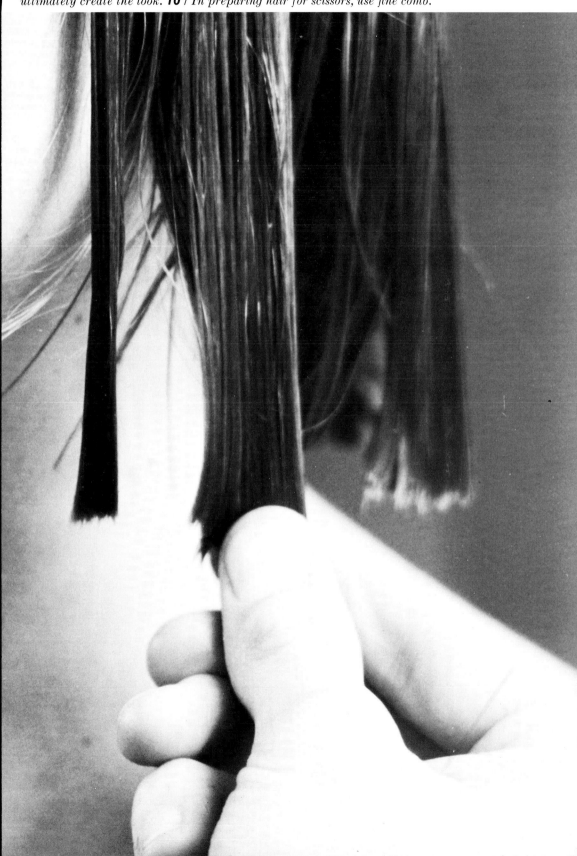

123

Battelle. You may be adding years by wearing too much hair, or too dark a shade of hair coloring. My standard rule on hair color, says Kenneth: Go lighter, rather than darker, as you get older. Of course, there are exceptions—such as brunettes who have very strong personalities! But generally, lighter is softer. And by lighter, we don't necessarily mean blond.

As a rule, straight or "down" lines in hair don't work too well. Again, there are exceptions. But I'd say, contain it, put it up, away from the face. And I've found that exceptionally curly hair is aging.

According to Suga, the most important consideration as a woman gets older is hair color. And what to do about going gray. Some women look wonderful with naturally gray hair—once you're gray, don't be afraid to wear your hair that way . . . if it looks good. Whether or not to cover up your gray—and how to do it—depends on two things, says Suga: the percentage of gray you have and your base color. If you have light-colored hair, blond or light brown, and you are less than half gray, Suga recommends that you keep the gray. If your base color is not too dark, you can highlight or frost your natural gray and it will look very beautiful. Women with darker hair can have reverse frosting—but whichever way you go, see a hair colorist or have a consultation with your hairdresser first. It is almost impossible to do this kind of coloring at home by yourself. In fact, the only kind of hair color you should ever attempt at home, says Suga, is one-process or semi-permanent color . . . nothing else you do yourself will look natural enough.

If you've been covering up your gray and you want to go "natural" . . . stop using permanent color. Switch to semi-permanent color in the same shade, which must be reapplied every five weeks. Keep on using this color until all of the permanent dye has grown out or is long enough to be trimmed off.

On an older woman, hair should not be more than shoulder-length, says Suga, who agrees with Kenneth that long hair tends to "drag" a woman's face down. You need to frame your face, adds Suga, with softness and volume. Beyond that, there are no special "rules." An older woman can wear bangs; she can even wear her hair slightly longer—if she can carry it off, the way Jackie Onassis does, for example. Another "don't" is: too-short hair—although, again, says Suga, if you can carry it off, you can wear it. The most important thing is to have hair that *moves*. (Nothing ages you faster than a hair "do.") And hair that is well cut . . . cared for . . . and groomed.

You need a certain height, says Suga, but to get it, it's not necessary to tease and spray. To achieve volume: get it through a cut, blow-drying, adding a few rollers at the crown. Be sure that your hair and the amount of volume it has are in proportion to your face—and your body. And the only way to judge that is by standing up and looking in a full-length mirror.

WIGS

Wigs are a great life-saver for women with thinning hair. If that's your problem, don't despair. There are options—in wigs and hairpieces. The best, the most natural are made-to-order with combinations of human and/or synthetic hair, sewn to a base. These are expensive, but worth the investment—they're practically undetectable, more comfortable (not as hot on the head as the machine-made variety) and will last you a lifetime. What wigs are not for: covering up a dirty head—there's no excuse for that!

HAIR COLOR Q & A

Q. *What's the best way to find a good hair colorist?*

A. The first thing to look for is a person you like and with whom you can establish a rapport. If you are basically conservative, for example, you won't be happy with a trendy colorist. It is important that you both have the same final result in mind.

Q. *Are there any particular trends in hair color?*

A. There is more blonding than ever before. But it's a new kind of blond look —a warm, textured play of light. Nothing harsh, nothing monochromatic about it.

Q. *When a woman decides to color her hair, how do you determine which color is right?*

A. Technically, the options are endless— there is a fantastic range of color available today. However, to choose the most flattering color, start by looking at the natural color tones in your hair. Stay close to these natural tones and emphasize one, or tone down another. But never make radical hair-color changes. No one should.

Q. *What kind of upkeep does going blond involve?*

A. A visit to your colorist once every four or five weeks should do it. But if you don't have the time or the money for this amount of upkeep (both important considerations in determining whether or not to go blond), there is highlighting or brightening. You get a lighter effect without too much change in your natural color—it brings out the full range of tones in your hair, and maintenance is minimal (touch-ups every three months).

Q. *Are there any special ways to care for colored hair?*

A. Absolutely. An acid-balanced shampoo helps keep the outermost layer of the hair the cuticle—smooth, so hair stays shiny. (If your hair becomes dry and the cuticle gets damaged, you will find that your hair color loses its shine—it simply looks dull.) And a deep-penetrating conditioner is a must after each shampoo—conditioning is very important for hair that has been chemically treated, whether it's colored or permed.

Q. *Is it true once hair has been permed it should not be colored?*

A. It's best to use only single-process coloring for permed hair, never double-process colors. The reason: when hair is permed, or dyed by a double process, each

> **Technically, the options are endless—there is a fantastic range of color available today . . . Stay close to the natural tones in your hair and emphasize one, or tone down another**

strand expands. If you do one chemical treatment on top of another, your hair is apt to become damaged—to dry out, to break. Most permanent hair-coloring dyes are formulated to work on ''virgin'' hair (in other words, hair that has not been permed). So, obviously, double-process coloring would be too strong to use on permed hair. Highlighting—a single process—is safe. And temporary color, which merely coats the hair shaft, rather than changing its natural structure, is safe, too.

Q. *What about caring for gray hair? Are there any special tips?*

A. Gray hair can be striking on certain people. But proper care is essential if you really want to have beautiful-looking gray hair. The hair must have texture, shine and be the right color—it should never be yellow or blue. You can highlight gray hair with streaks of white: It gives hair a lift.

Q. *What advice would you give to women who want to color their hair at home?*

A. Most hairdressers agree that it is best not to venture far from your natural color. It's OK to make small changes in your hair color at home, but if you want a major change, have it done professionally.

Q. *I'm losing all those gleaming summer highlights the sun put into my mousy-brown hair. Is there something subtle I can do?*

A. Try "painting your hair." If your hair is light brown or lighter, you can add sunny, natural-looking highlights in 15 minutes flat at home by simply stroking on strands of a special hair-painting mixture. Don't be timid. Be sure to apply the mixture thickly on thin strands.

Q. *Will a pastel toner work on natural hair?*

A. No. It will only deposit color on pre-lightened hair. It will not lighten natural hair.

Q. *I've always wanted to lighten my hair a few shades, but I'm afraid it will damage my hair. What should I do?*

A. Properly used, hair coloring will not hurt your hair. As a matter of fact, it will add body and manageability to your hair. Use a shampoo-in hair coloring that lightens, colors, and conditions in one step.

Q. *What can I use just to cover my gray?*

A. Use a hair-color lotion—the kind that washes away after four to six shampoos—in a shade just a bit lighter than your natural color. Your gray will be covered, your hair, highlighted; and a hair-color lotion can cover up to 100 percent gray. All you need do is re-apply when necessary.

Q. *I have dark-brown hair and want to go very blond. When I use a shampoo-in hair color, I always end up with brassy reddish results—never light or ash enough. What should I do?*

A. A shampoo-in hair color isn't meant to lighten dark hair to pale blond. Only two-step blonding using lightener and toner kits can do that. You first have to lighten your hair with a hair lightener, then follow it with a toner to add the desired shade of pale blond to your pre-lightened hair.

Q. *How do I apply a patch test before using hair coloring?*

A. (a) Wash a spot behind the ear or in the bend of your arm with soap and water.

(b) Blot dry.

(c) Mix equal parts of 20-volume peroxide and the tint selected.

(d) Cover the dry area with mixture.

(e) Do not disturb for 24 hours.

(f) Then check for any irritation.

(g) If irritated, you are allergic to that particular product and should try a different brand.

Q. *I use a hair coloring and mix the shades. Can I save the unused portion of coloring for my next retouch?*

A. Yes, you can save unused portions of coloring, but only if they have not been mixed with the developer. Save half-used bottles of color in a cool dark place. Keep them tightly capped and they'll remain fresh for up to six weeks. Never, never save color you've mixed with developer. Once it's mixed, use it up or toss it out.

Q. *May I do my permanent wave and hair coloring the same day?*

A. No. Apply your permanent wave and wait at least a week before applying your color touchup. If a tint is given first, the waving lotion may cause an uneven color; if the cold wave is given first, the tint may distort and weaken the wave pattern. So wait! Be sure you've shampooed at least twice before applying color.

Q. *Can I use a hair-color product when I have some blisters on my scalp?*

A. No. Do not apply color if scalp sores or eruptions are present. Wait until they heal. If they continue to be a problem, see your doctor.

Q. *May I use hair coloring to tint eyebrows and eyelashes?*

A. No. This would be most dangerous and lead to irritation.

Q. *How do I detect over-processed hair?*

A. This type of hair has been damaged by over-bleaching or over-perming. It is very curly when wet, frizzy when dry, and usually breaks off easily.

Q. *How do I treat over-processed hair?*

A. A series of treatments and conditioning is in order. Chemical aid to help mend split ends, oil treatments and other steps must be done by your hairdresser or with products suggested by a reliable cosmetician.

Q. *In what ways will climate affect the hair?*

A. Moisture in the air deepens the natural wave. Hair that has been lightened is always susceptible to the harmful effects of chlorine, salt water and sun.

Q. *When should I use a colorfast shampoo?*

A. When the hair has been tinted or toned or if the hair is in a damaged condition.

Q. *Depending on my hair coloring, how often do I need touch-ups?*

A. (a) For single process (shampoo-in hair tint), every three weeks.

(b) For double process, every 2½ to three weeks.

(c) For covering gray, every three weeks.

(d) For streaking and hair painting, every three months.

HENNA

To add the kinds of subtle red and rich brown tones you see in some of the prettiest hair around, the easiest, fastest, most natural way is henna—the natural vegetable dye that is obtained from the tropical henna plant. We're not talking about carrot-red henna coloring—that's not the direction hair and makeup are going today. The kind of henna you want now comes in a range of soft-reddened or burnished-brown shades, plus a natural no-color henna for body, condition and shine. What makes henna so healthy is the way it's applied to hair: with conditioners—oil, egg, protein treatment—added. The henna to go for at home is the natural, neutral henna, to use as a conditioning treatment—a hair shiner-upper! Mix neutral henna with boiling water; when it's cool, add two eggs for conditioning. Be sure the mixture is a paste/mud consistency—you don't want henna dripping down your face. Work henna through hair, the way you would a shampoo; if hair is thick, sectioning helps. Leave on for a half-hour to an hour, then rinse out. Henna doesn't dirty the hair; unless you want to, you don't have to shampoo. If you want to try colored henna, we think it's best to see an expert. If it's the first go-round, henna is left on for the longest time (this will depend on your natural color and the color you want to get). The second time it's applied (henna should be done every month or two), the time may be shortened—henna fades gradually and the time varies with individual hair.... If you've had hair henna'd with color in a salon and you want to try a follow-up coloring yourself, Christiaan's tips: At home, always use less color—he recommends ¾ neutral henna to ¼ colored. Always do a test strand first: clip a piece of hair from underneath, tape to a piece of paper—and test. Also, to protect skin from color stain, wear gloves and use petroleum jelly around the hairline.

When not to use henna: If you need to use a good protein conditioner on dry or damaged hair, don't use henna first. It may not give you the conditioning you need, and it coats hair, preventing other conditioners from penetrating. Other times not to use henna: if hair is permanent-waved; if you're blond—henna can turn hair green; if you have gray hair henna won't cover it, unless, says Suga, you are a brunette-going-gray and you like auburn highlights. Henna on brown hair turns the gray strands very red.

NAILS AND HANDS

Q. *Can nails be made to grow faster?*

A. Possibly. Although nail growth varies with the individual, it's fastest in summer, in youth, and decreases with middle age. Middle fingernails grow fastest, right-handed nails (on right-handed people—vice versa on lefties) grow faster than those of the left hand. Activities such as typing and piano playing increase nail production—it's the constant tapping of the nails against the keys that does it—rather like the development of calluses from a lot of rubbing against the skin. If your nails are slow to grow, begin to buff your nails, or massage fingers toward the tips to improve circulation.

Q. *Do hands always show the earliest signs of aging?*

A. Only if they have been neglected. The development of so-called "age" spots, for example, can be retarded by the regular application of a sunscreen. Existing spots can be partially bleached out with a depigmenting cream, or hidden with a waterproof cover-up. Dermatologists can lighten these spots and remove scaly bumps by different therapies, including cryotherapy (a "cold burn") or electrodesiccation (a "warm burn").

Q. *Does polish protect the nails?*

A. Except for people who are allergic to it, polish does, in fact, both strengthen and beautify the nails. Care must be taken, however, in using polish remover. It's largely composed of acetone, and excessive use could dry out some of the essential cementing ingredients of the nail plate and cause splitting. Better to touch up polish between manicures, rather than remove it every time there's a chip. For exceptionally weak nails, nail conditioners with protein or nail strengtheners (clear or colored polish containing microscopic fibers that invisibly build up the nail) can be of benefit.

Q. *Can brittle nails be helped?*

A. Try soaking them in warm olive oil—it gives a nice, soft gloss—or massage with hydrogen peroxide.

Q. *What causes splits and breaks?*

A. Improper filing is a common cause. A flexible emery board is far preferable to a stiff metal file. Never saw back and forth across the nail. Instead, file each nail in one direction—toward the center. Filing nails to a point is asking for breakage—if your nails tend to split, keep them as wide as possible at the base, making a slightly squared curve as

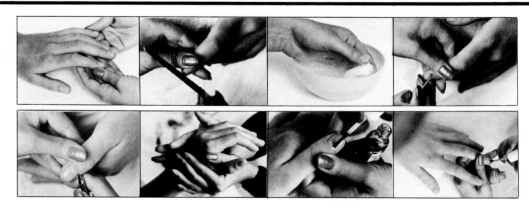

Keeping your nails as short as this, 1, is all the more reason to keep them pretty. Here a step-by-step how-to manicure. 2. A light filing to smooth edges—follow the natural line of the nail; avoid filing sides—the natural support of the nail comes from there. Use a diamond-dust nail file or a very fine emery board. 3. A few-minutes' soak in warm, sudsy water to clean nail area, soften cuticles. 4. Cuticle oil is applied and

they grow out. For weak nails, an additional strengthener is nail sealer or strengthener applied on the underside of the nail's free edge as well as on the top. White iodine applied at the base of the nail has long been thought to strengthen nails.

Q. *What causes soft nails?*

A. Chances are, it's using too much soap, water or cleansing agents—best to use rubber gloves when cleaning. Other causes could be nutritional—eat foods high in protein and calcium.

Q. *Do older nails need special care?*

A. Least aging: nails that are well groomed and don't call attention to your hands. As you get older, wear your nails shorter, rounder, with subtle nail coloring. It's attractive without being dramatic and attention-getting. Pale pinks, corals, berries look pretty. So does the whole range of pales. Avoid frosteds. To keep in mind: well-manicured nails simply buffed to a shine—or glossed with clear lacquer. Use plenty of hand lotion (it minimizes wrinkles). And don't forget a good dose of sunscreen out-of-doors. Another "trick": one wonderful "jewel," a ring, a bracelet, an eye-catcher.

FEET

Q. *How do I tell if a shoe has the right fit?*

A. First, make sure that calf muscles aren't overtight. The advantage of a flatter heel is that it helps stretch the calf naturally when you walk. A shoe that has too low or too high a vamp can cause constriction in the foot, leading to muscle or small-vein damage. Too tight a shoe can lead to vein damage not only in the foot but in the lower part of the leg. Too loose shoes—particularly prevalent with clogs—can result in corns and calluses.

Q. *Is it dangerous to wear high heels continuously?*

A. Since the calf muscles are insufficiently exercised with high heels, women who wear them should do daily exercise. To stretch calves: put your hands against the wall with your feet 16 inches away. Without moving heels from the floor, lean your chest against the wall, hold for three seconds. Do both morning and evening, repeating 10 times. To strengthen weak ankles and feet: Sit on a chair and hang a weight over your foot—a handbag weighing between five and 10 pounds is good. Raise the leg about six inches without straightening the knee, keeping foot pointed straight ahead. Do about 25 lifts on each foot.

Q. *How should stockings be fitted?*

A. Too-short stockings, like too-short shoes, can lead to foot problems. Stockings should not only be long enough, but they should be worn loosely over the toes. If they are too snug, the pressure that results when you stand can cause a number of painful conditions. Even with well-fitting shoes and stockings, it's wise to zip up your circulation by elevating your feet from time to time for as long as possible.

Q. *Is there a wrong way to buff toenails?*

A. Never buff them back and forth—the friction caused by that kind of motion builds up a great deal of heat, which is harmful to the nail. Rather, buff in one direction, out from the cuticle toward the free edge of the nail, with a rapid wrist movement and no real pressure against the nail.

cuticles gently pushed back—the nail grows from underneath the cuticle—too much pressure causes ridging. A cuticle "knife" is preferred to an orange stick —it exerts less pressure and lifts the cuticles as you push. 5. Any hangnails are trimmed with cuticle scissors—never pull off! 6. Lotion is massaged into wrists and hands— stimulating circulation, stimulating nail growth— then nails are wiped clean of excess cuticle oil and lotion, so polish will adhere. 7. A base coat is very important—it prevents nails from yellowing, helps polish stick, and gives an extra layer of protection to nails. 8. Two coats of polish—for short nails, use a light color, similar to your skin. A pale, translucent shade is especially pretty in summer; for winter, pale, pale peach or pale pink— plus a protective top coat.

167

BEAUTY SHAPE-UP

There's no doubt that each part of your face has its own potential for creative makeup. It's all in knowing how. Here are some essential tools, approved by *Vogue's* experts as a pro-quality kit. Fun to play with but not mere toys; perfect tools make all the difference.

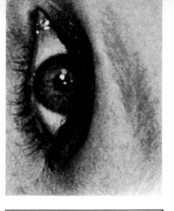 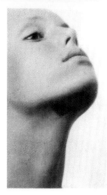

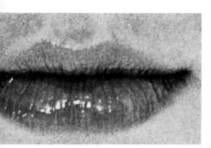

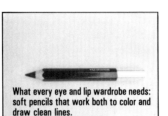

What every eye and lip wardrobe needs: soft pencils that work both to color and draw clean lines.

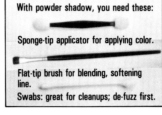

With powder shadow, you need these:

Sponge-tip applicator for applying color.

Flat-tip brush for blending, softening line.

Swabs: great for cleanups; de-fuzz first.

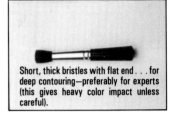

Short, thick bristles with flat end . . . for deep contouring—preferably for experts (this gives heavy color impact unless careful).

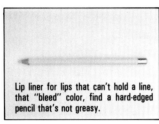

Lip liner for lips that can't hold a line, that "bleed" color, find a hard-edged pencil that's not greasy.

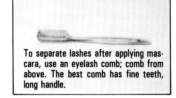

To separate lashes after applying mascara, use an eyelash comb; comb from above. The best comb has fine teeth, long handle.

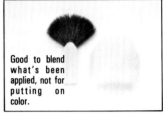

Good to blend what's been applied, not for putting on color.

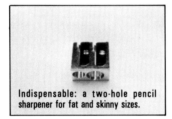

Indispensable: a two-hole pencil sharpener for fat and skinny sizes.

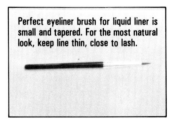

Perfect eyeliner brush for liquid liner is small and tapered. For the most natural look, keep line thin, close to lash.

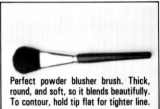

Perfect powder blusher brush. Thick, round, and soft, so it blends beautifully. To contour, hold tip flat for tighter line.

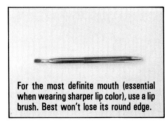

For the most definite mouth (essential when wearing sharper lip color), use a lip brush. Best won't lose its round edge.

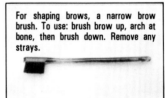

For shaping brows, a narrow brow brush. To use: brush brow up, arch at bone, then brush down. Remove any strays.

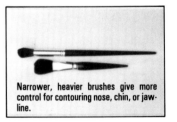

Narrower, heavier brushes give more control for contouring nose, chin, or jaw-line.

LIPS

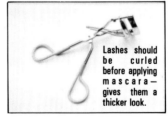

Lashes should be curled before applying mascara—gives them a thicker look.

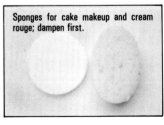

Sponges for cake makeup and cream rouge; dampen first.

CHEEKS

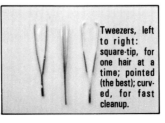

Tweezers, left to right: square-tip, for one hair at a time; pointed (the best); curved, for fast cleanup.

EYES

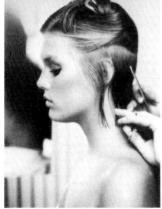

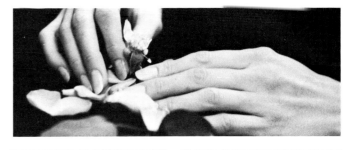

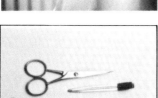

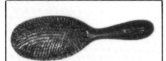

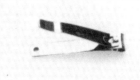

For trimming bangs: a small—controllable—scissors; to hold hair, aluminum clips that won't slip.

The basic brush: natural- and plastic-bristled (for thorough brushing without breaking), with a soft rubber base that is gentler on scalp.

You need at least one two-pointed wood stick . . . for cleaning under, around nails, pushing cuticle back, removing excess polish.

The toenail clip you want is long and big. It makes cutting the strongest nails easy.

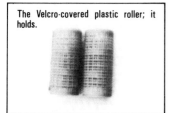

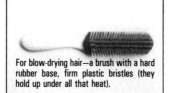

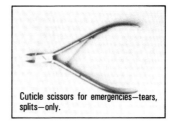

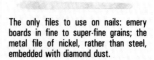

The Velcro-covered plastic roller; it holds.

For blow-drying hair—a brush with a hard rubber base, firm plastic bristles (they hold up under all that heat).

Cuticle scissors for emergencies—tears, splits—only.

The only files to use on nails: emery boards in fine to super-fine grains; the metal file of nickel, rather than steel, embedded with diamond dust.

NAILS

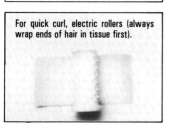

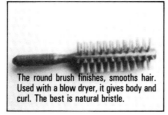

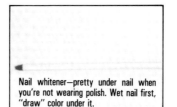

For quick curl, electric rollers (always wrap ends of hair in tissue first).

The round brush finishes, smooths hair. Used with a blow dryer, it gives body and curl. The best is natural bristle.

Nail whitener—pretty under nail when you're not wearing polish. Wet nail first, "draw" color under it.

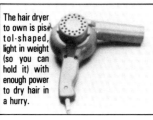

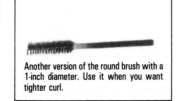

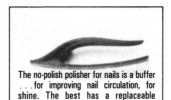

The hair dryer to own is pistol-shaped, light in weight (so you can hold it) with enough power to dry hair in a hurry.

Another version of the round brush with a 1-inch diameter. Use it when you want tighter curl.

The no-polish polisher for nails is a buffer . . . for improving nail circulation, for shine. The best has a replaceable chamois.

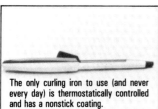

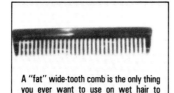

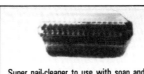

The only curling iron to use (and never every day) is thermostatically controlled and has a nonstick coating.

A "fat" wide-tooth comb is the only thing you ever want to use on wet hair to detangle and smooth it.

Super nail-cleaner to use with soap and warm water—a natural bristle nail brush with a row of firmer bristles along the top, angled to get under nails.

HAIR

The best hair comb for everyday: fine-toothed and tailed; for sectioning, too.

A fine-grain stone, stick-shaped and tapered, that is a natural abrasive . . . tapered end removes cuticle by pumicing; flat side smooths nail edge.

Edited by Alexandra Penney

RETARDING

This is just the beginning—the not-so-distant future holds endless possibilities for blurring the thin gray line between being young and feeling young

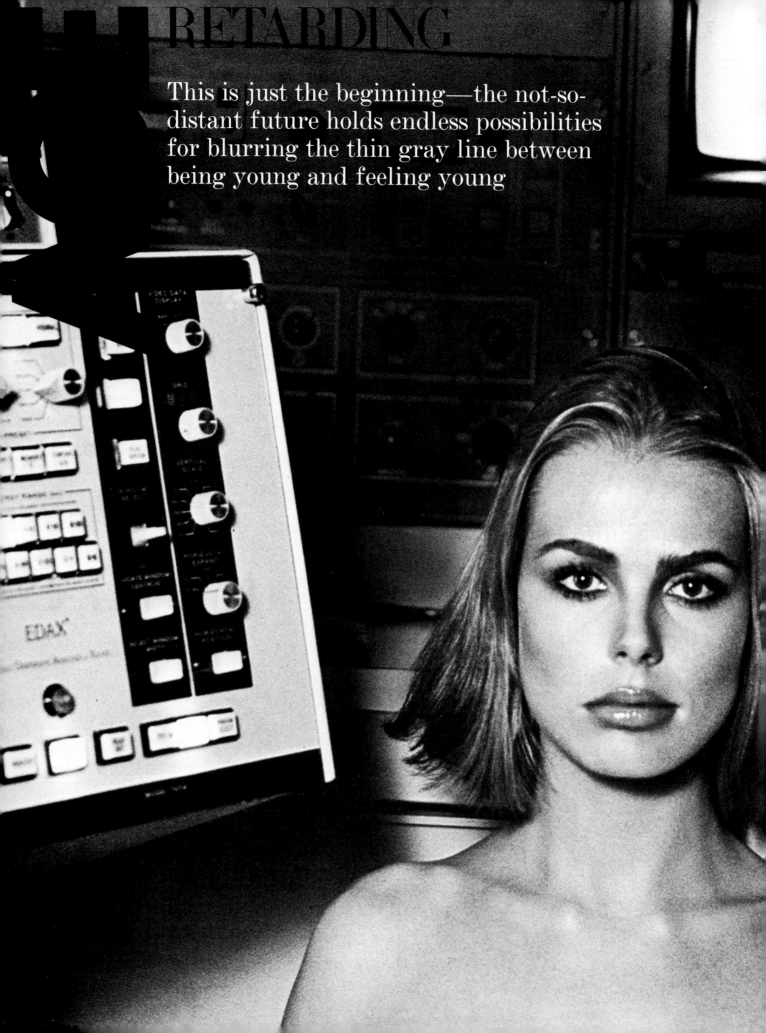

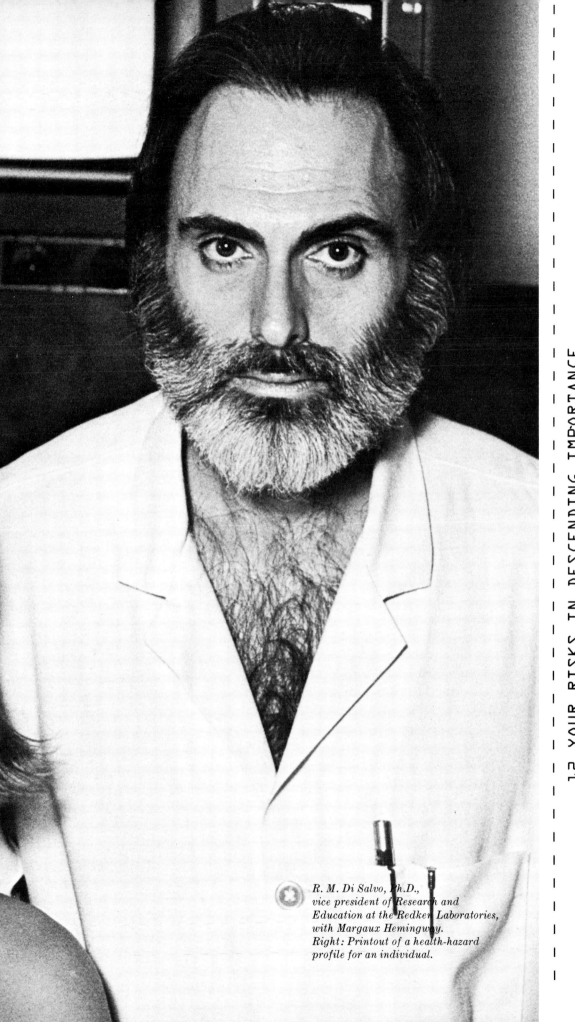

R. M. Di Salvo, Ph.D.,
vice president of Research and
Education at the Redken Laboratories,
with Margaux Hemingway.
Right: Printout of a health-hazard
profile for an individual.

12 YOUR RISKS IN DESCENDING IMPORTANCE

A RISK FACTOR OF 1.0 IS AVERAGE. A RISK FACTOR LESS THAN 1.0 CARRIES LESS THAN
AVERAGE RISK. A RISK FACTOR ABOVE 1.0 CARRIES GREATER THAN AVERAGE RISK.

12A ARTERIOSCLEROTIC HEART DISEASE   {HEART ATTACK}

13 AVERAGE   RISK   1,344 **********
14 YOUR CURRENT RISK   3,494 *************************   { 2.6 X AVG}
15 YOUR ACHIEVABLE RISK   968 ********   { .7 X AVG}

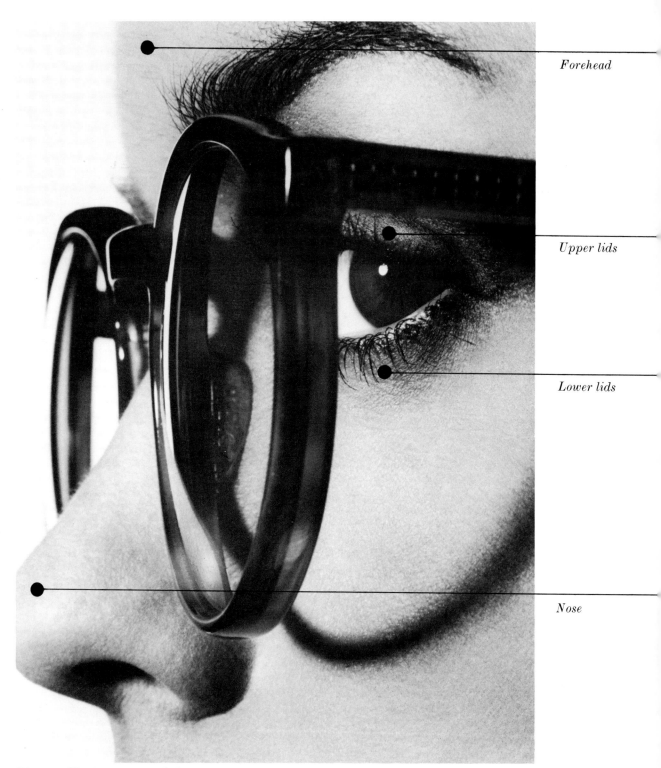

Forehead

Upper lids

Lower lids

Nose

Diagram illustrates some of the most common types of cosmetic surgery.

AGE RETARDING

by Marilyn Pelo

Medical progress is making it easier than ever to defy Mother Nature. Plastic surgery becomes more sophisticated every year, and, in the past decade, plastic surgeons, orthodontists and oral surgeons have made great leaps toward preventing the signs of aging. This is just a beginning—the not-so-distant future holds endless possibilities for blurring the thin gray line between being young and feeling young.

UNDERSTANDING PLASTIC SURGERY

When most people think of plastic surgery, the facelift immediately comes to mind, but this is only one operation in the plastic surgeon's repertoire of procedures that can be utilized to help us stay young- and healthy-looking. To help you understand what these various options are, here is an outline of plastic surgery techniques that work effectively to make us look and feel younger.

THE FACELIFT

The familiar term facelift actually describes a variety of techniques used to give the face a more youthful appearance. One must keep in mind, however, that a facelift will not make you look 30 years younger or like a new person; it will simply make you look like a somewhat younger you, taking off perhaps a dozen or more years.

The standard facelift procedure—the skin of the face and neck is separated from the underlying structure, then redraped and reattached—is frequently combined with one or more additional procedures—on the eyes, neck or nose—to achieve the desired results.

The period of time for hospitalization and for any swelling and discoloration to dissipate following the facelift depends greatly on the individual, but a standard procedure with standard results generally means less than a week in the hospital or at home. Makeup usually can be applied within a week and the return to an active social and business life, a matter of personal discretion, usually occurs about two or three weeks after surgery.

There are scars with facelifts, but most are hidden in the hollow behind the ear and in the crease in front of the ear. How obvious the scaring will be is simply guesswork. On most people the scars gradually become imperceptible and blend into the face.

Alas, a facelift does not always last a lifetime. To produce the most natural-looking results, the doctor will do as much or as little as he deems necessary, preferring to do the least amount. Those who are lucky never have to have the procedure repeated. But, depending on your skin, the procedure may have to be repeated, albeit in modified form, in as little as a year or, more likely, in five to eight years.

It is important to understand what a facelift cannot do. Crow's feet, the furrows that run from the base of the nose past the corner of the mouth and furrows between the brows will not disappear with a face lift. The lines may be temporarily diminished, but they will return because they are caused by muscular action beneath the skin's surface. They can be eradicated with direct injection of liquid silicone, which, as of this writng, is still pending FDA approval.

The fine lines on the face, such as crow's feet, can be eliminated through dermabrasion, chemical peeling or chemabrasion, a combination of dermabrasion and chemical peeling. With dermabrasion, a common treatment for acne scars, the skin is "frozen," then abraded or "sanded" with a wire brush or diamond fraise. About three weeks or a month later, when the skin is completely healed, it should be perfectly smooth. With chemical peeling, the abrasion is caused by chemicals; chemabrasion is a combination of the two methods.

THE FOREHEAD

Today, the forehead is lifted to eliminate the deep furrows that run across the brow. This is, in effect, a partial facelift: the skin of the forehead is detached and redistributed over that area. However, one must have a hairline of average height for this procedure to be done, because it may raise the forehead as much as an inch. The scars are hidden in the hair and, if one has a very high hairline, the result might not be worth the expense.

THE NOSE

Nasal reconstruction, or "rhinoplasty," can decrease the size of the nose, retailor an awkwardly shaped nose, build up an undersized nose or reconstruct one which has collapsed because of a severe infection of the tissue, an accident or excessive use of cocaine.

One of the most frequently performed plastic surgeries, nasal reconstruction also has a splendid success rate. Even when the operation is performed on a young person, its effects will usually last a lifetime. Scarring, too, is almost always insignificant.

THE EYES

The surgical technique used to improve the appearance of the skin around the eyes is called blepharoplasty or simply eyeplasty. The ability of this procedure to change the appearance of a person is truly phenomenal. Those with an excess of skin and/or fat either above or below the eyes—or both—can have it trimmed away and eliminate this condition which, due to heredity, may appear at a painfully premature age.

The success rate of this surgery is very high. Most operations on the lower lids never have to be repeated, though the upper lids sometimes require a second operation after a period of time. The scarring that it creates can be hidden deftly in the natural creases of the upper and lower lids.

It is interesting that many men opt for eyeplasty ahead of facelifts and find that it solves their problems for a lifetime.

THE EARS

You can reshape the ears to reduce their size, to make them lie closer to the head or otherwise to be more attractive in relation to the rest of your features. This surgery, too, has a good success rate and rarely requires any follow-up surgery as time passes.

ORTHODONTICS AND ORAL SURGERY

The bone structure is the foundation of your face. The soft tissue—muscle and skin—is draped over and attached to these structural elements like upholstery fabric on a chair frame. The teeth give shape to the mouth in the same way that cartilage defines the shape of the ears and nose. In short, these structural elements are the architecture of the face, and

174

the skin is a decorative covering which will manifest the passage of time in much the same way that upholstery on a chair fades, stretches and frays.

The ability of these structural elements to support the soft tissue has a profound impact on the way we look and the rate at which we age. For example, some people with receding lower jaws, sometimes called "weak" chins, may find that, even as young people, they acquire so-called double (or even triple) chins. Crooked teeth and an improper bite not only look unattractive but also may cause undue stress on the soft tissue, causing it to stretch or wrinkle prematurely. An upper lip inadequately supported by a receding upper jaw may sag and wrinkle. An improperly aligned bite creating an asymmetry of the face can cause an inappropriate strain on the soft tissues of one side of the face, causing it to age more quickly, making the asymmetry more obvious.

Each of these problems can have a deleterious effect on general health and appearance, but all of them can be corrected.

THE ORTHODONTIC OPTION

Although many people consider orthodontics to be primarily for children, these dental specialists now can also help those who did not get the treatment that they should have had as children. They can eliminate gaps between teeth, respace overcrowded teeth and realign crooked teeth, even change an awkward profile caused by poor occlusion. In short, they can inspire you to smile from ear to ear.

Hundreds of people each year are taking advantage of this progress in dentistry. Many orthodontists, at least those in metropolitan areas, are now seeing a flood of adult patients, who have concluded that late is definitely better than never. Their ranks include both men and women of all ages and professions.

A primary reason for the parade of adults on their way to the orthodontist is the advent of removable braces (dentists call them appliances), which you can take off when you would feel more presentable without them. These braces are best used for closing gaps between teeth, easing crowding or straightening a turned or otherwise crooked tooth. According to several specialists, these problems usually can be treated in short order—over the course of perhaps six months or a year—with permanent braces; the option of removing the appliance usually requires a longer period of treatment and the results using removable appliances may not be as close to the ideal as application of the permanent variety.

The costs for orthodontic work and the number and length of visits all vary depending upon your problem and the specialist you choose, so it is important to discuss this during the initial consultations. Some medical insurance programs do cover orthodontics, but far more do not—or only do so under special circumstances—so it is wise to check the specifics of your coverage and discuss them with your orthodontist prior to beginning treatment.

While orthodontic procedures usually net permanent results, once the braces are removed, Mother Nature takes control once more. As a result, though braces may no longer be necessary, one may still be required to wear a retainer—usually a small plastic plate or a band of wire—at night for a year or more to keep the teeth from drifting back into their old familiar position.

THE MAGIC OF ORAL SURGERY

In the late 1970s, an internationally known makeup artist appeared on a national television show where a panel of people were discussing their experiences with plastic surgery. During the course of the show, the artist, who had had his face lifted, said that he believed anyone considering plastic surgery should first consult an oral surgeon. During the course of his work, he had seen many

175

clients who had had facelifts in attempts to correct or compensate for problems that were structural—unattractive jaw lines, unbecoming profiles. These problems, said the makeup artist, could have been dealt with better through oral surgery than plastic surgery, which had treated the symptom rather than the major problem.

One of the best-known practitioners of this aristocracy of dentistry is Dr. Stanley J. Behrman, director of oral surgery at the New York Hospital-Cornell Medical Center in New York City. He agrees with the makeup artist and believes deeply that the techniques which he and other pioneers have developed can help us stay younger-looking longer.

He explains, "The changes we can make not only make people look younger and better and make them feel young, but the surgery can also retard the aging process. An abnormal relationship of the bone structure inevitably creates strain on the soft tissues, causing them to sag, wrinkle and furrow. We can eliminate this. The faces will age, but more gracefully."

The amazing technique that accomplish these wonderful results are called maxillofacial surgery; methods devised in recent years allow the surgeon to cut apart the facial bones, then reassemble them—like a jigsaw puzzle—to redesign the bones that are detracting from otherwise attractive faces. Such procedures usually do not produce visible scars because the incisions are made inside the mouth. Postoperative swelling or bruising is relatively insignificant. Hospital stays for maxillofacial surgery are rarely more than a week, and patients can often return to work within just a few days. No bandages, no casts are necessary, and the risk of infection is minimal, for the surgeon is working on bones that are almost impervious to bacteria that could be a formidable threat to other parts of the body. Best of all, maxillofacial surgery lasts a lifetime.

With most maxillofacial procedures, it is not necessary to detach the soft tissues from the bone. As result, the muscles and skin attached to the bone will move right along with the bone, which, according to Dr. Behrman, "can have very salutary effects. In fact, patients may look as though they have had facelifts instead of oral surgery."

Finding a surgeon to discuss your specific problems does not require a trip to New York or Los Angeles, for these specialists are found all over the nation. To find one in your area, contact the American Association of Oral and Maxillofacial Surgeons, 211 East Chicago Avenue, Chicago, Illinois 60611.

THE NECK

There's much good news in this area for people whose necks age more quickly than the rest of their faces or bodies. A recently developed technique is now being used to re-shape the neck and under-chin. The most prominent cause of aging in this area involves the platysma muscle, which spans the neck from the under-chin to the clavicle or "collarbone." Oddly enough, this muscle performs no function except to record the passage of time by creating vertical lines or bands along the neck. (To understand the effect of this muscle, stand before a mirror and tense your lower lip.) In the past decade, surgeons have discovered that they can solve this problem by cutting this muscle and simply ignoring it or by turning it into a kind of sling (called a muscle flap) to support the tissue. In either case, the technique, often combined with a redistribution of the neck skin or a facelift, can eliminate this unsightly condition in a way that a simple lifting of the skin in the area cannot do. While the long-term results of this surgery are not known, the short-term indications are very promising, the scarring minimal and well hidden, and if the muscle does not reattach itself (which it rarely does), the operation will not have to be repeated.

THE BREAST

A woman unhappy with the appearance of her breasts need not live with what she was born with. Those who have breasts that are droopy, rather than too large or too small, can have an operation called mastopexy, a process which uplifts the breasts. Others who think Mother Nature has been too generous with them can undergo reduction mammoplasty, which reduces the amount of breast tissue and uplifts the tissue that remains. Those who have small, but not drooping, breasts can have augmentation mammoplasty, which introduces an implant into the breasts. Today the most common inplants are packaged silicone gel, inflatable implants filled with saline solution, or a combination implant that is silicone gel surrounded with the inflatable variety. If you seek this operation, the type of implant used will largely depend on the physician. It remains true that an implant sometimes causes a hardening of the tissue around it, because of the body responding to a foreign substance. These problems can often be dealt with in the doctor's office; more severe cases may require surgical correction.

Scarring from these types of surgery can most often be tucked under the breast. In those cases of breast reduction where the nipple must be moved to a more natural location, hairline scars will be apparent for a time around the nipple and areola, and between the nipple and the bottom of the breast. As with other surgeries of this type, the scarring will usually diminish as time passes.

THE ABDOMEN

Keeping one's stomach in shape may be one of life's larger trials, but if the problem is truly severe, a plastic surgeon can help. In cases where childbirth or extensive weight loss has left a woman with hanging skin, she can turn to the surgeon for help. Two words of warning: First, this operation cannot be used to make fat people thin; the weight must be lost before the operation to remove loose skin can be performed. Second, it will produce scars in the creases of the lower abdomen that can be hidden under a swimsuit but that may be visible when one is undressed. As a result, while the surgery is very successful, many doctors will not do the surgery unless they are sure that the problem they are solving is far greater than the scarring problem it may cause.

OPERATIONS TO THINK TWICE ABOUT

THE THIGH AND BUTTOCKS LIFTS

It is true that plastic surgeons have developed what are called body sculpturing techniques that can be used to reduce the excess flesh of the thighs and buttocks. However, you may have a difficult time finding a respectable surgeon who will perform them. The reason: scars. Says Dr. Victor I. Rosenberg, director of plastic surgery at Beekman-Downtown Hospital in New York City, ''The scarring is so severe, so deforming, that few doctors will perform [these operations] on a person who simply wants to look better. This skin simply does not heal as well as other parts of the body, and the scars are very difficult to hide. Most people will say that they will trade the baggy flesh for scars, but they usually have no sense of what bad scarring is—hideous. And these scars cannot be hidden under a swimsuit.''

ARM LIFTS

The problems of the thigh and buttocks lifts are equally true with the so-called arm lift, which reduces the baggy flesh on the underside of the upper arm. Says Dr. Rosenberg, ''Again, the scarring, which runs the length of the upper arm—is so severe that surgery has no aesthetic value. If you have it, you'll be wearing long sleeves the rest of your life.

Attempts to make the incision serpentine and thereby reduce scarring have not made any significant difference.''

THE "MINI" LIFT

Dr. Dicran Goulian, Jr., attending surgeon in charge of plastic surgery at The New York Hospital-Cornell Medical Center: ''There is no such thing as a mini lift. A properly executed facelift requires that the skin be separated from the underlying structure and repositioned. The implication of the term 'mini lift' as a simple stretching of skin, taking a tuck, without going through the essential reordering of the skin in relation to its supporting structure, is simply stupid. It is a shortcut to nothing. And because of the location of the scars with the 'mini lift,' it is often not possible to go back and do it right.'' However, modified face-lifting procedures can be performed, usually on your second time around, when adjustments are being made a year or several years after your original facelift.

FINDING THE RIGHT SURGEON

Word-of-mouth is the best method. Friends or friends of friends who have had plastic surgery that looks good to your eye are usually the best sources. Local hospitals and medical centers may also be of help. It is best if you can get several names and then take the time to interview each doctor, recognizing that they will be interviewing you at the same time, deciding whether they will take you as a patient. And they may refuse if they do not think that you need the surgery you are asking for, if they question whether they can produce the results you are looking for, if they believe that you are expecting the surgery to solve emotional or other problems unrelated to the surgery at hand, if you are not adequately healthy to undergo surgery or if you are seeking plastic surgery as a means of eliminating problems caused by ongoing obesity.

If several surgeons refuse to take you as a patient, you should certainly examine your reasons for requesting the surgery.

In the course of the consultation, there are several points to look for. First, if you are offered a menu of procedures (like the one above) and asked which you are seeking, go elsewhere. This is surgery, not an assembly line. Every operation must be specifically tailored to the patient's face. Some people believe that they want ''the works'' when they only need their eyelids altered. A good doctor will not give you a procedure that you do not need.

A good doctor will also let you know exactly what he or she plans to do and what results you can expect. This is not the time to deceive yourself in any way. Listen carefully, because what the surgeon thinks you need is what you will get. When the surgery begins, you are not in charge.

You should also be told where the scars will be (do not believe anyone who says there will not be any), and what the possible complications are. You should also be told what kind of anesthesia will be used, how long your hospital stay will be, when you should expect to resume a normal business and social life.

If the doctor plans to operate in his office, a practice that is becoming more common, be sure to ask what the doctor's system is for getting you to the hospital quickly if there is an unforeseen emergency. After all, this is surgery, not a haircut or a facial. Advises Dr. Rosenberg, who does not operate in his Sutton Place office, ''Any in-office surgical procedure should be done as though you were in the hospital. No one should lead you to believe that any of this is lunch-hour surgery.''

Be sure that the doctor talks with you about postoperative care, which is equally as important as the consultation and surgery, for this is when complications (severe swelling, infection, bleeding), if there are any, will be dealt with. Your physician should assure you that he or she will be available anytime, day or night, should you have a question.

THE PRICE OF SURGERY

Do not be leery if the doctor asks for full payment of his fee in advance of the surgery (the consultation fee is separate). Advance payment is standard procedure for plastic surgeons doing cosmetic work. Explains one prominent surgeon, "These are people having surgery they don't really need in terms of physical health. If they are unhappy with it for any reason, they tend to refuse payment. Those who have a reasonable gripe can take legal action."

Prices for plastic surgery vary greatly. The trend toward in-office surgery is an attempt to reduce these costs against the across-the-board escalation of medical care costs coupled with galloping inflation. In general, one can expect to pay more in large cities, where costs are generally higher for any business. In 1980, the costs for plastic surgery varied from $2,000 to $8,000 for a facelift with eyelid reduction. A "nose job" started at about $1,500 and ran as high as $4,000. In addition, there are usually separate charges of several hundred dollars for anesthesia and operating-room facilities.

Of course, not all costs are monetary. With any of these surgeries you will be out of circulation for a period, depending on the surgery you have, and depending on how keen you are about having other people know you have had it. Initially, life will not be the same. Your doctor will most likely recommend that that part of the body on which he operated not be exposed to the sun for periods ranging from a couple of weeks to six months; this is to avoid undue swelling and burning. You may have to avoid any manipulation of your face or breast—such as a facial or caressing of the breast as part of lovemaking—until the tissues mend. But these restrictions are quickly lifted.

LOOKING AHEAD

Every doctor involved in these areas of age retardation looks toward the future with great hope for progress. While plastic and oral surgeons continue to add to their repertoire of procedures that diminish the telling signs of aging, dermatologists and other medical specialists are increasing their research to keep the signs of aging from registering so quickly. For example, several are exploring the area of cell renewal, the skin's natural process of surface cell replacement, which naturally slows down with time. The dry, rough, even gray look that older skin develops, particularly in times of low humidity, is directly attributable to a slowdown in this process of old cells' sloughing off to make way for new ones. Doctors involved with cos-

> **" Word of mouth is the best method to finding the right surgeon "**

metics firms and with general dermatological research are now deeply involved in studying cell renewal in order to create products that keep this process functioning to maintain a youthful appearance. And they have achieved some success, developing products for major cosmetic firms—Elizabeth Arden and Estée Lauder to date—that increase the rate of cell renewal. (This is not to be confused with so-called cell therapy—a fad that is purported to provide the skin with restorative and regenerative catalysts—in which most doctors have no belief.)

Remember, too, that there will always be charlatans peddling what they want us to believe is the true Fountain of Youth. So far no one has found it, but with the great strides that are being made in all facets of medicine, its modern-day counterpart may be just around the corner.

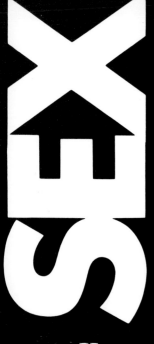

SEX

Your sexual style is yours, and, as you change, so should that style. It is important to recognize this natural process

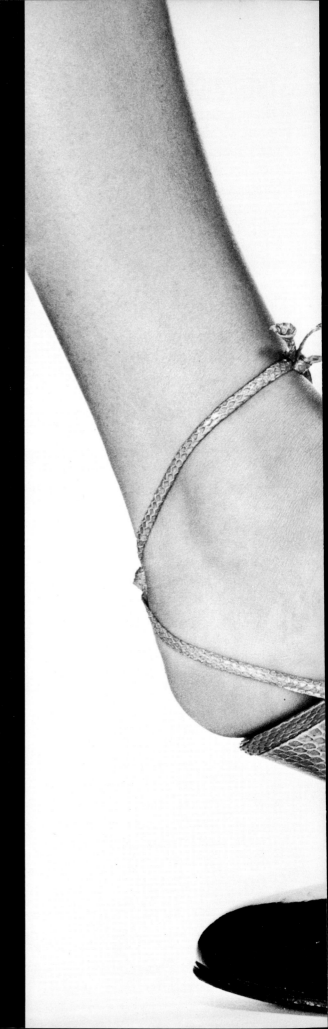

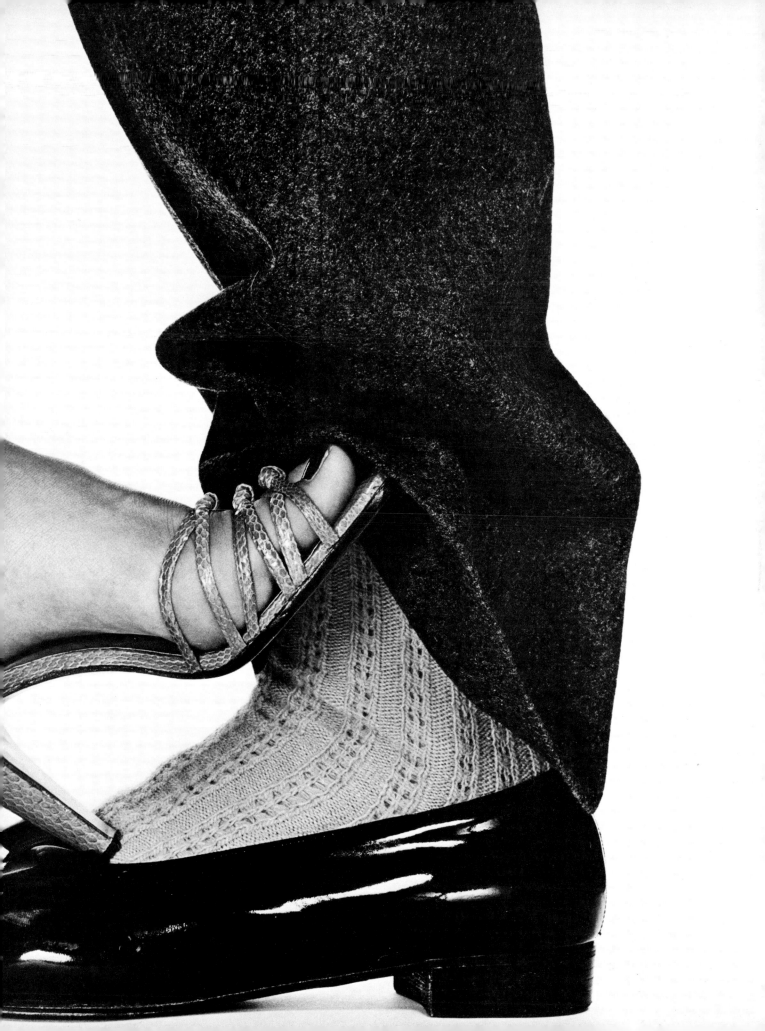

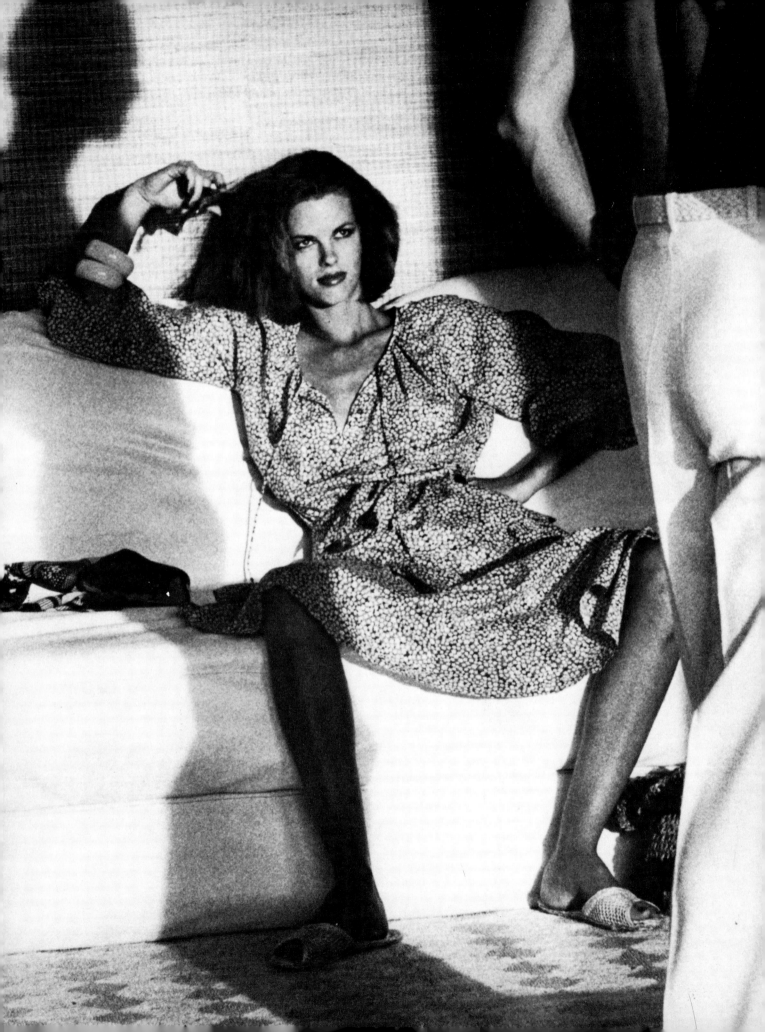

LOVERS WHO LAST

by Mimi Avins and Jane Greenberg

Lovers who last give themselves and their partners permission to change. They have a positive attitude. If a man for some reason experiences impotence, he and his wife can look at the problem as being unable to have intercourse the way they are used to, not as being unable to have sex. When couples have developed as people, it is reflected in their sexual satisfaction. A woman can adjust more easily to a hysterectomy or the appearance of some wrinkles if her sense of self-worth is adequate. She and her partner realize she is more than just the sum of her parts.

In the long-running sexual fantasy of popular fiction, two perfect bodies spontaneously unite to have rip-roaring orgasm on cue without much stimulation. The fantasy single woman is the insatiable swinger, sexually in demand, easily comfortable with strangers who instantly bring her peaks of pleasure.

The ideal married woman so satisfies the husband she unfailingly adores that he never looks at another woman. Don't base your personal expectations on other people's fantasies.

When it comes to sex, it seems like the superlatives always live next door: Our neighbors have sex more often, and it's more fun,

Lifelong lovers all seem to have one thing in common: they have been able to maintain high levels of sexual activity throughout their lives.

more exciting, more daring . . . better. We expect sex to be in life as it is in fiction.

A problem is always a felt discrepancy between the way things are and the way we would like them to be. We'll always fall short of the fantasy models. When reality doesn't measure up to our expectations of what we think we're supposed to be, we think we have a problem.

Good sex is good sex. It doesn't have to be love, a measure of your values as a woman, a political statement or a fountain of youth. It does not make you wiser or even necessarily happier. It can be a part of a full life—just a part. Sex may be a high priority in your life at one time, less important at another. Losing perspective only brings that well-known killjoy, pressure, into our lives.

The complement to that old line, "If it feels good, do it," must be "If it doesn't—stop!" The best pattern is your own pattern. If it's working for you, don't feel pressured to be different. If it's not working for you, give yourself permission to try something new.

Sexually, we have come a full circle. Thirty years ago, a woman entering marriage minus her virginity was afraid of being found out. Today, that woman's virginal daughter is as afraid her inexperience will be discovered. Someone else dictating what is and what isn't okay is still tyranny. Your sexual style is yours, and as you change, so should that style.

183

It is important to recognize this natural process: Realize that different times in your life make for a healthy outlook, one that makes you a good lover to your lover, and to yourself.

SEX WHAT TO EXPECT

by Paul E. Cohen

"Nothing could be further from the truth," Masters and Johnson assert, "than the often expressed concept that aging women do not maintain a high level of sexual orientation." Nevertheless, most women fear that the menopause will drastically change their ability to enjoy sex. This fear no doubt stems from the fact that "change of life," or "menopause" does refer to a phase in a woman's life when the body undergoes significant changes. It is interesting to note that the advent of the menopause comes about a decade later now than it did less than a hundred years ago. When the cycle of menopause does begin, the ovaries start gradually decreasing their production of the hormones estrogen and progesterone. Ovulating and menstrual periods cease once the cycle is complete. As these changes are taking place—and the entire process could take 20 or 30 years—the vagina becomes shorter and narrower, the major labia shrink, the walls of the vagina become thinner and much of their elasticity is lost. The ability to lubricate when stimulated may also decrease, but in general sexual desire, the ability to have sexual intercourse, and the capacity to reach orgasm will not be affected, though the orgasms themselves will probably be somewhat shorter.

Many women sail through menopause hardly realizing that they have done so. The trouble, for those who do feel discomfort, can usually be traced to the reduction of estrogen levels—particularly from a very sudden lowering of the estrogen level in the body. Generally, the physical problems are not serious —headaches, fatigue, hot flashes and some brief periods of emotional instability.

There are solutions to many of the ailments of menopause. The one which most quickly comes to mind is hormone replacement. It can alleviate much of the distress, but a potentially dangerous side effect may be uterine cancer. However, until scientists come up with a satisfactory verdict on replacement hormones, sexual activity itself remains the best remedy. The simple fact is, as Masters and Johnson stress, "if opportunity for regularity of coital exposure is created or maintained, the woman suffering from all of the vaginal stigmas of sex-steroid starvation still will retain a far higher capacity for sexual performance than her female counterpart who does not have similar coital opportunities."

Sexual activity also helps maintain the size and elasticity of the vagina after menopause. A young women's vagina has remarkable expandability—after all, it can accommodate the body of a baby. After menopause, elasticity lessens. Regular sexual intercourse keeps the vagina from shriveling and exercises the muscles which "grip" the penis. Some women also do exercises to tighten these muscles— one of the best methods is to practice stopping and starting the flow of urine by flexing and releasing the muscles which surround the vagina. *Continued on page 193*

Thirty years ago, a woman entering marriage was afraid of being found out. Today her virginal daughter is as afraid her inexperience will be discovered.

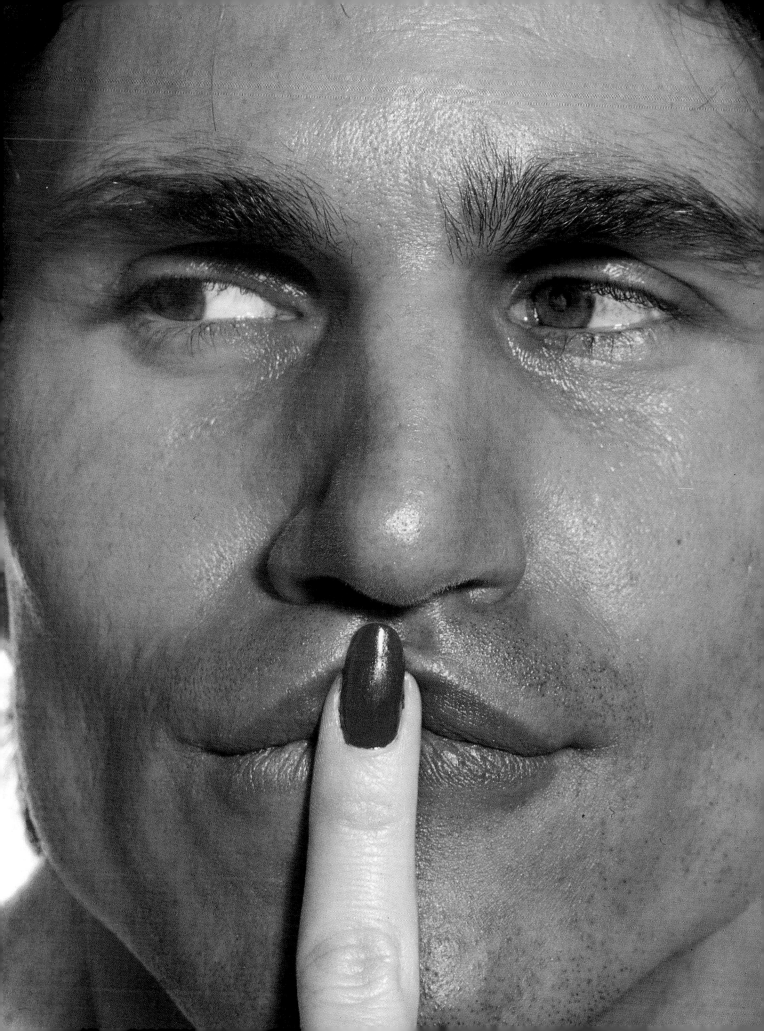

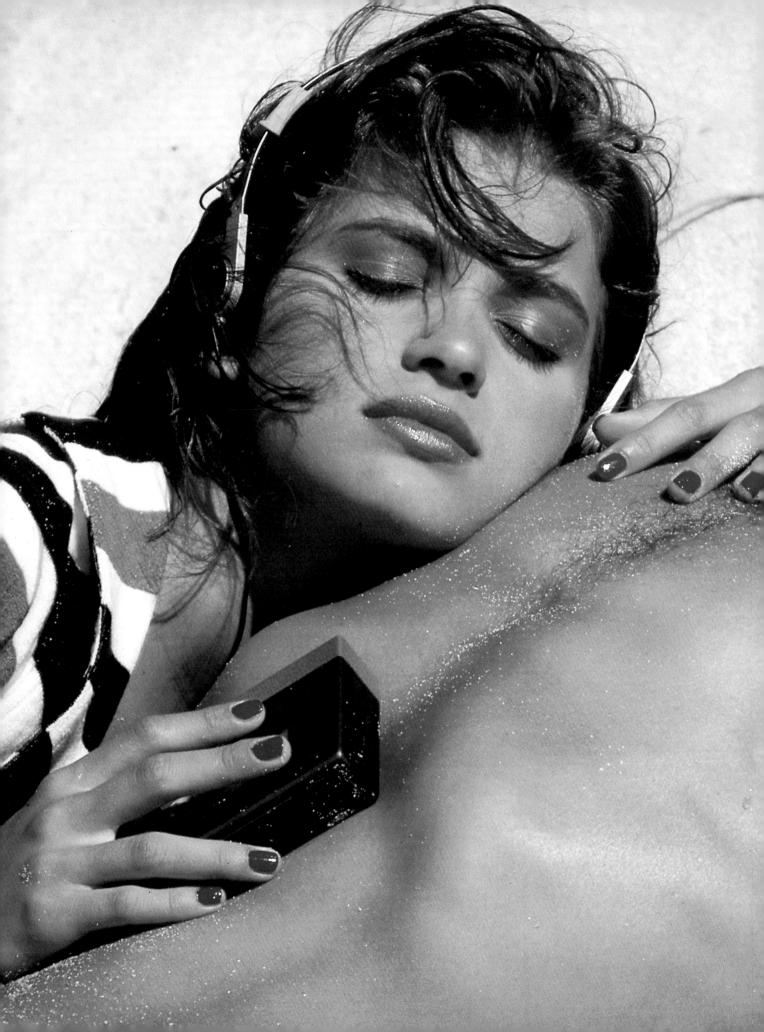

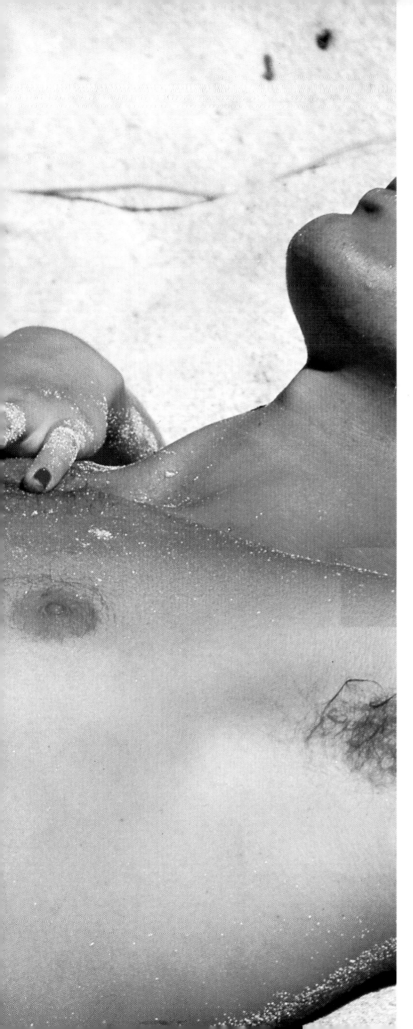

L*ifelong lovers all seem to have one thing in common. They have been able to maintain high levels of sexual activity throughout their lives.*

Following pages: Good sex is good sex. It doesn't have to be love . . .

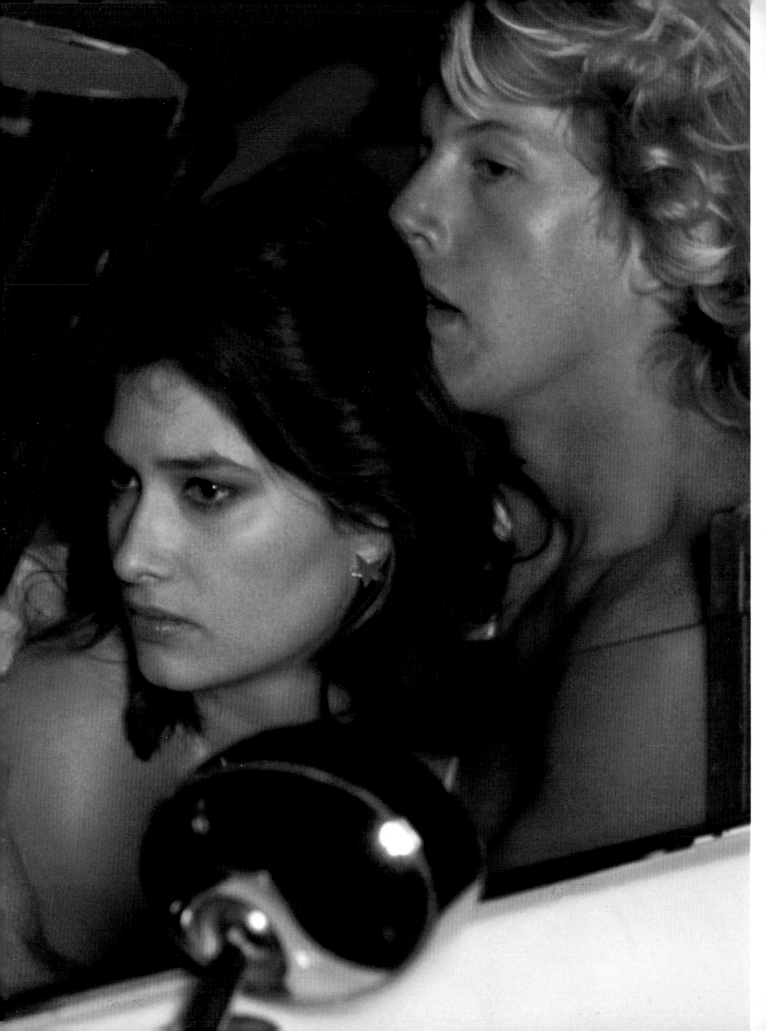

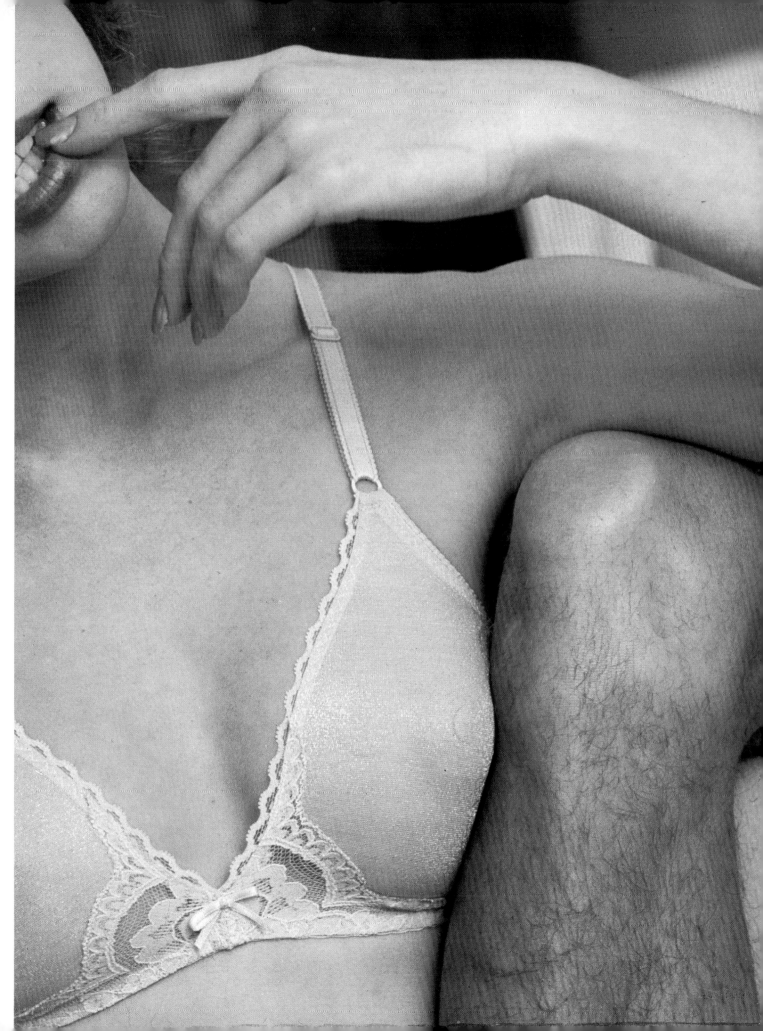

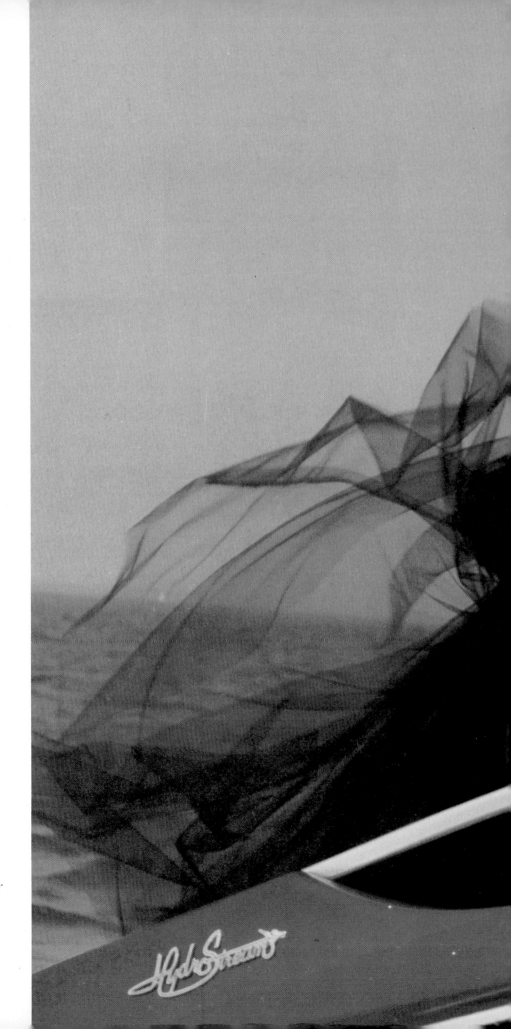

"Of course there is biological aging," says Dr. Alex Comfort. "But if you exercise you won't slow up much physically." Proper functioning of the body and of sex organs requires continuous and systematic activity.

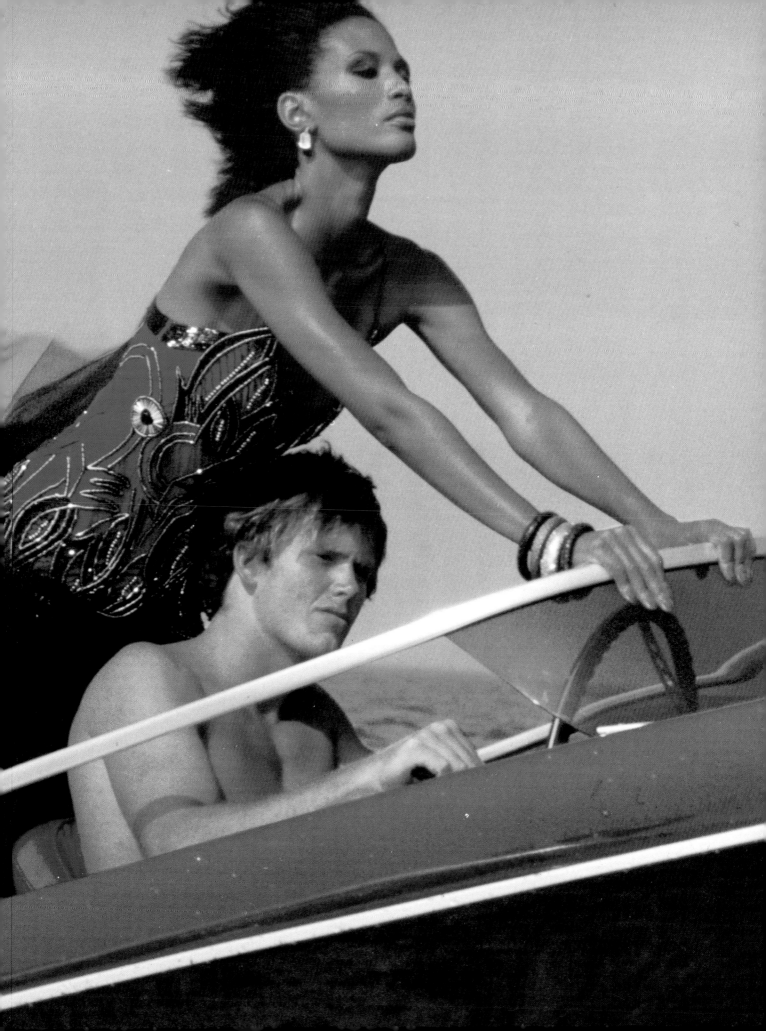

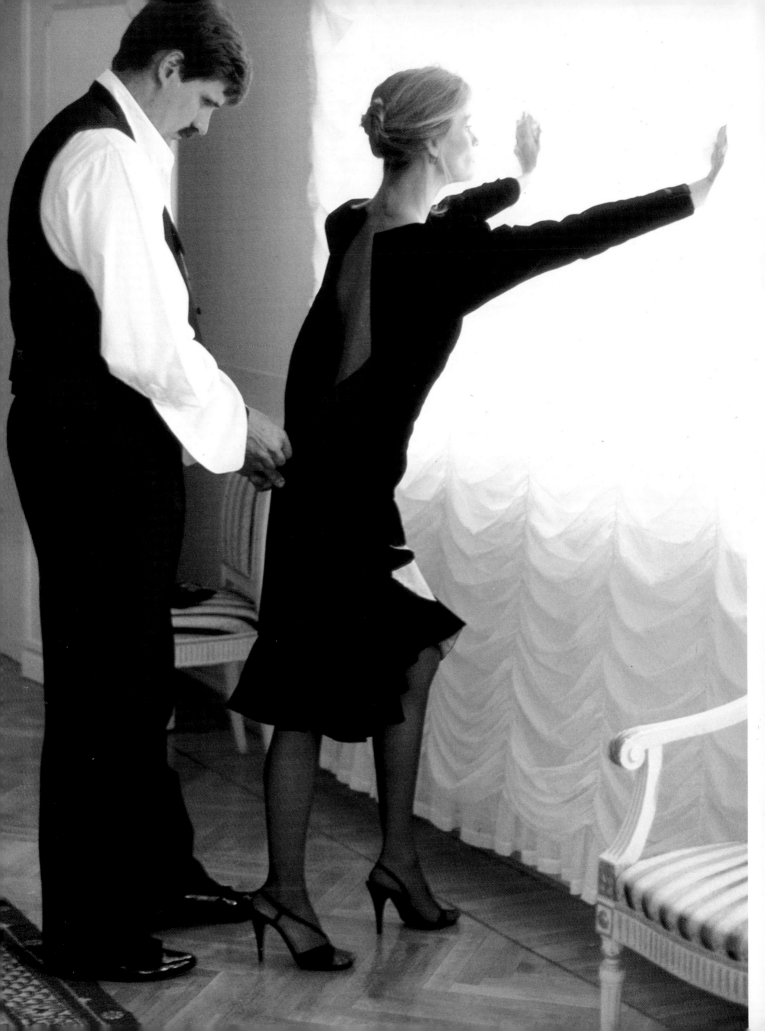

Continued from page 184

Despite the changes which occur during menopause, Masters and Johnson have reported the good news that there is absolutely "no limit drawn by advancing years" to female sexuality. In fact, the end of menopause often marks the beginning of a period of peak sexual satisfaction. Twenty-one percent of a group of women aged 55–66 who were tested by the University of Chicago's Committee on Human Development revealed that "after the menopause, the woman is more interested in sex than before." After menopause, a woman loses her fertility, but she need not ever lose her libido.

If a woman reaches middle age and finds her sexual desires gone, she is less likely to be suffering from hormone starvation than from an emotional problem associated with menopause. Depression with the loss of the reproductive function is one of the commonest psychological problems. "The ability to conceive," writes Dr. Michael Daly of Temple University, "whether a child is wanted or not, is at least a motivation of the libido in women."

Women often value themselves primarily for their biological contribution to society—largely, perhaps, because our society does still hold that sexuality is primarily for procreation. Women who stay at home bearing and raising children are especially prone to postmenopausal depression. "Her ego is threatened," observes Dr. Nathaniel Wagner, "and she feels depressed when reproductive function ends." The feeling of loss may be compounded and the depression more severe if their husbands are reaching the peak of their careers—as men often do in their fifties—at the same time that menopause ends.

Depression has a profound effect upon both

The single woman's fantasy is the insatiable swinger, sexually in demand, easily comfortable with strangers, who instantly brings her peaks of pleasure.

sexual interest and performance, just as sexuality and self-esteem are closely related. A woman's feelings about herself can be tied to any number of ways of winning approval from men. Whether this is the ability to conceive or lies in the idea of youthful attractiveness, when these vanish, a depression can set in which might make a woman feel isolated and dull her interest in sex. Depression, however, can be the most curable of psychological problems and a competent counselor or physician will certainly be able to help.

" *21 percent of a group of women aged 55-66 who were tested revealed that, after the menopause, the woman is more interested in sex than before* **"**

The best cure for anxiety or depression over sexuality is perhaps the most pleasurable one : Regular sensual stimulation not only keeps interest at high levels, but it ensures effective sexual performance throughout one's lifetime.

Lifelong lovers all seem to have one thing in common: They have been able to maintain high levels of sexual activity throughout their lives. "Of course, there is biological aging," concedes Dr. Alex Comfort, author of The Joy of Sex. *"But if you exercise, you won't slow up much physically." Proper functioning of the body and of sex organs requires continuous and systematic activity.*

The slower responses to sexual stimulation that naturally occur in both sexes can be a true advantage, and the growing numbers of those who claim that sexual intercourse gives them more pleasure as they age often account for the improvement by citing this reason. Not only does it take more time to reach a high pitch of sexual excitement, but once that peak is attained, a person in the 50–70-year range can maintain it almost indefinitely.

193

HOW MEN MATURE SEXUALLY

It is well known from the findings of such famous researchers as Alfred Kinsey and William Masters and Virginia Johnson that men reach the peak of sexual interest and responsiveness in their early or mid-twenties, about 10–20 years before women. However, when a male is stimulated to high sexual output during these formative years, Masters and Johnson have pointed out, "and a similar tenor of activity is established for the 31–40-year range, his middle involutional years are marked by constantly recurring physiologic evidence of maintained sexuality." Nonetheless, it must be kept in mind that "maintained sexuality" greatly varies from man to man.

The physiological changes which the male undergoes are numerous but do not affect the enjoyment of sex. The angle of the erect penis of a 60-year-old points down, not up as in the younger man. "Psychic" erections—those inspired by fantasy or reading titillating material—occur less frequently, though tests on 90-year-old men revealed that nocturnal erections continue, indicating a lingering physical potency even though the men may have abandoned sex.

Testes loose their firmness, and the lubricating fluid emitted from Cowper's gland before ejaculation may disappear after 60. Seminal fluid will decrease and reduced ejaculatory pressure will result in shorter, less intense orgasms, young men's lasting perhaps two to four seconds and older men's only a second or two.

The physiological changes which the male undergoes are numerous but do not affect the enjoyment of sex.

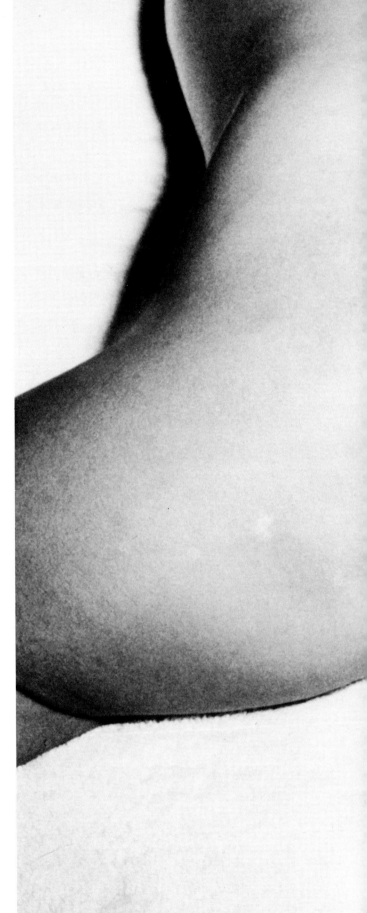

194

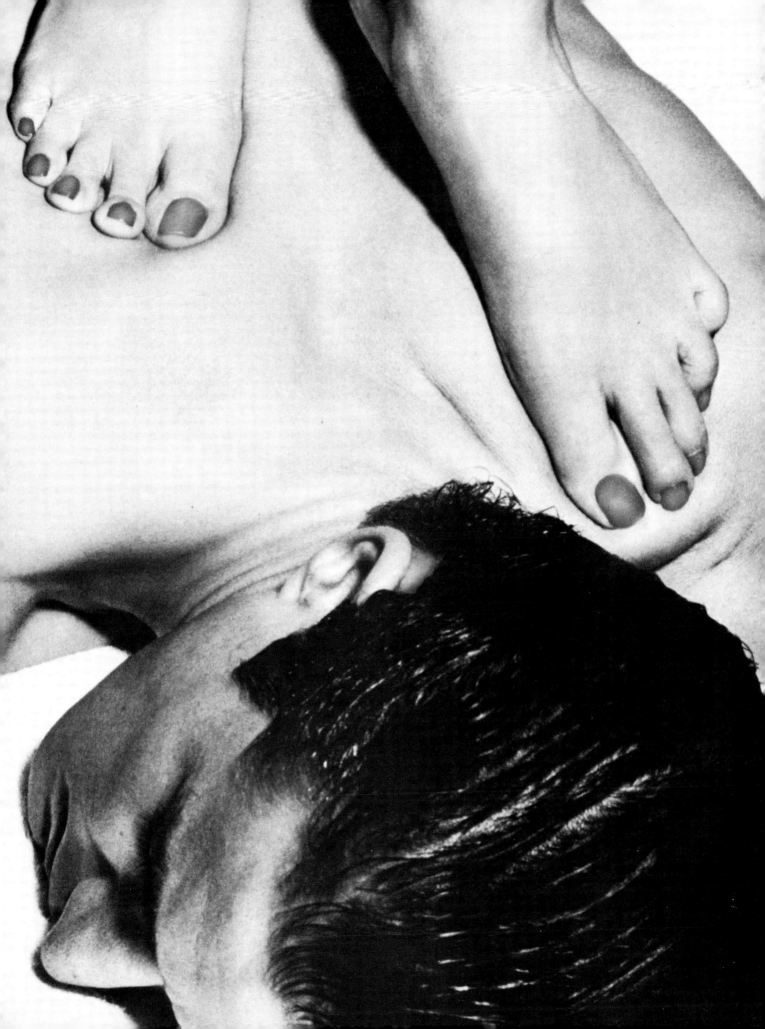

Because of these physiological changes, all of which are a natural part of the general slowing up of the body, a man's response to sexual stimuli is slower. It may take as long as three or four minutes of manipulation of the penis and other sex play for a 50–70-year-old man to reach an erection less firm and less full than one a younger man (20–30) takes just seconds to achieve. Orgasms occur less often —a refractory period of from 12 to 24 hours is usually necessary before another can be reached.

" Sexually, we have come full circle . . . The complement to that old line 'If it feels good, do it,' must also be 'If it doesn't, stop' "

Retirement generally has the most devastating effect on a man's self-image and his sexuality. After the transition from contributing member of society to retiree, writes Dr. Comfort, "people are rendered unemployable, useless and, in some cases, impoverished." With the sudden loss of status, boredom, financial worries and perhaps ailments of aging come depression, tension and fatigue which can very easily make a man temporarily impotent.

Another major factor which can have a destructive effect on a man's sexuality is the fear of impending impotence as a result of age. Impotence in men, in fact, has nothing to do with age: It is usually caused by anxiety. Masters and Johnson discovered that the factor contributing most often to the loss of potency is the fear of failure itself: "The fear of inadequacy is the greatest known deterrent to effective sexual functioning, simply because it so completely distracts the fearful individual from his or her natural responsivity by blocking the reception of sexual stimuli

either created by or reflected from the sexual partner."

Despondency caused by boredom with sex is another problem facing males as well as females. Masters and Johnson believe it to be the main reason most people give up sex. Often confused with biological dysfunctioning, the decline is usually "affected by a psychological fatigue," notes Dr. Kinsey, "a loss of interest or repetition of the same sort of experience, an exhaustion of the possibilities of exploring new techniques, new types of contacts, new situations."

David Gutmann, Ph.D., a professor of psychiatry at Northwestern University Medical School in Chicago, recently conducted a test on Mayan Indian men. Showing a group of the men a picture of a man climbing a rope, he asked them what they saw. More than 90 percent of the younger men described a man working very hard to ascend the rope and ultimately falling, while half of the older men saw him playing and enjoying himself—a thought that occurred rarely to the young men. In sex, too, a grit-your-teeth-and-prove-you-can-do-it attitude often gives way to a free-flowing and joyful willingness to take pleasure in whatever may happen as men leave their late teens and early twenties, shedding sexual conflicts that often accompany these years.

LIFE EXPECTANCY

The following statistics are based upon the findings of the United States Bureau of Census and the United States Department of Commerce. The annual collection of death statistics began in 1900. The statistics were based upon a sampling of 10 states and Washington, D.C. The collection of birth rates began in 1915 and was also based on this 10-state area. It was not until 1933 that the collection of vital statistics included the entire United States. The following statistics show average life expectancies for men and women beginning in 1901. In 1940, for example, men lived to an average age of 60.8 years while women lived to an average of 65.2 years. By 1978, these averages had increased to 70.2 years for men and 77.8 years for women.

1901–1978
AVERAGE YEARS FROM BIRTH

YEAR	MEN	WOMEN	
1901–1910	49.32	52.54	• Sources: Statistical Bulletin of the Metropolitan Life Insurance Company
1909–1911	50.23	53.62	
1920	53.6	54.6	
1930	58.1	61.6	• Statistical Abstract 1950 Edition
1940	60.8	65.2	
1950	65.6	71.1	• Statistical Abstract 1979 Edition
1960	66.6	73.1	
1970	67.1	74.8	
1975	68.7	76.5	
1978	70.2	77.8	

" Impotence in men, in fact, has nothing to do with age: it is usually caused by anxiety "

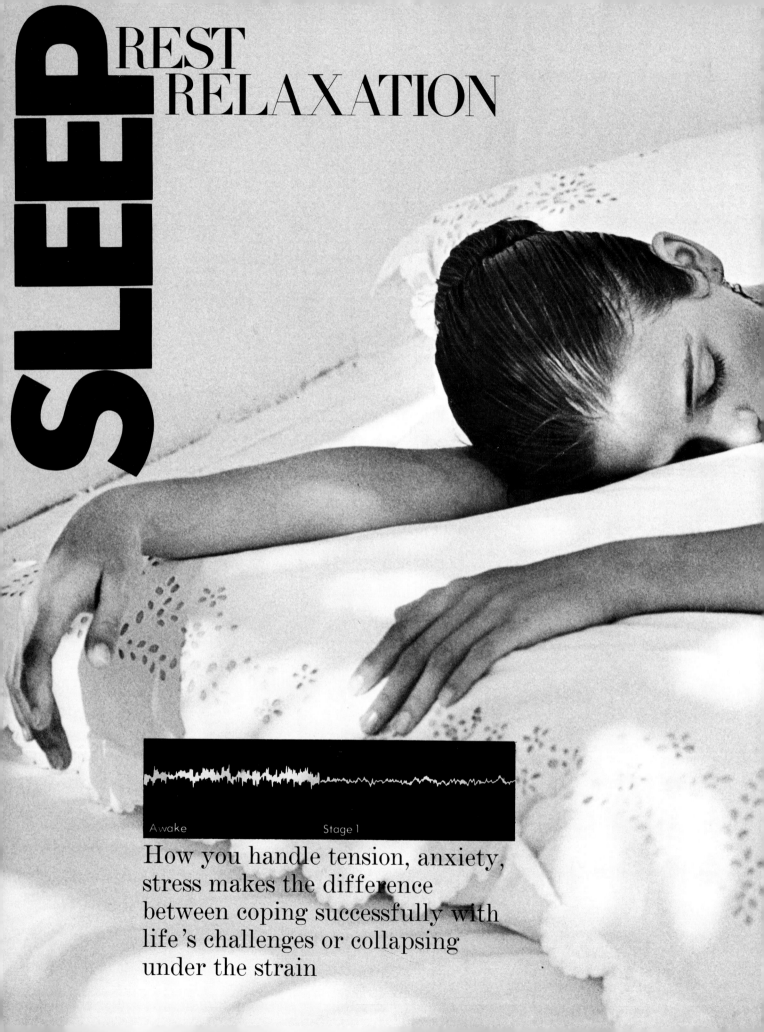

SLEEP REST RELAXATION

Awake   Stage 1

How you handle tension, anxiety, stress makes the difference between coping successfully with life's challenges or collapsing under the strain

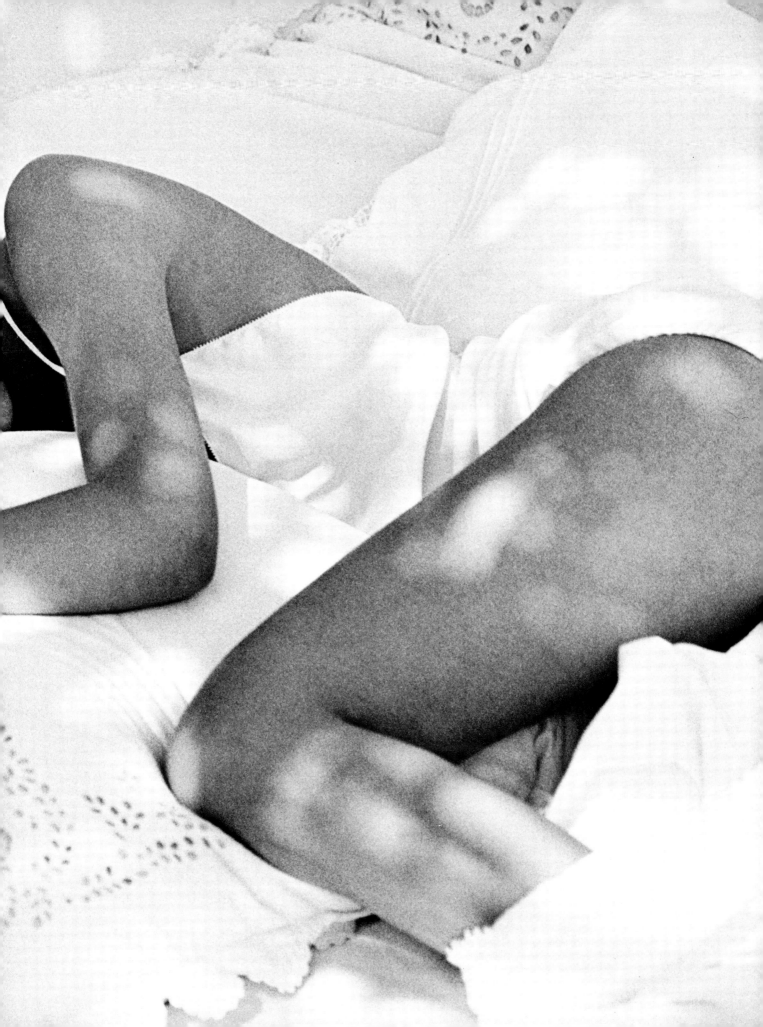

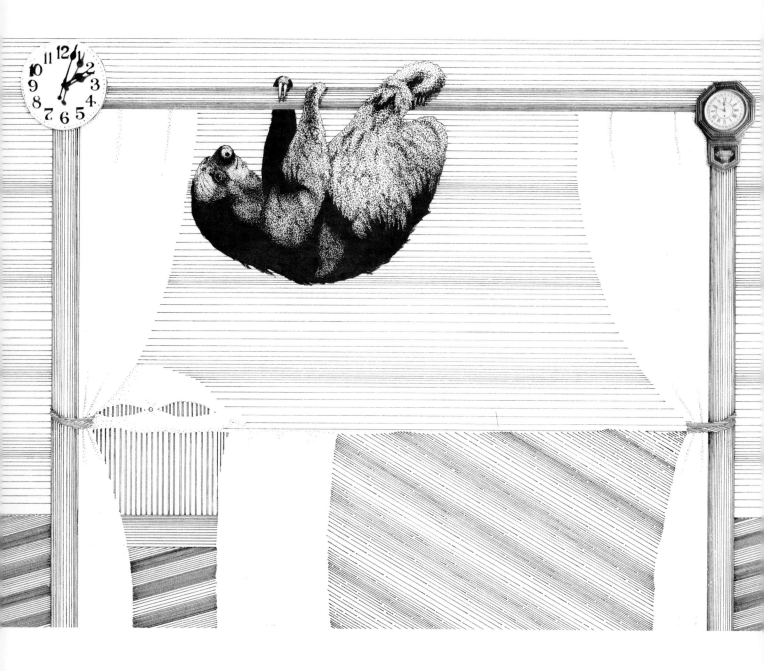

REST, RELAXATION AND SLEEP

by Carol Kahn

To wake up after a good night's sleep, feeling totally refreshed, ready to take on the world, is surely one of life's greatest pleasures. Perhaps no other bodily activity is so associated in our minds with feeling fit and looking good. We speak of "beauty sleep," ask our house guests *how* they slept, announce with the pride of accomplishment that we have "slept like a log."

Sleep is a restorative, the gift of oblivion after the wear and tear of the day's activities. But sleep is not the only way to turn off the mind and slow down the body. Rest and relaxation are just as important in renewing energy and combating fatigue. Unfortunately, as our lives have become more complex and stress-inducing, the opportunities for just letting go seem to have become fewer. Many of us are unwilling to take the time to unwind. Or we have simply forgotten how to do it.

Yet what is most natural can be learned. We can *learn* how to de-tense, to be passive, inactive, receptive and to heed the great psychologist Fritz Perls's invitation to "lose your mind and come to your senses." In this chapter, we will look at how to get the most

The sloth lives up—or down—to his reputation: he sleeps 20 hours a day, a mammalian record. By contrast, Dall's porpoise and the shrew do not sleep at all. Human beings usually sleep about eight hours.

out of doing the least. This includes techniques for sleeping well, obtaining rest that is equivalent to sleep, breathing deeply, meditating, relieving tension in both mind and body and, finally, indulging in the ultimate lift for sagging spirits and frayed nerves—the relaxing bath.

SLEEP FUNCTIONING AND CHEMISTRY

Interestingly, the latest scientific research seems to bear out our instinct that sleep is nature's balm. Although the function of sleep has yet to be determined, many researchers agree with Edinburgh biochemist D. J. Bruce Durie, Ph.D., that "sleep is an absolute necessity to repair the ravages of the day."

The two kinds of sleep—dream sleep, or REM sleep (named for the Rapid Eye Movements made by the dreamer), and non-REM sleep, or non-dreaming sleep—both appear to be involved in cell repair and recharging our batteries. There is evidence that growth hormone production and protein synthesis are stepped up in non-REM sleep. Some of these products are then used for repair of brain tissue during REM sleep, according to a theory set forth by Ernest L. Hartmann, M.D., director of the Boston State Hospital Sleep and Dream Laboratory, in his book, *The Functions of Sleep.*

If scientists don't yet know the *why* of sleep, they are starting to get a handle on the *how* of it. In the past few years, no less than three research groups, in Japan, Switzerland and the U.S., have isolated small protein chains called peptides from the fluid surrounding the brains of animals that are sleep-deprived. When these peptides are injected into the cerebro-spinal fluid of wide-awake animals, slumber soon follows.

These peptides are neurotransmitters, that is, they carry chemically coded messages from one part of the nervous system to receptors on the cells of another part. In this case, the message is ''go to sleep.'' In other words, says Harvard sleep researcher J. Allan Hobson, M.D., ''the brain manufactures its own sedatives.''

SLEEP AND AGING

There is a clear-cut link between sleep and growing older, although the reason for this is not known. ''Nothing that scientists can measure changes as much with age as do sleep patterns,'' says Irwin Feinberg, M.D., former director of the sleep laboratory and professor of psychiatry at New York University. ''And there is nothing that changes sleep patterns as much as normal aging.''

The newborn baby sleeps an average of 16–18 hours a day, with fully half that time spent in REM sleep. By the time a child is five years old, REM sleep has declined to 25 percent of total sleep time, where it remains through most of adulthood until dropping sharply again in old age.

The folk wisdom that older people have trouble sleeping has been amply borne out in studies by Dr. Feinberg and others. One takes longer to fall asleep, wakes much more frequently, and has far less Stage 4 sleep, the deepest slumber of all.

Our biorhythms also change with age, according to Elliot D. Weitzman, M.D., director of the Sleep-Wake Disorder Center at New York's Montefiore Hospital Medical Center. Instead of the dominant circadian (literally, around the day) rhythm of youth in which you sleep all night and are up all day, you move into a cycle in which the 24-hour day is divided into ''multiple sleep-wake segments.'' This means little naps in the daytime and many awakenings at night. ''People develop a shorter sleep time,'' says Dr. Weitzman. ''Instead of waking at seven o'clock, they wake at five or six. But they do not stay up as late at night as they used to—they want to go to bed at 10 instead of midnight. So there is a definite phase shift here.''

By understanding these changes in sleep patterns and biorhythms with age, we can adjust ourselves accordingly. Rather than resort to pills or alcohol to get the sleep we think we need, we should realize, as Dr. Weitzman puts it, that ''this is simply one of the things that happens when you get older.''

HOW MUCH SLEEP SHOULD YOU GET?

''The night and day is 24 hours. It is enough for a man to sleep one third of them,'' wrote the 12th-century physician and philosopher, Maimonides. In the light of modern sleep studies, does this prescription still hold? Yes and no.

Looking at two of the largest U.S. surveys of lifestyle factors related to mortality statistics, it appears that there is a correlation between sleeping seven to eight hours a night and living longer. One study, carried out by the American Cancer Society, involved more than a million persons who had died from all causes over a six-year period. In evaluating

Awake   Stage 1   S

the sleep data that had been collected incidental to the study, Daniel F. Kripke, M.D., head of the sleep disorders clinic at the Veterans Administration Hospital in La Jolla, California, found that short (less than four hours) sleepers and long (more than 10 hours) sleepers had two to three times the death rate of those who slept an average of seven to eight hours.

> **"** . . . It appears that there is a correlation between sleeping seven to eight hours a night and living longer **"**

Dr. Kripke's findings are essentially confirmed by the second study of almost 7,000 persons in Alameda County, conducted by Lester Breslow, M.D., M.P.H., dean of the School of Public Health at the University of California in Los Angeles, and his colleague, Nedra B. Belloc. The Breslow-Belloc study, which began 14 years ago and is still going on, found that maintaining a regimen of seven good health habits, such as eating breakfast, not smoking, getting moderate exercise and sleeping seven to eight hours a night, was positively related to being healthier and living longer.

The problem with these and other studies of lifestyle factors, as numerous critics have pointed out, is that they do not sufficiently resolve the chicken-and-egg dilemma of which came first. That is, do people live longer because among other things they are sleeping seven to eight hours a night, or are people who get a ''normal'' amount of sleep healthier to begin with?

In addition, sleep needs can vary enormously from one person to another and even within the same person at different times of life. The record sleep sprinter, according to laboratory studies, appears to be a 70-year-old woman who, since the age of 14, has been sleeping about 52 minutes a night!

Your mood can also influence the amount of sleep you require. Greater stress, anxiety and life changes step up our demand for sleep, says Dr. Hartmann. On the other hand, when we are content with our lives, we can get along on less sleep.

There even appears to be a personality difference between those who sleep less than six hours and those who average more than nine hours. Short sleepers, says Dr. Hartmann, tend to be extroverts who breeze through the day taking life in their stride. Long sleepers are the worriers who take things and themselves very seriously.

To figure out your own sleep needs, go to bed at the same hour for several nights, note what time you awaken, and how you feel throughout the day. If you awake feeling rested and are not excessively sleepy during the day, you are probably getting the right amount for you.

For a more complete picture of your sleep habits, Charles Pollak, M.D., co-director of the Sleep-Wake Disorders Unit at Montefiore, recommends keeping a record of your sleep time, including naps, for a month and then averaging it out. ''You can assume that the average is pretty much a reflection of your natural tendency.''

Once you have determined how much sleep you need, you can try cutting down if you wish. One way to do this is to set your alarm back 15 minutes every week. Another way is

REM sleep (Rapid Eye Movements, made by the dreamer) and non-REM (or non-dreaming) sleep both appear to be involved in recharging our batteries.

Stage 3   Stage 4   REM

to cultivate the art of the catnap (see the section on relaxation). If you have flexible hours, you can try Dr. Hartmann's special sleep formula for those who want to get in as much work as possible: Go to bed at 11:00 PM and sleep for two hours. This gives you most of your deep sleep. Then get up, work for six hours and go back to bed at 7:00 AM for three more hours of early morning sleep when the REM period is at its height.

While not all sleep researchers believe that reducing sleep is a good idea, they do agree that a skipped night of sleep is no more serious than a skipped meal. Even prolonged periods of no sleep are relatively harmless. It is true that experts in brainwashing techniques have combined sleep deprivation, isolation and emotional turmoil to weaken their subject's hold on reality. But under normal circumstances most people, including Roger Guy English who spent 12 weeks awake in one stretch, are perfectly fine after one night's makeup for the missed sleep.

HOW TO FALL ASLEEP

If you have trouble sleeping either chronically or just once in a while, here are a dozen different things you can do for yourself. Remember that sleep is a very individual matter so you may have to try several techniques before finding the one that works for you.

1. AVOID SLEEPING PILLS

The sad, shocking truth about insomnia is that one of its main causes is chronic use of sleeping pills. While pills may tide you over a crisis situation for two or three nights, they are definitely not for longer use. Almost all of them are habit-forming, suppress REM sleep, and lose their effectiveness after two weeks. In a classic series of studies, husband-and-wife psychiatrists Anthony and Joyce Kales, director and associate director, respectively, of the Sleep Research and Treatment Center of the Pennsylvania State University Medical School, found that pill addicts took as long to fall asleep and awakened more times than insomniacs not on medication. Furthermore, when the pill popper tried to go "cold turkey," a rebound effect occurred in which the insomnia worsened and sleep, when it came, was racked by vivid, disturbing dreams.

At this point there is no hypnotic that is completely effective or safe. The Food and Drug Administration has proposed new standards for ingredients used in all over-the-counter sleep aids. And prescription drugs, including the older barbiturates and the newer benzodiazepines (Dalmine, Valium, Librium, etc.) have side effects ranging from death due to overuse in the first group to interference with coordination and alertness in the second group.

2. FOLLOW GOOD SLEEP HYGIENE

No coffee, strong tea, or alcohol at night. Caffeine-sensitive people should also limit their breakfast coffee to one cup. A recent study also showed that chronic cigarette smoking adds to sleep difficulties. Except for sex, avoid stimulating mental or physical activity several hours before bedtime. Most important: Don't take your work to bed with you.

3. CHOOSE A CONDUCIVE SLEEP ENVIRONMENT

Insomniacs generally have a lower threshold of physiological arousal. Cut down on sensory stimulation by having an uncluttered bedroom, drapes or shades to make it as dark as possible, and some way to screen out noise. The low hum of an air conditioner or a sound-tranquilizing machine with settings for surf or rain can block out noise as it lulls you to sleep. Keep the room at a comfortable, coolish temperature; vaporize if necessary. It is extremely difficult to sleep in a stuffy, dry, overheated room.

4. MAINTAIN REGULAR HOURS

Put your biorhythms to work for you by sticking fairly close to a sleep schedule. "Timing is critical," says Dr. Pollak. "If you go to bed too late or get up too early, you shift the timing of sleep and move it into hours when it ought not to occur."

5. FIND A SLEEP RITUAL

Unconscious ceremonies at bedtime, such as closing doors and making lists keep some people awake for hours. But a conscious ritual that becomes inextricably associated with drowsiness can be a sleep aid. Choose a pleasant, not too stimulating activity, such as reading a light book (or a boring one), doing a crossword puzzle or watching TV.

6. EXERCISE

A half-hour of vigorous exercise a day is one of the best assurances of sleep at night. According to Lenore Zohman, M.D., director of the cardiopulmonary unit at New York's Montefiore Hospital and Medical Center, many people who start a walking or jogging program find they not only sleep better but need to sleep less. While strenuous exercise is best done in the morning or afternoon, mild activity in the evening, such as an after-dinner stroll, can help you unwind and loosen your muscles, a big plus for bedtime.

7. EAT A WELL-BALANCED DINNER

Researchers at St. George's Medical School in London found that meals high in carbohydrate and low in fat reduced non-REM sleep and increased dream sleep. The reverse—high fat and low starch—also caused more dreaming but did not affect non-REM sleep. A well-balanced meal produced the most balanced sleep pattern.

8. TRY NATURE'S SLEEPING PILL

L-tryptophan, an amino acid found in high concentrations in protein-rich foods, such as milk, meat and fish, has sedative properties.

Hence the rationale behind the old-fashioned sleep remedy of hot milk before retiring. At this point you have to eat your L-tryptophan because the pill form has not yet been approved for use by the Food and Drug Administration.

9. RESET YOUR BIOCLOCK

All sorts of things can throw your body out of kilter: jet-lag, late-night cramming, working night shifts. But some people have inborn body rhythms that are out of sync with the rest of society: the so-called larks and owls. If, for instance, you tend to stay up later and later on days off from work and find it terri-

> **"** *A skipped night of sleep is no more serious than a skipped meal; even prolonged periods of no sleep are relatively harmless* **"**

bly difficult to adjust to a routine schedule, you may be suffering from Delayed Sleep Phase Syndrome. The way to deal with this, according to Dr. Weitzman, is to shift your body clock *ahead* by going to bed three hours later rather than earlier. If you keep rotating your sleep schedule in this manner, eventually you reach the point where you are maintaining conventional hours. The reason you move forward rather than back is that you can force yourself to keep awake but not to go to sleep. A similar approach can be used for jet lag. If you are planning to fly across more than two time zones, phase-shift yourself ahead for a few days before your flight so that you are closer to local time when you reach your destination. Unfortunately, expe-

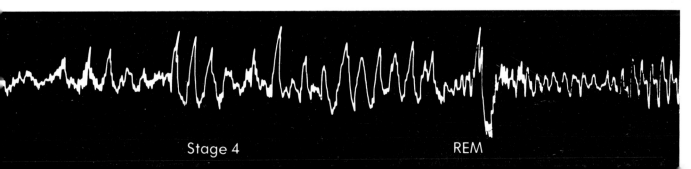

Stage 4   REM

rience has shown that there is little you can do to adjust to night work, except to find another job if your body continually rebels.

10. DECONDITION YOURSELF

This behavior-modification self-help program was developed for chronic insomniacs by Richard Bootsin, Ph.D., a psychologist at Northwestern University. About 60 percent of those who have tried it—including people who have been on sleeping pills for years—have found it very effective, according to Dr. Bootsin. If you attempt this program, keep it up for several weeks. "It feels awful, the first night," he says, but it gets easier as you go along. The six rules (no cheating allowed) are as follows:

- *Go to bed only when tired.*
- *Don't use your bed for anything but sleep. (Dr. Bootsin does bend the rules to allow sex.)*
- *If you can't fall asleep after 20 minutes, leave the bedroom and read, watch TV or do your worrying in another room.*
- *Return to bed when you're ready to sleep. If you still can't go off in 20 minutes, go back to the preceding step. Keep this up all night if necessary until you fall asleep.*
- *Set the alarm for the same time every day and get up when it rings regardless of how tired you are. Don't sleep for more than one extra hour on the weekend.*
- *Cut out all naps.*

11. PRACTICE RELAXATION

Unwind after a busy day by trying one of the techniques or the relaxing bath, all described in the next section of this chapter.

12. DON'T PANIC

The greatest enemy of sleep is worrying about not getting enough of it. Regardless of how much sleep you miss, your body will make up for it. If you're lying in bed wide awake, read a book and let sleep sneak up on you. Or give up altogether and use the extra hours for doing something that you never seem to find time for during the day. Just bear in mind the words of Dr. Pollak: "Nobody dies of insomnia and no one can stay awake forever."

REST AND RELAXATION

Tension, anxiety, stress—these are the hallmarks of modern life. To avoid them completely is not to live. It is how you handle them that makes the difference between coping successfully with life's challenges or collapsing under the strain. And you must learn to do this in your own way. The highly competitive workaholic usually relaxes best with a demanding activity, such as playing chess or a hard game of squash. For these people, the more inactive they are, the tenser they get.

Unfortunately, Western culture gears us for working, competing, thinking on our feet, meeting the demands of a hurry-up society. Only recently have we become aware of the need to cultivate the nonverbal, nonrational side prized in the Orient. Through Eastern techniques of yoga, meditation, deep breathing, as well as adaptation of these methods for Western use, many people are learning to tap new sources of energy, liberate the mind and body and achieve a sense of renewal. The health benefits of the techniques described below are well documented. All of them can help you attain a more relaxed state, revive your energy, focus your concentration, and contribute to a longer, healthier life.

DEEP BREATHING

Inspiration. It is no accident that the same word refers to stimulation of the artistic and creative impulses as well as the physiological act of breathing. The double meaning is contained in the Latin root, *spiritus*, which signifies both mortal breath and the breath of a god.

To reach the height of your own inspiration, you must learn to breathe fully and deeply. Complete breaths that expand and contract the lungs benefit both mind and body. As Gay Gaer Luce notes in her book, *Your Second Life,* "When breathing becomes deeper and slower the heart does not have to beat so fast. Heart rate may drop from 72 beats a minute to 50 or 40. The heart is no longer having to work so hard . . . the blood pressure drops, the body relaxes and the nervous system becomes calm."

The extra oxygen to the muscles and nerves also releases tension and energy, making available hidden sources of inspiration. "Our bodies store all the history of our experience and so we may experience memories and stored feelings as we make contact with our muscles," writes Luce.

There are two forms of deep breathing, one from the West and one from the East, that are the exact opposites of each other and yet accomplish the same results: release of muscular and emotional tension. The Western technique of deep abdominal breathing is simply an extension of the way most of us breathe normally. To do it, sit comfortably erect with both feet on the floor and take a few long, relatively slow deep breaths. Make sure each time to exhale fully before inhaling. Try to draw the breath way down into the lower abdomen, advises Luce. "Your chest will only move at the very end of the breath. This means that your lungs extend fully and fill completely with air."

If you start to feel dizzy, stop! You are hyperventilating, that is, you're exhaling too much carbon dioxide. But with practice, your body automatically adjusts to the new levels of oxygen and carbon dioxide generated by deep breathing.

The second technique is the Taoist method of reverse breathing developed in China more than 2,000 years ago for advanced students of Tai Chi. In this form of deep breathing, the abdomen moves *in* rather than out with each inhalation, allowing the chest to balloon with air. As Korean-born Tai Chi Master Don Ahn explains it: "If you want to expand the lungs to their maximum, you have to let the abdomen pull in. As that happens, you not only see the chest expanding, but you can see that you are moving your entire spine and exercising each vertebra along its length. The internal energy moves up to the neck and head.

"When you're actually doing reverse breathing, the inhale is one relaxed but active movement. You then let out your breath in a totally inactive, relaxed exhale, which should last only half as long as the inhale, but still expel all the air."

What does Taoist reverse breathing do for you? It helps stretch and straighten the spine, unblock muscle tension and release strong, locked-in emotions, says Ahn, whose school, the Ahn Tai Chi Studio, is located in SoHo in New York City. "These are not things you want to do suddenly without understanding or supervision," he warns. "I think people trying reverse breathing on their own should limit themselves to about five minutes. The emotional as well as physical results can be hard to handle."

DE-TENSERS

Tension isn't just a feeling in the muscles or moist palms. Think of those wind-up toys in the five-and-ten-cent stores: little men beating drums for all they're worth, tin bears turning tight circles, waddling ducks endlessly flapping their hinged wings. If you ever feel like you're one of those toys at the end of a tightly coiled spring, going nowhere fast, out of control as though someone else were turning the key—that's tension!

It's a robber of sleep, a depleter of energy, an anti-beautifier, an underminer of health and well-being. We all suffer occasionally from its effects and we all should learn ways of dealing with it that are constructive and beneficial. Sometimes small changes in lifestyle can have a ripple effect, widening your perspective and opening up new channels for self-discovery and awareness. Here are some time-honored de-tensers:

1 Take a tea break. Emulate the English and enjoy the mild stimulation of a cup of tea in the late-afternoon hours when most people's biorhythms are ebbing.

2 Take a walk. Get out, leave your environment, enjoy new sounds and sights, feel the pulse of energy when you move.

3 Work it out. In most instances, writes stress pioneer Hans Selye in his book, *Stress Without Distress,* "diversion from one activity to another is more relaxing than complete rest." Oddly enough, when you feel overburdened and overworked, throwing yourself into a task like cleaning your drawers or painting a bookcase can do wonders for relieving tension.

4 Cultivate the art of the catnap. When you're feeling knocked out, sit—don't lie down—and let yourself slowly nod out. Try counting backwards from ten letting your breath come slower and head drop lower with each count. The trick is to keep the nap shorter than twenty minutes. The shorter, the better. After waking, sit a few minutes until your head clears. Once you have the knack, you can go into the deepest sleep for the briefest period of time and wake with new-found energy.

5 Do something different. Walk a new way to work, explore another neighborhood, experiment with a daring hairstyle, but something that is not "you." Breaking out of your old routine can revitalize your jaded senses.

6 Let go. There are two keys to letting go, says psychiatrist R. W. Shepherd, M.D. First is the readiness to do nothing. Second is the acceptance of its effortlessness. "Letting go means simply letting things happen, not making them happen," says Dr. Shepherd. "This means surrendering to not doing, or, better said, to letting something else do for you." Shut off your mind, he advises, and let your nonrational, nonverbal side do the work. Try giving in to your impulses rather than being afraid of them. Gain control by giving it up.

7 Take a vacation. Dispense with the idea of your indispensability. Try going away on a moment's notice. Take a weekend, a week, whatever you can manage. Tell yourself you deserve it. Pack your bags and leave your guilt at home.

8 Learn to play. Play is liking what you are doing and doing what you like, It may be a competitive game of tennis, carrying out an exacting experiment, winning a contract. "The person who faces life with a play spirit sees the world as a toy," says Laurence Morehouse, Ph.D., professor of kinesiology at UCLA and author of *Maximum Performance.* "Life is very exciting. It's something to explore."

You are never too old or too dignified to play. "The qualities of childhood carried into adulthood keep us young and healthy," says anthropologist Ashley Montagu. "The tremendous capacity for learning, the endless curiosity, open-mindedness, the need to experiment, the imagination, sensitivity, sense of humor and playfulness—all these qualities are designed to develop as long as we live."

THREE RELAXATION TECHNIQUES

1. DEEP MUSCLES RELAXATION

This anti-stress technique slows heart and respiration rate, lowers blood pressure, and leaves you as rejuvenated as after a good night's sleep. It takes about two weeks to do it well and after that fifteen minutes once or twice a day is ideal. With practice, you can go limp for the minute and a half that it takes the traffic light to change.

● *Sit or lie down on your back in a quiet place. Close your eyes.*
● *Starting with your right side, tense hand and relax it. Tell it to feel heavy, limp, warm. Continue doing the same thing up forearm, upper arm, shoulder, then foot, lower leg, upper leg.*
● *Do same progression on left side. Once you have a secure awareness of all your muscles, you can skip the tensing.*
● *Go on to relax muscles from hips up through abdomen to chest (no tensing). Tell muscles to feel heavy, limp, warm. Your breathing should slow and come more from diaphragm than chest.*
● *Now let relaxation flow into shoulders, neck, jaw, face muscles, especially around eyes and forehead. Final touch: tell your forehead to feel cool.*

2. RELAXATION RESPONSE

This 20th-century, Western form of meditation was devised by Herbert Benson, associate professor of medicine at Harvard Medical School and director of the Division of Behavioral Medicine at Boston's Beth Israel Hospital. The age-old practice of repetitive prayer, mystical meditation and chanting, Dr. Benson found, all elicit an altered state of consciousness he calls the "relaxation response." A sense of calm, peace of mind and complete relaxation generally accompany this response. A few individuals even experience ecstasy. But regardless of the subjective feeling, the astonishing fact is the physical benefits are the same: a decrease in blood pressure, heart rate and respiratory rate and a rise in Alpha waves, the brain wave associated with relaxation and a sense of well-being.

Here's how to do it: Sit in a comfortable position and close your eyes. Beginning with your feet, deeply relax all your muscles finishing with your face. (You can use the previous exercise to do this). Keeping your muscles in a relaxed state, become aware of your breathing. (Breathe through your nose only.) Silently repeat a syllable, word or phrase on each exhalation. Let your breath flow easily and naturally. Maintain a passive attitude throughout. If distracting thoughts occur, don't dwell on them. Return to repeating the word you have chosen. Do this for 10–20 minutes, checking the time if you wish, but don't use an alarm. After you have finished, sit quietly for several minutes, first with eyes closed, then open. Do not stand up for a few minutes.

Don't worry about how you're doing, says Dr. Benson. After a while, you should be able to evoke the response quickly with little effort. He recommends doing it once or twice a day, but not within two hours after eating. To learn more about this technique, read Dr. Benson's book, *The Relaxation Response.*

3. PROGRESSIVE RELAXATION

Developed 50 years ago by Edmund Jacobson, M.D., Ph.D., this granddaddy of all modern relaxation methods is as popular today. It detenses all the body's approximately 1,000 skeletal muscles and can be used for going to sleep as well as conserving the body's energies during waking activities.

"If you are as limp as a rag doll, you are then truly relaxed," according to Dr. Jacobson. The opposite state is tension, which he defines as "the shortening of muscle fibers, which can be reversed." The more muscles contract, the higher the discharge activity in the nerves leading to and from the muscles. Signs of nervous tension include tightness in the neck, shoulders back and chest; headaches; constipation, diarrhea, and "chronic indigestion"; feelings of uneasiness and phobias. Nervous tension contributes to high blood pressure, peptic ulcer, spastic colon and heart attacks. "It seems not too much to say that tension disorders are the modern plague," says Dr. Jacobson.

The essence of Dr. Jacobson's technique is to develop a fine sense of muscle awareness that allows you to detect hidden tension and then let it go. He calls his technique "progressive relaxation" because you systematically learn to isolate and then relax the muscles in each group, going from muscle group to muscle group, until you reach the ultimate goal of total relaxation. Here is the progression (the technique is practiced lying down and then in a sitting position): Right arm, right leg, left arm, left leg, trunk, neck, forehead, brow, eyelids, eyes, visual imagery (the eye muscle tension accompanying visual imagination), cheeks, jaws, lips, tongue, the speech apparatus (includes the muscles of the tongue, lips, jaws, chest and diaphragm).

Remember that every effort is accompanied by tension. The trick is to "go negative," says Dr. Jacobson. For the same reason, you do not give yourself suggestions, such as "my arms are becoming heavy." "Learn to relax as you might learn to dance or swim," he says. Complete relaxation of the eye and speech apparatus usually leads to sleep within half a minute. And, claims Dr. Jacobson, the sleep of a trained relaxer is the most restful of all.

The full course—which takes an hour a day, every day, for two months to learn in its entirety—is outlined in Dr. Jacobson's book, *You Must Relax*. If you wish to study the technique with a qualified professional, write to the National Foundation of Progressive Relaxation, 55 East Washington Street, Suite 311, Chicago, Illinois 60602.

THE RELAXING BATH

From the Roman baths of Caracalla to California hot tubs, a luxurious soak has been synonymous with the ultimate in pleasure and relaxation. Of course, a bath need not be a social ritual, but rather the essence of privacy, the chance to get away from it all and go into a world of your own making.

A bath can be healing, restorative, soporific or invigorating. Use the bath time to mull over the day's positive events, plan the evening, fantasize or meditate. To make the most of your bath experience, try some of the suggestions below. Remember, the more total the pleasure, the more you can let go. And that, of course, is the idea—to indulge yourself, to give in to your hedonistic tendencies, to do something that is just for you.

THE BATH ENVIRONMENT

Begin by choosing the right setting. Even a small bathroom can be made inviting. Fill the space with flowers and plants that love a moisture-filled room. Grow-bulbs can substitute for sun, but turn them off while bathing since they are not particularly attractive. Rugs or a carpet are warm, absorbent, silencing, a touch of softness in all that tile.

Bring all your senses into play. Enlarge the space artfully with mirrors. Hang paintings, prints, collections of pretty things to delight the eye. Color the water yellow with lemon slices and lemon-scented bath oil the way they do in Japanese inns, or Mediterranean blue-green or milky white. Scent your bath with oils, crystals or powders. Or use various herbs in and around the tub to suit your mood. Jean Rose, an expert on aroma-therapy and author of *Herbs & Things* recommends sassafras, cedar and hemlock (the nonpoisonous variety) for meditation; carnation as an aphrodisiac; rose and sandalwood for tranquility. Keep a cassette recorder or small portable radio (at a safe distance) so that you can hear

WARM-UPS

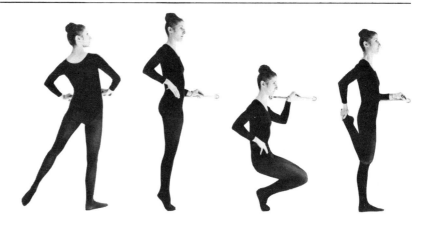

● *Use towel rack as a bar for support. There should be no tension in shoulders. Left: Raise one leg behind, tightening muscles in back of thigh and buttocks. Lower leg. Repeat with other leg. Center left and center right, with one hand on bar for support, rise on toes, then lower body* *slowly, moving hips in bump-and-grind motion. Keeping on toes, slowly return to standing position. Right: Supporting yourself with one hand on towel rack, lift outside leg back with knee bent. Grasp foot with free hand and pull. Turn around and repeat on other side.*

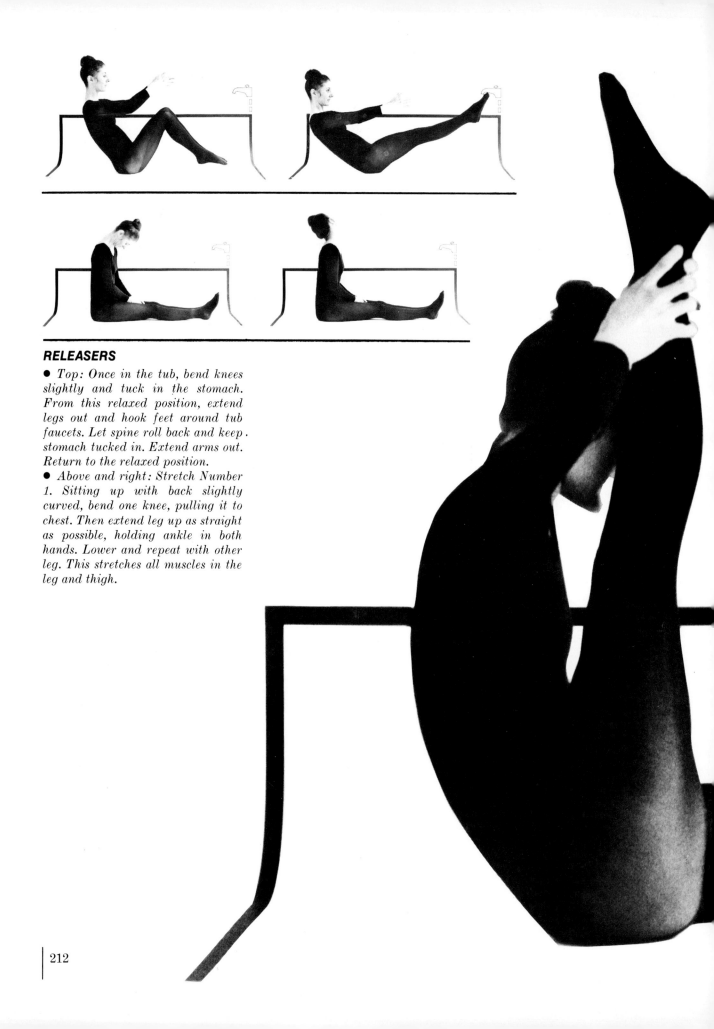

RELEASERS

● *Top: Once in the tub, bend knees slightly and tuck in the stomach. From this relaxed position, extend legs out and hook feet around tub faucets. Let spine roll back and keep stomach tucked in. Extend arms out. Return to the relaxed position.*

● *Above and right: Stretch Number 1. Sitting up with back slightly curved, bend one knee, pulling it to chest. Then extend leg up as straight as possible, holding ankle in both hands. Lower and repeat with other leg. This stretches all muscles in the leg and thigh.*

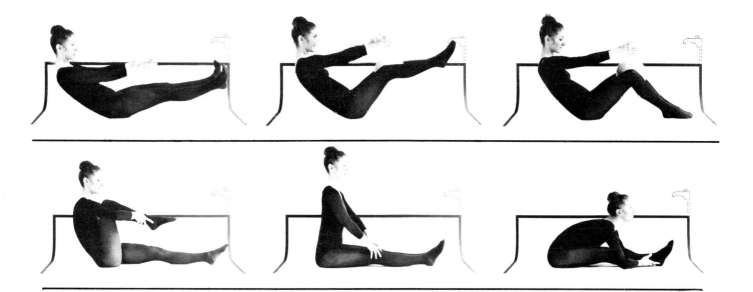

- *Top left: An Isometric. Press heels against end of tub and push. This works muscles of the entire leg. Shoulders should be rounded, as this stretches the lower back and abdomen. Stretch arms out and tense the body except for the shoulders and neck. Release.*
- *Top center and right: Place a small beach ball between your knees, squeeze the ball, holding in with inner thigh muscles; feel the pull through buttocks and stomach (if you need to, hold onto your knees for support). Release. Next, hold the ball tight between knees again and extend legs out as far as possible. Don't exceed your endurance.*
- *Above, opposite and left: Neck Roll. For relaxation after stretches. Sitting up straight, let head roll around from front to side to back, feeling the tension released in the neck and shoulder area.*
- *Above center and right: Stretch Number 2: Sit normally, lifting up from the hip to get back completely straight. Extend arms out to grasp ankles and pull chin down to the knees.*

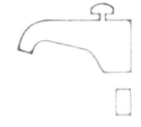

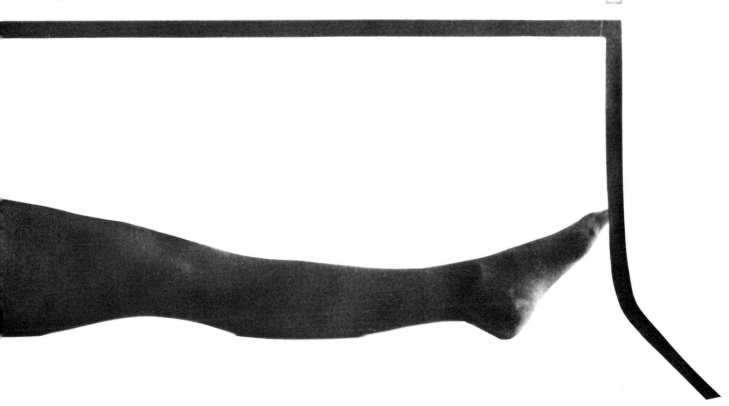

your favorite music. Add slim shelves or a small table to keep magazines and books within reach. These can also hold a cool glass of water—a good idea for replacing body water lost in perspiration and dehydration in a warm tub—or a goblet of wine. The last sense is the sense of touch. Stack a goodly supply of sponges, loofahs, scented soaps and gels nearby and then just mix with warm water to complete one of the most sensuous of experiences.

HARD VS. SOFT WATER

If your bath water leaves a ring of soap around the tub, it is hard. Hard water is healthier for drinking than soft, which has been associated with increased incidence of heart attack, but it is a poor rinser, produces less lather and is unkind to skin. Try softening your water by adding bath salts containing sodium derivatives rather than Epsom or rock salts. Use a synthetic soap that can be completely rinsed off, rather than a medicated soap (unless you're under doctor's orders). Bubble baths, gels and oils can also help soften bath water and skin. For best results, install a water-conditioning device to remove minerals.

BATH TEMPERATURE

Be as finicky with the bath water as Goldilocks with her porridge. Too-hot water dries out your skin, causes spidery looking capillaries to form, exhausts rather than relaxes, and can be dangerous for anyone with pulmonary or circulatory problems. Too-cold shocks your system. For a just-right feeling, envelop your body with water at your own internal temperature: between 98 and 99 degrees Fahrenheit. Elbows are good, but a water thermometer is better to ensure a temperature that soothes without putting to sleep. For a quick pick-me-up at the end of the bath, let water temperature slide down to a cool 70° to 85°F.

BATH TIME

Fifteen minutes is all you need to put yourself back together again. Never stay more than 20–25 minutes or your skin will pucker

like a prune. Water is nature's moisturizer, but, like too much of any good thing, oversoaking has a detrimental effect, in this case dehydrating the skin.

SPECIAL BATHS

THE UNWINDER

On really stressful days, let the water gently trickle into the tub, so it has the restful sound of a Moorish fountain in the garden of the Alhambra. Ease yourself into the warm water and then sit up straight, letting your head loll front to side to back. Next, slowly stretch, submerging the tight muscles of neck, shoulders and spine until the water comes right to your chin. If you are really weary, rest your neck on a towel wrung out in cold water. Just lie back and do nothing. (Don't forget to unplug the phone.)

THE INSOMNIAC'S BATH

This one time, raise bath water a few degrees to get the full soporific effect. Try sipping a glass of warm milk while you're in the tub or reading a light book. Do everything you need to do before the bath, so you can take your drowsy body right to bed. Remember, don't stay in too long; the tub is not for sleeping.

THE SEA BATH

For a sea change, try pure sea salt from the health food store or mineral bath salts containing sulphur or algae. One such product is Algemarin Foam-Bath, which turns the water Adriatic blue and is filled with algae to revive your skin. Or try this bath recipe from *The Royal Swedish Longevity Diet + Weight Control Program* by Zina Provendie: Put one cup of packaged seaweed from your local herb shop into a heat-proof glass jar, cover with boiling water and steep for an hour. Strain and pour into bath for make-your-own seawater.

AFTERBATH

For the perfect afterbath glow, rub your body all over with a good moisturizing cream, lo-

A pleasure ritual: the bath. If your schedule keeps you constantly on-the-move, take a breather—with the sensuous revitalizing pleasures of the bath.

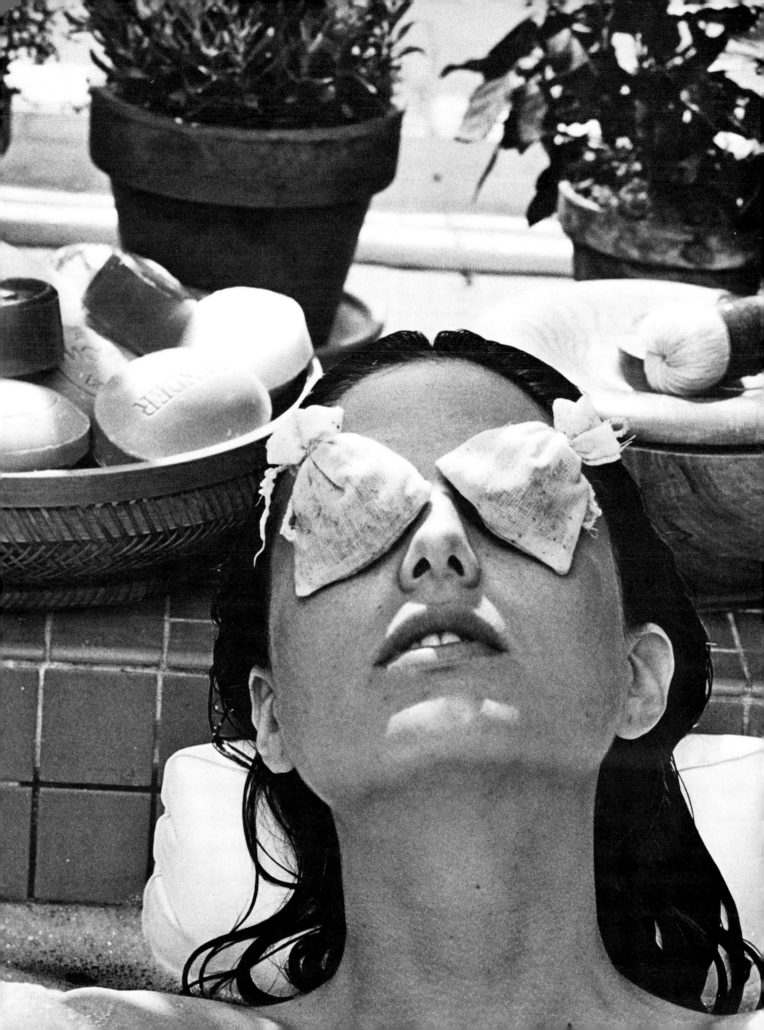

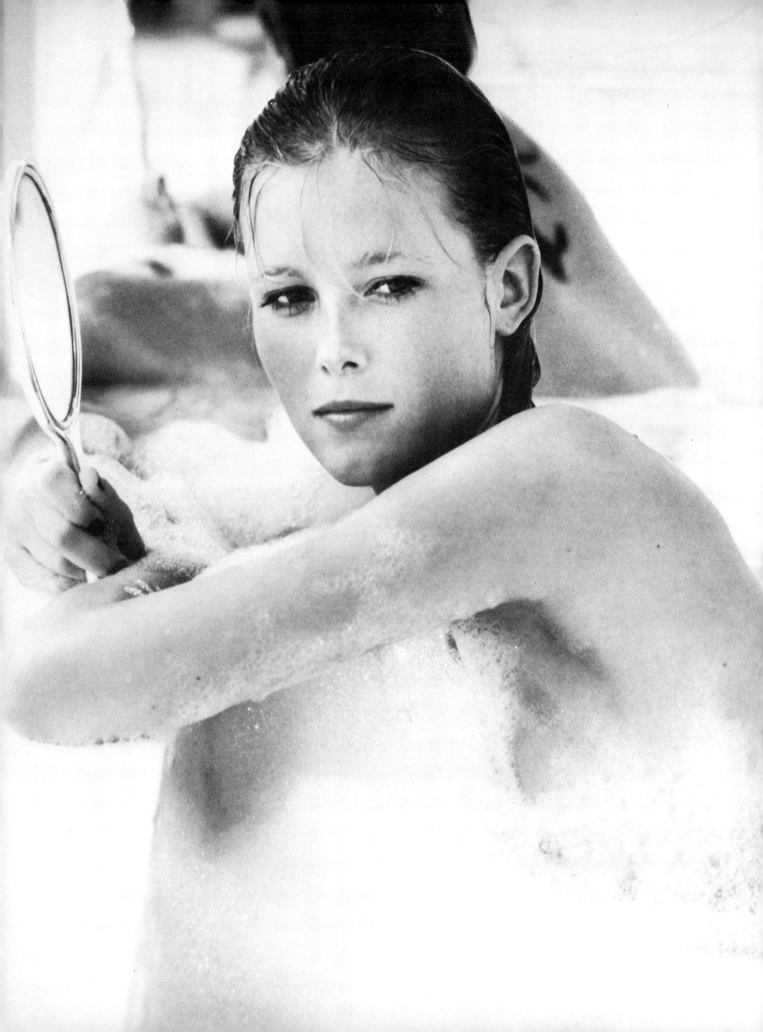

STRENGTHENERS

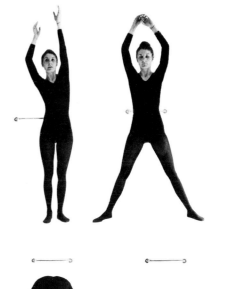

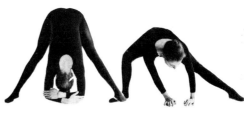

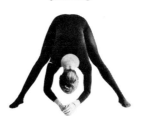

Final stretches and tension releasers after bath, out of tub. Stand up straight, stretch first one arm, then the other in an overhead reach. Then, with legs slightly apart, bend over from the waist, letting head and arms drop. Bend one knee and extend the other leg and stretch. Return to center position and repeat with other leg. Finally, straighten back with head and arms still dangling over. These are all excellent beauty revivers since they bring circulation coursing to the head and face, promoting a healthy flush.

217

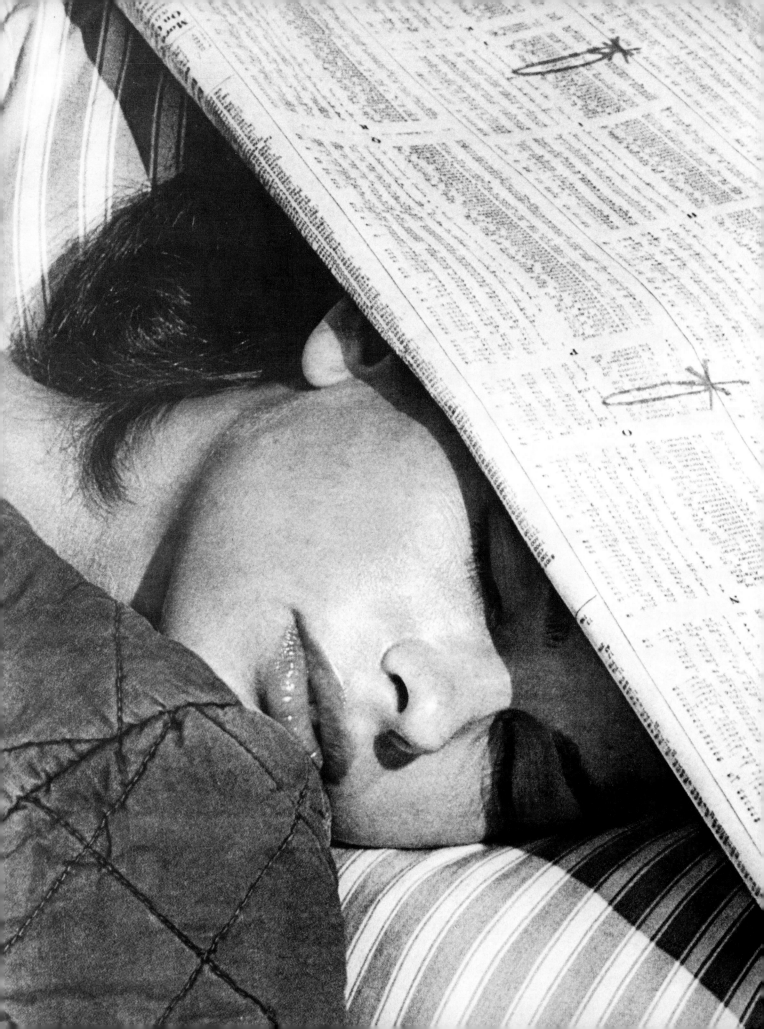

tion or oil. Do it while you're still damp to seal in the moisture, leave your skin soft and supple and enhance the relaxed feeling.

As a final touch, try a few of Andrea Hanson's stretches before leaving the bathroom. 1. Standing up straight, stretch first one arm then the other in an overhead reach. 2. With legs slightly apart, bend over from waist, letting head and arms drop. Then bend left knee and stretch. Straighten left leg and repeat stretch with right knee bent. Finally, straighten back with head and arms still dangling over. This will bring the blood coursing to your head and face and give your skin a rosy, healthy glow.

Make the six o'clock bath a daily ritual. It will cleanse your spirit as well as your body, rid you of the cares of the day and leave you rested, relaxed and refreshed for the evening to come.

CATNAPS

We all have our ups and downs during the day in which periods of sleepiness alternate with periods of alertness. Some sleep researchers believe that a Basic Rest Activity Cycle (BRAC) occurs every 90 minutes, which accounts for the successive phases of REM and non-REM sleep during the night and continues unnoticed throughout the day. "Presumably we become more active at 90-minute intervals both day and night," writes sleep pioneer Dr. William C. Dement in his book, *Some Must Watch While Some Must Sleep*. Fluctuations in body temperature and other biorhythms also contribute to how wide awake we feel at any given point during the day.

You can get through these low points by simply waiting for the upswing of the activity cycle or by sleeping through the worst of them. If you're not a natural napper, try this simple self-hypnosis, sleep-inducing technique. Sit—don't lie down—and say to yourself: "I am going to count from 10 to one and by the time I reach the count of one I will fall into a deep, restful sleep. I will sleep 15 minutes and when I awake, I will feel refreshed, alert and ready to go." Then begin counting, letting your breath come slower and head drop with each count. Once you get the knack, you can dispense with the ritual and go off at the drop of an eyelid.

The secret of a good catnap is its brevity. Too long a nap may cut into your normal sleep pattern. On the other hand, a quickie at your desk or in your armchair will provide a second wind that can carry you straight to bedtime.

Edison, Churchill, Muhammad Ali and Eleanor Roosevelt all made good use of short snoozes, but perhaps the most artful napper of them all is Salvador Dali. According to Dr. Dement, the Spanish surrealist sits in a chair beside a tin plate on the floor, holding a spoon over the plate as he starts to doze. "At the precise moment of sleep," says Dr. Dement, "the spoon slips from his fingers, clatters onto the plate and he is snapped awake. Dali claims he is completely refreshed by the sleep that accumulates between the time the spoon leaves his hand and the time it hits the plate."

" Cultivate the art of the catnap. . . . Once you have the knack, you can go into deepest sleep for the briefest period of time and wake with a new-found energy "

In the midst of a hectic day a catnap can revive sagging spirits and leave you feeling refreshed, alert.

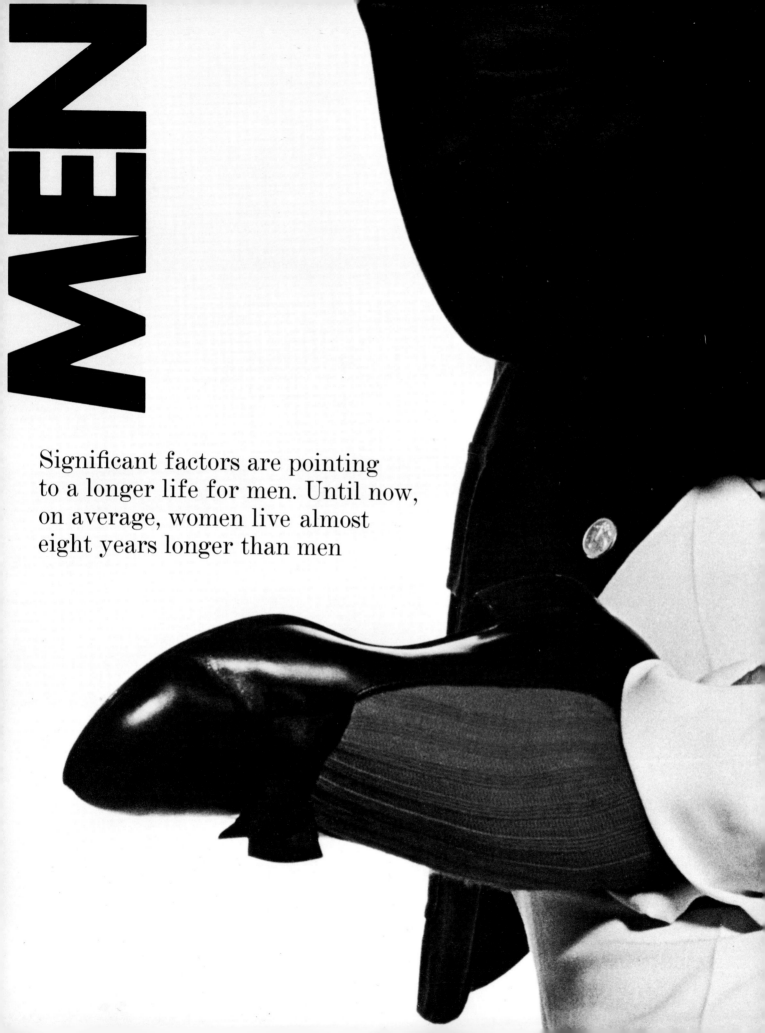

MEN

Significant factors are pointing
to a longer life for men. Until now,
on average, women live almost
eight years longer than men

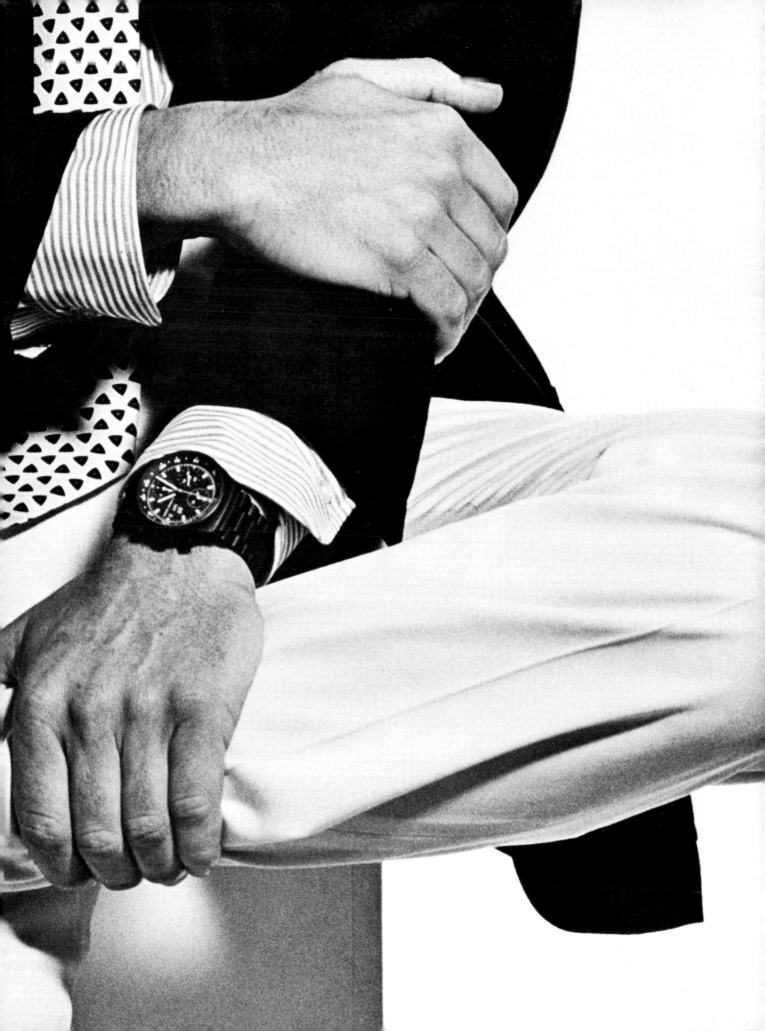

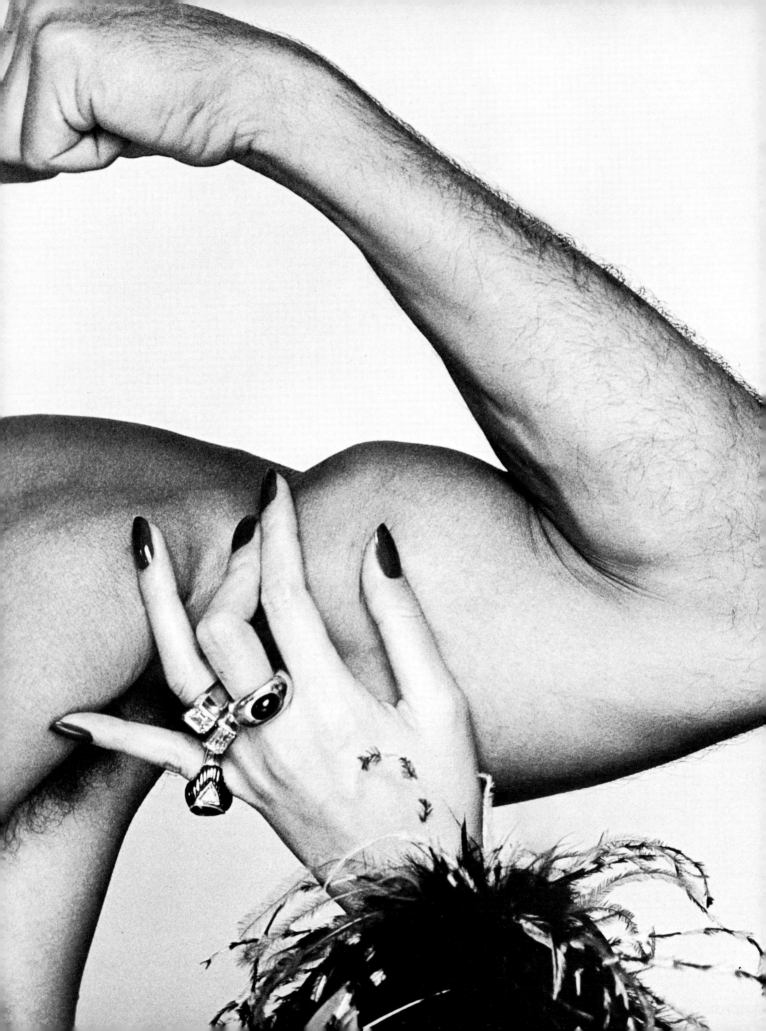

MEN: WILL YOU OUTLIVE THEM?

by Dr. William Bennett

Most men would disagree with A. E. Housman's congratulation to an athlete dying young. "Smart lad," he wrote, "to slip betimes away"—better to leave the field before the victory laurels could wither or the sound of cheering give way to silence.

Yet the poem captures a kind of truth about men and aging. There is a common image of the man who, after a burst of adolescent glory, settles in for a long period of relentless physical and sexual decay. Professional success comes in the middle years, but it often seems to be purchased at the price of bodily well-being. And, when all is said and done, men do die young. The overall mortality rate is 60 percent higher for men than women; on average, women live almost eight years longer than men.

Could it simply be men's fate to die young? It has often been argued that women have stronger constitutions than men, are better protected against illness by a strong immune system, for example, and suffer less from heart disease because female hormones seem to prevent atherosclerosis. Both of these factors probably do, indeed, play a minor role, but differences in the behavior of the two

It has often been argued that women have stronger constitutions than men and are better protected against illness by a strong immune system.

sexes appear to be more important by far, to the difference in their life expectancy. In effect, "men kill themselves off," as Dr. John S. Rowe, director of the Division of Gerontology at Harvard Medical School, puts it.

The single most important reason for early death in men is cigarette smoking. From the beginning of this century until the mid-1960s, the number of men who smoked cigarettes steadily increased. Few women smoked until after World War II. This difference in cigarette use alone, it is estimated, could account for one-third to one-half the difference in mortality.

Of the illnesses caused by smoking, heart disease begins to separate the men from the women after the age of 40; then, after age 60 cancer, especially cancer of the lung, becomes increasingly important in the mortality difference, as do the chronic lung diseases.

This picture can be expected to change, however, as men have begun to give up smoking in fairly large numbers. At present, a third of adult men smoke, as opposed to one-half of them just 15 years ago. Meanwhile, tragically, the rate of smoking among women has been climbing. As a result, by the end of this century, we may well see a relative increase in the number of old men and somewhat fewer old women.

Smoking is not the sole reason for the higher rates of heart disease in men. Aggressive, competitive behavior, which has traditionally been more typical of American men than women, also appears to be an important predisposing factor. One student of the subject, biologist Ingrid Waldron at the University of Pennsylvania, has "very roughly" estimated that this masculine trait may account for as much as one-sixth of the difference between male and female death rates.

Over 20 years ago, Dr. Meyer Friedman and Dr. R. H. Rosenman described a personality type in which aggression and competitive drive were dominant features, and they found that this personality ("Type A," as they called it) was associated with a high risk of heart attacks. According to Dr. Friedman, who is now director of the Harold Brunn Institute at Mount Zion Hospital in San Francisco, people of Type A depend excessively on the opinions of others for their own self-esteem. They thus become caught in a game they can't win; they push to achieve more and more, though not necessarily better and better, but satisfaction never comes. (Shakespeare, as you might have expected, provides one of the most vivid expressions of the Type A outlook; it is in Ulysses' famous speech to Achilles in *Troilus and Cressida:* "beauty, wit, high birth, vigor of bone, desert in service, love, friendship, charity," count for nothing, he says, after only a brief time has passed; what matters is new victories, not old virtues.)

Dr. Friedman observes that the dominant emotions of people who engage in this unending struggle become "irritation, impatience, aggravation and anger." The nervous and endocrine systems, in response to these feelings, bathe the heart and its blood vessels in a sea of adrenaline and other stress-related hormones, and the toll which must eventually be paid is a heart attack.

Proof that Type A behavior causes heart disease has yet to be found, even though the statistical association is quite strong and the physiological explanation is plausible. As Dr. Friedman points out, to prove that Type A

behavior causes heart attacks, it will be necessary to modify the behavior in a large number of patients and show that they suffer fewer heart attacks than they would have if left to their own devices. Such a study is under way with a group of patients who have already had one heart attack, but they must be followed for several years before the results can be known.

Will women entering the work force begin to suffer from Type A behavior and its consequences, just as men seem to have? A study of working women, reported early in 1980 by Suzanne G. Haynes and Manning Feinleib from the National Heart, Lung and Blood Institute, indicates that working women are more likely than housewives to display Type A behavior—and they complain more about job-related and other stresses than either men or housewives. But so far, working women have not shown a significantly greater rate of heart attacks than housewives. It is possible that all women are partially protected by their hormones from coronary heart disease,

" The single most important reason for early death in men is cigarette smoking. Meanwhile, tragically, the rate of smoking among women has been climbing "

and it is certainly true that women in general have a rather low rate of heart attacks before menopause. Increasingly, laboratory evidence indicates that the heart is capable of responding directly to both male and female hormones, but at the moment the story is getting more, not less, complicated.

Accidents, especially automobile accidents, also kill men more than women. To be sure, this is partly due to the fact that men drive more than women, but mile for mile, men have more accidents and more of the accidents are

224

fatal. Although traffic deaths involve fewer men than either heart disease or cancer, accidents happen to younger men; as a result, about as many years of life are lost to dangerous driving as to either of the main killer diseases.

Other types of accidents also take more male than female lives. Work hazards, though diminishing as time goes by, still affect more men than women, because more men work and they are exposed to more dangerous occupations. Shootings kill five times as many men as women, and many more men than women die from drowning. Dr. Waldron concludes that macho behavior is a significant risk factor for men. Being brave, taking risks, refusing to back out or back down—all of these classically "masculine" traits exact their toll of lives.

Taking a drink to provide false courage— or just taking a drink—is also more common among men than women. Alcohol contributes heavily to the accident rate and also leads to one major fatal illness: cirrhosis of the liver. Twice as many men as women die of cirrhosis, but this statistic, too, may change as alcoholism is becoming increasingly prevalent among women.

Suicide is also a distinctly male way to die —even though three times as many women as men attempt to kill themselves. Men are simply a great deal more successful at it: Twice as many men as women actually commit suicide, many of them in older age groups.

Dismal as this statistical landscape on first glance appears to be, it conceals a thoroughly optimistic prospect. If so much of the excess mortality of men is the result of their own behavior, and not just biological fate, we can look for relatively rapid change in the overall statistics, and individuals can hope to separate themselves from the statistical pack. The fall in cigarette smoking alone should have an enormous impact on mortality rates. Indeed, the death rate from heart attacks is already falling rapidly. It may take another 10 or 15 years before lung cancer begins to diminish, but in principle this is a disease that could virtually disappear if cigarette smoking were to go out of fashion.

Other social and psychological changes are harder to define, but they could make a large, if diffuse, contribution to lowering male death rates. A gradual de-emphasis of stereotyped masculine behavior could help men to abandon such trappings of machismo as the cigarette and the stiff drink. Recognition that Type A behavior usually is less productive than it appears to be may reduce the incentive to participate in "rat races" that lead mainly to an early grave. Less cheerful is the possibility that women will take up a number of these bad habits as part of their continuing emancipation.

“ Heart disease begins to separate the men from the women after age 40 ”

Changes in the pattern of marriage and divorce may also affect the mortality rate of men. Married men have, in the past, been much longer-lived than single, divorced or widowed men. By contrast, the life expectancy of women is little affected by marital status. It is simply not clear why married men live longer, although a number of rather obvious explanations leap to mind: Men are poorly trained to take care of themselves; men with self-destructive habits are unlikely to form stable relationships; men are more likely than women to benefit from psychological support in a marriage. Yet, despite a high divorce rate, the death rate of men is unlikely to rise for the reason that remarriage is common and relatively few men remain single for long periods of time.

Although aging gracefully may seem less important to men than sheer survival, knowing how to live well can lead to longer life. That, at least, is the conclusion reached by psychiatrist George E. Vaillant of Harvard

University. Late in 1979, Dr. Vaillant reported a new finding from a 40-year study (described in his book, *Adaptation to Life*) of 200 men who had been closely followed since they were in college. Dr. Vaillant and his coworkers measured the mental health of these men in a variety of ways. Independently, and with no knowledge of the men's psychological status, an internist assessed their physical health. When the two evaluations were compared, the investigators discovered that men with relatively poor psychological adjustment were the ones who went on to suffer most heavily from chronic illness or early death.

Using statistical methods to isolate the probable effects of alcohol use, smoking, obesity and heredity, Dr. Vaillant learned that the mental health rating was still highly significant as a predictor of physical health. Men who had not only been reasonably successful in their work but also knew how to enjoy leisure time, whose marriages were satisfying to them and who had no history of abusing

" Dismal as the statistical landscape on mortality may be at first glance, it conceals a thoroughly optimistic prospect "

drugs or alcohol, experienced few of the ailments that troubled men with poor psychological health.

Also in 1979, two other studies with similar results were published. One of them had followed graduates of Johns Hopkins Medical School over a 30-year period; it found that an "irregular and uneven" temperament was associated with a much higher rate of major illness than either the "slow and solid" or the "rapid and facile" personalities. The other study followed a sample of adults living in Alameda County, California, for nearly a decade. The investigators there found that peo-

ple who were poorly connected with networks of family and friends had mortality rates two to three times higher than those who cultivated relationships with other people, and this result stood up even after it was subjected to a fair amount of statistical testing to eliminate possibly confusing factors.

In summarizing, Dr. Vaillant observed of the men in his study, "chronic anxiety, depression and emotional maladjustment, measured in a variety of ways, predicted early aging, defined by irreversible deterioration of health. Put differently, the data suggest that positive mental health significantly retards irreversible midlife decline in physical health."

Decline in physical well-being must and does occur in midlife but, as Dr. Vaillant's remark indicates, with a great deal of potential variability. Apart from certain behaviors that we might just as well call "bad habits" —smoking, abuse of alcohol or drugs—and the less easily defined qualities of mental health or psychological adjustment, perhaps the major influence on the rate of aging in men is physical exercise.

Youthful involvement in sports gives way, in most men, to a much more sporadic pattern of activity—or nearly complete inactivity— by the mid-to-late twenties. The effect of this pattern on health has been hard to measure. Some occupational groups, say construction workers, are more active than others, such as public accountants, but myriad other differences between the occupations and the people in them make comparison impossible. And, when all is said and done, one individual's need for exercise may be markedly different from another's. There is a great danger in looking at one case—or a few of them—and trying to generalize.

The best studies—and the most widely cited—have been conducted by Dr. Ralph S. Paffenbarger, Jr., of Stanford University. In one study, following nearly 17,000 alumni of Harvard University, for 6–10 years, he found that men who used more than 2000 calories a

FITNESS BENEFITS OF SELECTED SPORTS

H=High, M=Medium, L=Low, M-H Depends whether recreation (M) or vigorous (H)

Sports	Circulo-respiratory Endurance	Muscle Strength				Muscle Endurance				Flexibility			
		Arms	Legs	Abdomen	Back	Arms	Legs	Abdomen	Back	Shoulder	Hip	Elbow	Knee
Cross Country Running	H	M	H	M	M	M	H	H	H	L	M	L	H
Cycle	L	L	L	L	L	M	L	L	L	L	L	L	L
Diving	L	L	L	H	M	L	L	L	L	H	H	L	L
Marathon	H	M	H	M	M	H	H	H	H	L	H	L	H
Parachute Jumping	L	L	L	L	L	L	L	L	L	L	L	L	L
Scuba Diving	M	M	M	L	L	M	M	M	M	H	M	M	M
Soccer	H	L	H	M	M	M	H	M	M	M	M	M	H
Softball	L	M	M	M	M	L	M	L	L	H	M	H	H
Surfing	L	L	M	L	L	L	L	L-M	L-M	L	L	L	M
Tennis	H-M	M	H	M	M	M	H	M	M	H	M	H	H
Walking	H	M	H	M	M	M	H	H	H	L	H	L	H

From *Rating the Exercises* by Charles T. Kuntzleman, and the Editors of *Consumer Guide.*® Published by William Morrow & Co., Inc. Copyright © 1978 by Publications International Ltd.

week in physical activity (sports, climbing stairs, walking) had 40 percent fewer heart attacks than men who were less active. To spend 2000 calories a week, it is necessary to run between two and three hours, swim a slow crawl or play basketball between three and four hours, play squash for about two-and-one-half hours, or walk between five and six hours. In other words, half an hour to an hour a day of exercise has to be budgeted to reach the goal of 2000 calories a week. Dr. Paffenbarger found that activities requiring participants to keep on the move and including bursts of more intense effort were most likely to protect the men from heart attacks. Sports such as golf, bowling, baseball, softball and volleyball were much less effective. (Indeed, playing volleyball requires less than two-thirds the effort of walking for the same amount of time.) The value of tennis depends very much on how the game is played; the harder the game, the better.

Dr. Paffenbarger also studied a group of 3700 San Francisco longshoremen over a period of 22 years. Again, he found that those men who did the most physical work were least likely to have heart attacks. Studies of this type clearly indicate that better cardiac health and longer life are associated with lifestyles that include a reasonable amount of physical exertion. But it remains to be proved that individuals who begin physical conditioning after a period of inactivity can, in fact, reduce their chances of getting a heart attack. Much of the evidence available to date could be interpreted to mean that people who tend to live longer, perhaps because they are genetically sturdier, are also the people who tend to be physically active.

Yet, as Alexander Leaf, an expert on aging, formerly chief of medicine at the Massachusetts General Hospital and now at Harvard, points out, there are indications that deterioration of the cardiovascular system can be reversed. He cites as one example a program conducted in eastern Finland, which has one of the highest heart-attack rates in the world. After five years of intense effort to eliminate smoking, lower blood pressure and reduce dietary animal fat, this population is beginning to respond with a fall in the rate of heart attacks. Another case in point, he says, is the Dutch people at the end of the German occupation. Presumably owing to poor diet—and perhaps other aspects of wartime austerity—the rate of death from heart attacks declined markedly, and autopsy studies of people who had died for reasons other than heart disease showed that there was less atherosclerosis than before the war.

"I think what remains to be proven, and what we ought to look at," Dr. Leaf comments, "is whether you can take a given individual with risk factors and intervene to make a difference. It's all being done on faith at the present time." To provide a more certain basis for recommendations to people who want to stay literally young in heart, Dr. Leaf

THE HEART RATE CHART

Age	Threshold for training (70% of Maximum Predicted Beats/Minute)	Limit not to be Exceeded FOR PEAKS (85% of Maximum Predicted Beats/Minute)	Maximum Predicted Beats/Minute
20–24	140	170	200
25–29	140	170	200
30–34	136	165	194
35–39	132	160	188
40–44	128	155	182
45–49	124	150	176
50–54	119	145*	171
55–59	115	140*	165
60–64	111	135*	159

* Limitations for persons over 50 must be rigidly followed.
130 limit for 60-year-olds is less than 85% level, but preferable.

is now setting up a careful study that will examine the effects of diet and exercise on people who have already experienced heart trouble. Although he is extremely cautious, Dr. Leaf is clearly optimistic about the potential for this program.

A major reason for believing that exercise will contribute to prolonged life, and better health along the way, is that exercise improves various aspects of bodily function and chemistry that are known to affect the rate of aging. For example, the body's ability to use oxygen declines with age. At rest the difference is hardly detectable, but when someone pushes himself to maximum effort, the diminished ability to take in oxygen and convert it to energy becomes conspicuous. The maximum ability to use oxygen puts a ceiling on strength and endurance, and the fact that it falls with age is the major reason why we all say to ourselves, from time to time, "I just can't do what I used to, I get out of breath sooner than I did."

But for people who exercise regularly, the rate of decline is much slower than for sedentary people. Indeed, active men in their sixties have a greater capacity to use oxygen than inactive men 10 years their junior and are nearly the equal of sedentary men in their forties. "Active" in this case means men who at least do the equivalent of jogging only three miles a week—let us say by playing handball, squash or tennis. The payoff, for the men, is that they are hardly more limited in their activity than those men 20 years younger who are still coasting on the remnants of youthful vigor.

In addition, two very recent reports offer evidence that exercise confers protection from certain kinds of biochemical aging. One study showed that exercise raises the level of sensitivity to insulin. This is important because the common type of diabetes that begins to appear late in middle age is primarily a disorder of insensitivity to insulin (and not a lack of the vital hormone). The other investigation produced data indicating that men who run at least six miles a week raise their levels of HDL-cholesterol. Although excess cholesterol in the blood contributes to clogging of the arteries, it is now known that the HDL form is actually beneficial and may even aid in reversing damage that has already been done. Both these studies offer persuasive evidence that it was exercise alone, and not other differences between the lifestyles of joggers and sedentary men, that led to biochemical improvements. On the other hand, the possibility still cannot be completely ruled out that there is some basic biological difference between people who choose to jog and those who do not—unlikely as it may seem.

For purely practical reasons, jogging or running is the activity likely to offer significant health advantages to most people. Nearly all other forms of exercise require equipment of some sort, cooperation of a partner or team, or time spent traveling to a proper location. Running can often commence at the front door, calls for no special equipment other than a properly fitted pair of running shoes, and can be done at almost any time of day, alone or with company. Running also requires no special skills, although novices may find that they take a little while to get the hang of running with an efficient and comfortable stride.

Naturally, people who take up a more active lifestyle after a sedentary period run certain risks. It is a standard recommendation that people over the age of 35 check in with a doctor before beginning their program. This is good advice, but it is important not to overdramatize the hazards. People who set out on a program of gentle conditioning, who don't begin by competing with others, and who don't try to prove anything to themselves, have little to fear. The most important protection is not a doctor's go-ahead, but the ability to pay attention to signals from one's own body and to pace things accordingly. In a small group of men who died during or shortly after running, as reported in a 1979 study from Stanford University, virtually every one had some indication of ill health which he appears to have ignored. In other words, it is important to approach exercise not with a ''do-or-die'' outlook, but rather with the expectation that it should make one feel *better*, not worse.

One aspect of life that physical conditioning is said to improve is sex. Little systematic evidence has been collected on the matter, although testimonials from evangelistic joggers abound. Some, more ''scientific,'' support for the belief comes from a 1969 study, now over 10 years old, in which normal men at high risk of a heart attack entered an exercise program. As their level of conditioning improved, the men became more sexually active. (In fact, the increase in sexual activity was correlated with a lowering of cholesterol in their blood —another index of physical fitness.)

Sexual aging is extremely variable among men, and relatively little is known about it. For virtually all men, the peak of sexuality,

" Older men who retain the ability to be visually stimulated are the ones who maintain a more active sex life "

as indicated by frequency of sexual behavior, is in the mid-twenties. From the age of 40 on, the amount of sexual activity in healthy, normal men diminishes by about half with each passing decade. But the rate of decline for any individual may be considerably faster or slower. Some evidence indicates that men who live to great old age are likely to retain their sexual responsiveness, perhaps as an aspect of their general physical vigor.

Investigators have concluded that testosterone, the male hormone, does diminish with age, but the finding could be questioned on two grounds. First, the majority of studies have used men of various ages and compared the results rather than following the same group of men through life. Second, levels of testosterone go up and down during the day, and it is important to be sure that one man's high level is not compared to another man's low. Very recently, independent studies of

229

two different groups of men, followed over a number of years, have shown that, on the whole, levels of testosterone do not go down with age, nor do levels of female hormone rise —provided a man remains in good general health. In other words, there appears to be no biochemical equivalent of the female menopause in healthy men.

The relationship between testosterone levels and sexual activity is not, however, a simple one. One normal man can have a testosterone level over three times higher than another, equally normal man, and yet their level of sexual activity may be very similar. In other words, a man whose hormone level is in the normal range is very unlikely to respond to treatments with extra testosterone by becoming sexier. Of course, psychological factors play an enormous role; a man who believes that any treatment is going to help him may well respond to his belief with restored vigor.

Clyde Martin, Ph.D., a sociologist at the Gerontology Research Center in Baltimore (a division of the National Institute on Aging) who collaborated with Alfred Kinsey on his famous studies of human sexual behavior, has for 12 years been collecting and analyzing the sexual biographies of men enrolled in the Baltimore Longitudinal Study of Aging. This research project has been going since 1941; its subjects are male volunteers between the ages of 25 and 90 who come to a research center every year and a half for various tests and interviews. The object is to determine how normal men age. Dr. Martin has explored the sexual experience of these men, partly in an attempt to learn how sexual activity changes with aging, and partly to see whether he can identify factors that lead to greater or less sexual activity as time goes by. To date, he has been able to find certain correlations, but no definitive causes. Men who were sexually more active at an earlier age than their contemporaries are the ones most likely to maintain a relatively high level of sexual activity into old age. Interestingly enough, as Dr.

Martin observed in an interview, older men who retain the ability to be visually stimulated are the ones who maintain a more active sex life; men who lose this capacity are quite likely to lose interest in sex and to become relatively inactive.

Dr. Martin's findings are consistent with data from another survey of aging men conducted by Eric Pfeiffer and his colleagues in the Department of Psychiatry at Duke University. Dr. Pfeiffer also found that men in his group were most likely to be sexually active in later years if they had a background of being interested in sex, enjoying it and engaging frequently in sexual behavior. Their level of interest and enjoyment was also strongly influenced by the men's evaluation of their own health; those who complained of being unwell—regardless of the actual situation—were unlikely to report much enthusiasm for sex. But the frequency with which these men had intercourse was much more strongly determined by their true state of health, as evaluated by the physicians examining them. Sexual activity of older women, on the other hand, was mostly influenced by whether they had a sexual partner and much less by subjective or objective changes in their health. Dr. Pfeiffer also found that, as a rule, responsibility for terminating sex in a marriage rested with the man and not the woman.

True though it is that declining sexual activity is a normal part of aging in men, and often seems completely acceptable to the individual, impotence is not necessarily normal, and men who are troubled by it should not take a fatalistic attitude. Episodes of impotence are, of course, common and their frequency increases with age. Often failure to obtain or maintain an erection results from fatigue, anxiety or other temporary circumstances. But more frequent impotence, particularly in men who have not previously experienced it, may be due to more serious psychological or medical causes. At present, though, it is quite unclear what proportion of cases are purely psychological. The common teaching has been that only a very small number of impotent men have a medical reason for their condition, but recent research by Dr. Richard Spark of the Beth Israel Hospital in Boston has called the whole matter into question. He studied a group of impotent men, ranging in age from 18 to 75, and found that more than a third had hormonal problems, and all but a few of this group could be successfully treated with hormone therapy.

Perhaps the greatest hindrance to the treatment of impotence is a man's reluctance to talk about it. Yet any man who experiences impotence is most likely to recover if he does discuss it. He should begin with his sexual partner, because anxieties about failing the

❝ There are indications that deterioration of the cardiovascular system can be reversed ❞

partner's expectations may be rather easily cleared up, and with them the impotence. But if impotence persists beyond a few episodes and seems to be establishing itself, early consultation with a sympathetic physician should be the next step. Dr. Spark's discovery suggests that a hormonal cause should be very carefully sought, and for this purpose a specialist in the field—an endocrinologist—should probably be consulted. If no hormonal or other medical cause is found, a psychotherapist, preferably one with current experience in treating disorders of sexual function, should be asked to help. Impotence is more likely to be treatable—regardless of the cause—if it is dealt with early. The longer it is established, the more refractory it becomes, as a rule.

Distressing as it may be for a man to suffer from lack of the male hormone, testosterone, virtually all men, as they age, experience one disadvantage from having it: a condition

known as "prostatic hyperplasia," "prostatism," or "enlarged prostate." The prostate gland surrounds the urinary channel where it leaves the bladder to enter the penis. It contributes secretions to semen, and by doing so presumably enhances the fertility of sperm. As years go by, the prostate begins to enlarge; then, at some point, in many older men it narrows or closes off the urinary passage. Virtually no other species suffers from prostate enlargement, except the dog, which develops a very similar condition. Working chiefly with dogs, Dr. Jean Wilson and his colleagues in the Department of Internal Medicine of the University of Texas Southwestern Medical School in Dallas have been able to establish a cause of prostatic hyperplasia. During a lifetime of exposure to testosterone, they find, the prostate accumulates a metabolic by-product of the hormone. This by-product, perhaps assisted by small amounts of female hormone (which can be found in all men, especially late in life), appears to cause the abnormal growth of prostate tissue that eventually leads to urinary obstruction. Dr. Wilson theorizes that the same process works in human males, but he acknowledges that there are other viewpoints on the matter.

Surgery for prostate enlargement is now highly effective and very safe, but Dr. Wilson would like to find a way to use drugs or hormones to prevent the discomfort and the urinary obstruction that make surgery necessary. Medical prevention, however, is a long way off, in his view. Meanwhile, unfortunately, there is no sound evidence that anything can be done to prevent prostate enlargement. Popular ideas—such as adding zinc to the diet or increasing the level of sexual activity—cannot be shown to have produced any benefit. The most important thing is to be aware of changing bodily function and to see a physician when urinary changes are first noticed.

Following pages: For purely practical reasons, jogging or running is the activity likely to offer significant health advantages to most people.

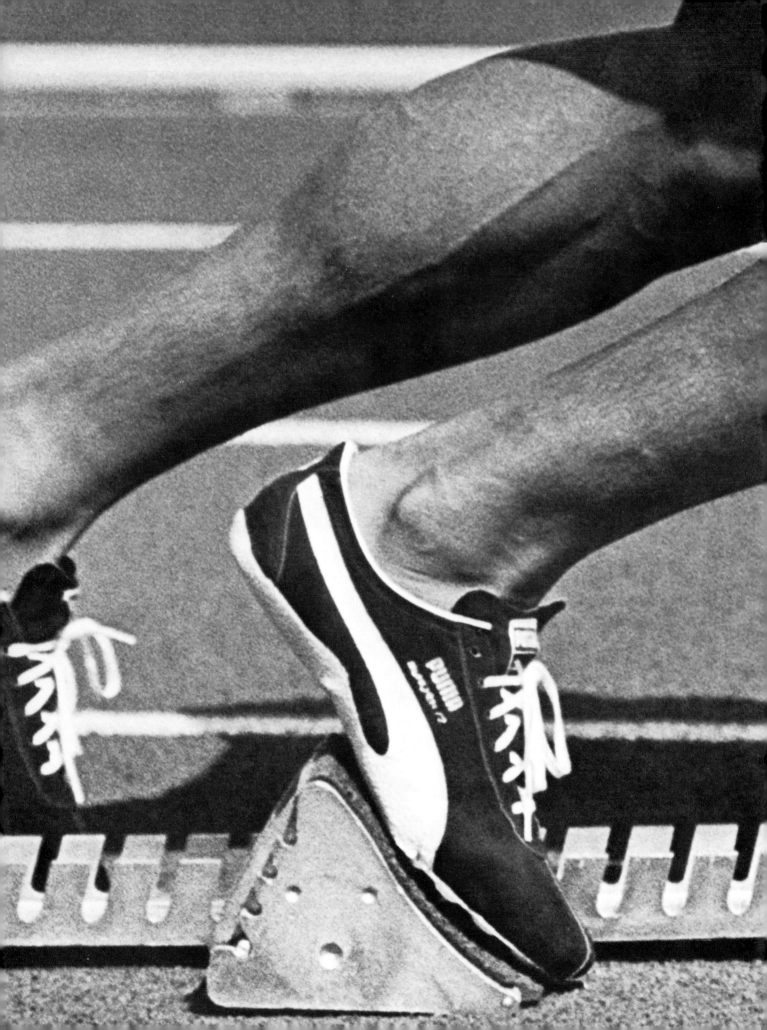

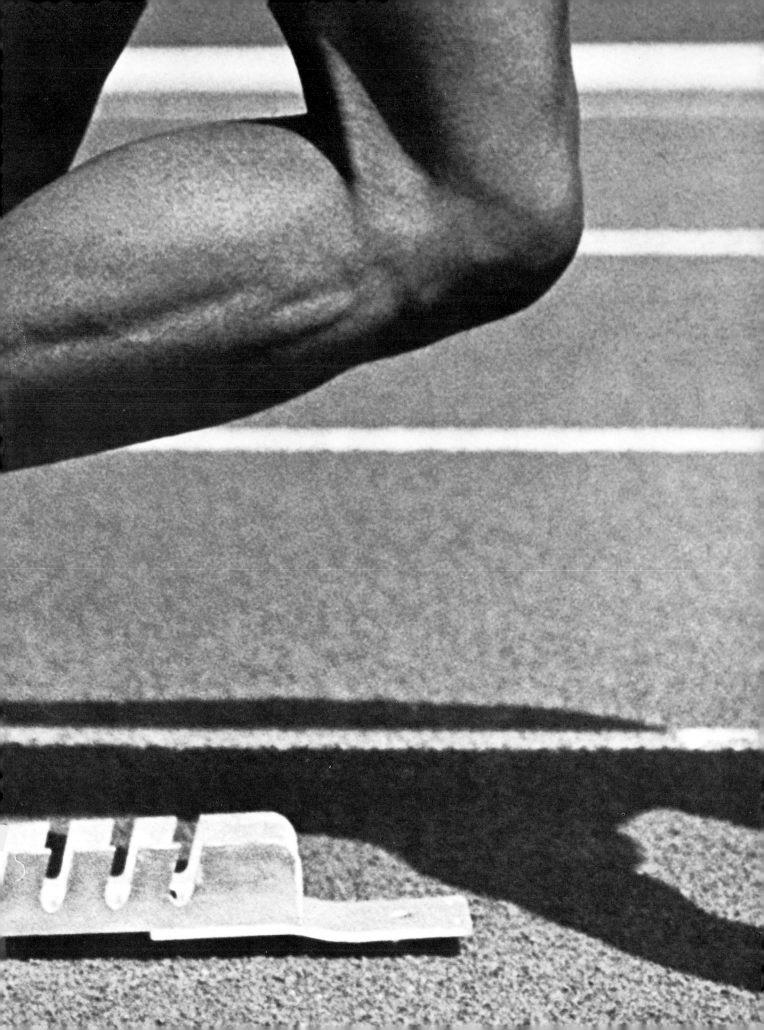

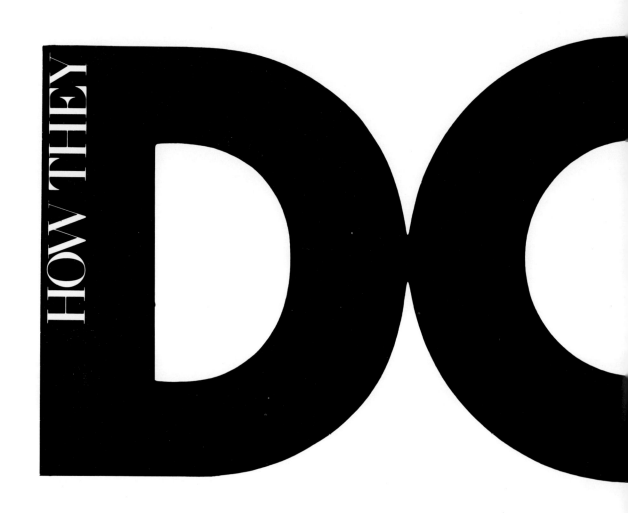

HOW THEY DO

by Amy Gross

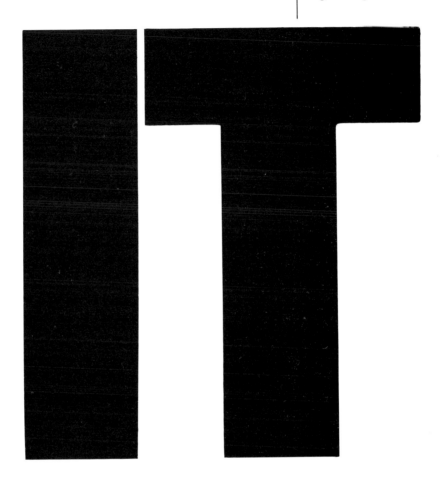

Some people stay young—they are young at 70, at 80. The seven people profiled here are outstanding examples of youth continued into age. They come from the most disparate circumstances, from distant parts of the world, and remote fields of work (there's a ballet coach, an architect, a nightclub owner, a pioneer in sexual rights), and yet the seven have much in common. They have all taken leaps, breaking with their past or expected future, inventing their own lives. They have a receptivity to the new, an appetite for change, a talent for adaptation. Their lives have all been rattled by history, by the Russian revolution, Nazism, McCarthyism, the Depression. They lost all or much and yet somehow emerged with no residue of bitterness. They just went on; that's what made sense to them. The seven all thrive on their work, considering themselves fortunate, if not blessed, to have work that can be continued as they continue. They relinquish to age what they must and are conspicuously thrilled by their present powers, enthusiasms, vitality. Their capacity for pleasure appears to be enormous, which is, perhaps, why meeting them is such a very great pleasure.

235

"My pupils—they are young girls. They come bubbling, and you have to bubble with them."

ALEXANDRA DANILOVA

Alexandra Danilova has an hour between classes, so we meet in the faculty lounge of the School of American Ballet, breeding ground for the dancers of the New York City Ballet. Mme. Danilova is one of the legends of this legendary company. In 1924, a soloist with the Maryinsky Theater (now the Kirov), she left post-revolutionary Russia, where at least one million people were dying of starvation. With George Balanchine and two other dancers, she went to Germany, and then to Paris where Diaghilev swooped up the émigrés for his company, the fantastic Ballets Russes. Danilova became a prima ballerina, Balanchine choreographed, and the two lived together for four years. ("Living with genius," she says, "is difficult. All I wanted was to go dance tango in the evening, like all the kids. I was dying, 'Please take me. I want to dance Charleston.' He say, 'No, you can't see, it's full of smoke, why you want to go?' He was so serious.")

Danilova danced to the end of the fifties, then turned to teaching, staging, choreographing, coaching leading dancers of the company, and a few years ago, appeared as the dance coach in *The Turning Point*. "The marvel of Danilova," said Holly Brubach, *Vogue*'s dance critic, "is that she spans the history of 20th-century ballet, from the Maryinsky to the New York City Ballet. Somehow she kept pace with all the changes—nobody else has

done that. The famous line about Danilova is that she was 'champagne on stage.'"

Now in her mid-seventies, Danilova is still champagne. Her laugh could be bottled as the sound of delight. She is thin, limber, long-legged like all Balanchine favorites. Even in corduroy pants and a sweater, she has an elegance of line. Her coloring is wonderful—honey-blond hair, large blue eyes as amused as they are in her early photographs, and skin so amazingly smooth and peachy. I ask if she's had cosmetic surgery. "I had my eyes done a long time ago," she says, "like everybody else. I could lift face but it would be ridiculous to look suddenly 25. I don't want to look, at my age, like a girl and I try not to overdress, but on the other hand, I don't want to put drab old dresses on, you know," she laughs. She speaks slowly, enunciating heroically to transcend her Russian accent. She is as conscious and responsible about her work, the way she lives, the way she is aging, as she is about her speech.

"The artist wants to age gracefully. You can't help it—everything gets old. The carpet. The car," she laughs, "the people. But not to fall apart. Not to be ashamed of it, or think it is a *disahster*—it is not. What I did when I was 50, I don't want to do when I am 70. I see all my friends getting older and some get older ugly, get more demanding and walk around like wise men giving all the time advice when one doesn't ask them—a little bit tiresome, don't you notice? I no-

tice because all my friends," she giggles, "are getting old with me. So I think it's a great work, to work with oneself and be agreeable and nice-looking."

She is not for letting oneself go, or drawing away from the rituals of femininity. She exercises every day for 10, 15 minutes, "always under protest, but I do it," she laughs. "And I always put creams on my body after bath, which is boring." Boring? "Of course it's boring!" She thinks she keeps her figure by never eating lunch ("I don't eat a lot but I eat well—breakfast, a good dinner"). She takes herself to the hairdresser regularly for a proper coloring: "I would hate to be my age and have someone say, 'Oh look at that terrible dye job.'" Grooming for her is a sign of dignity ("First thing off the bed in the morning, I comb my hair. Some people walk half a day without combing hair.") It is also a self-imposed requirement of her job. "I demand my pupils are nicely coiffed and look groomed and I hope I look that way." She is setting a standard of the dancer.

To be useful, she thinks, is essential ("Tribes leave old women to die with a cup of water saying they are no longer useful"), and "to find the interest"—to find both what interests you and the motivation to go after it. Asked what interests her, she answers, "Everything. Politics. I read everything. I love music, Broadway, I go to ballet when new companies come—it's my business. And of course my pupils—they are young girls: They come bubbling and you have to bubble with them. They ask questions and you better have the answers. . . .

"To get interested," she says, "you have to do a little work with yourself. You know, sometimes you say, 'I don't want to do *anything*, what's the matter with me?' And the other voice—I always have two voices—says, 'Come on, take the bag and go.'" The bag? "My body." She keeps herself very disciplined, she thinks, "but also reasonable. If you're tired...people say, 'but I can't go to bed at nine o'clock.' I can," she says blithely. Staying flexible is staying young.

There is something else about Danilova that offers a clue to long-running youthfulness; a relentless realism that keeps her gripped to the present. Asked about the importance of the past to her now, she goes not to nostalgia for former glories but to lessons learned. "My past was wonderful. It was hard times, but I wouldn't change anything. Because during the revolution, I had good schooling, I understood the price of life, I had hunger...so I appreciate hot water and soap. A lot of other people take everything for granted."

Her training in appreciation and self-reliance began before the revolution. Orphaned at the age of two, Danilova was raised by two aunts. "One was not interested in me," she says simply. The other was "wonderful and very strict for my good. When I was to clean my room, she'd say, 'Make it nice. It's your room. No one will help.' I was brought up always to do the best I can, whatever I do. I have pride in everything I do, cleaning my house or teaching class."

I wonder if it was difficult to move from the stage to behind the scenes. "I'm very proud of myself, if you want to know the truth. I never thought I could do what I'm doing. I always ask, 'Can I do that?' Mr. Balanchine always encourages: 'Of course you can do that.' I am always worried about my teaching. I poke myself with fork," she laughs again, "you know? To be alert to what my pupils need. If I don't do my best," she says, "they can always get somebody else."

Making a point about how dancers are evaluated, she says, "It's like it doesn't matter how long it takes you to do interview: You have to get good article. You can complain to your friend, how hard you worked, and he'll say, 'So did I!'" Her tone is breezy. "So did everybody else." This merciless streak of hers must spare her many of the disappointments of illusion.

I ask if religion means anything to her. "No. I think that the world is very big and consists of different people that fulfill all kinds of different missions. Some are wonderful philosophers. Some are in the arts and give us to forget our sorrow, you know? All different designations. And some," her voice turns crisp, "are just stupid and waste everybody's time and you drop them. They say, 'Oh I'm so worried,' worrying what can't be helped. Drop them. Look for people that will feed you."

"Seventy should be a declaration of the most enormous joy. At 40, I wondered if I was getting old. At 70, it's all clear, marvelous, a release. You just wait."

PHILIP JOHNSON

The architect Philip Johnson, who was born on July 8th, 1906, resembles one of the Cycladic marble figures that influenced Brancusi. Johnson is similarly pared down to essence, a simple carving, a slim perfection. In his 37th-floor office in the Seagram Building on Park Avenue (designed by Mies van der Rohe and Johnson), in the clean white eastern light trumpeting into every corner, Johnson reigns as the small ticking motor, the impetus. His eyes are devilishly bright. His movements are dartingly quick—a twitch, for instance, to check his watch. Time counts. A visitor speeds up around him, talks faster; one does not loll. But then Johnson has always been "madly energetic," according to Calvin Tomkins, writing in a New Yorker profile; always running—never walking—down the corridors of the Museum of Modern Art, where he founded the Department of Architecture.

And what is the secret behind all that energy? Was he born with it? "Oh yes. It's just accident," he says. Good genes? "Yes, Father was 98 when he died, mother was 85. One grandmother was 80."

His own health? "Good. Open-heart surgery, yes. Except for that, I'm all right."

Does he take particularly good care of himself? "No, I don't. I eat everything, drink everything. I hate exercise. I hate any manner or means of care-taking. You live longer if you pay no attention. It's an American disease, this taking-care-of-yourself business." His tone is playful and provocative. "American values...I can't understand them."

His values then are...? "I don't know...I was a student of Greek most of my life so I suppose I inherited from the pre-Socratics my Weltanschauung, but my way of life is more medieval, where the love of God (though I'm not religious) might be of more interest than sex and consumer goods.''

And what substitutes for love of God? ''Art. That's what keeps me going of course.'' A devilish smile: ''Art has a tremendous advantage. Look at Sophocles. He did his best work after he was older than I am. I look forward''—he grins—''to my best work.''

The worst time in his life, he says, was the period before he became an architect. ''I wandered around doing all sorts of silly things, farming and politics. I made so many mistakes. One does.'' (Johnson's public mistake was sympathizing with Nazism in the thirties. By way of reparation, Tomkins suggests, Johnson designed a synagogue years later and returned his fee to the congregation.) ''And then for a couple of years, I did nothing, because I had plenty of money and didn't know what to do. That's really death: inactivity.

''But once you're engaged, that's the only thing that matters. The work never gets any easier,'' he says. ''You still anguish. You still feel inadequate, but that's the way it is. It's a constant continuing.''

Nine in the morning until six at night, five days a week, Johnson works in Manhattan. Weekends, he gets away to his famous glass house in Connecticut. ''It saves my life. That's where I work. I built a studio and closet myself in there without telephone, water, music, for maybe four, five hours a day. Evenings I no longer work. That's one change with age.''

He used to run ''a sort of restaurant-hotel at the country house on weekends,'' he laughs. ''But now, people are not so important to me. The architecture is more important. I only wish I could do more.'' He grins, a flame happy to consume itself. Johnson seems both proud and delighted to have such a passion,

such devotion. ''I felt kind of tired and told my doctor I was losing my grip, and he said, 'When was your last vacation?' And I said, 'I've never had one. So I took one and read War and Peace. It was great. My third time. It's just an unbelievable joy.''

Johnson has always been considered inconoclastic in his use of stone, and he is still startling. He shocked multitudes recently with his choice of a Chippendale-like broken pediment atop the new AT&T building on Madison Avenue. He is ''crazy about the new architecture,'' he says. ''We're having a battle now with one of the leaders of the profession because he thinks a building we're helping to sponsor in Portland is awful. But that's good, isn't it? I mean, it's nice to have battles still.'' His ''prejudice for the new,'' his enthusiasm for the younger generation of architects, cuts him off from his contemporaries. ''They are getting smaller, I know them as little as possible.''

Has he changed with age? ''I'm much nicer. Life begins at 70. Because then you no longer have anything to prove to yourself or the world. See: You're not pushing, you don't have to break any new frontiers, you either have it made or you haven't. In either case, it's all freewheeling. So 70 should be a declaration of the most enormous joy. At 40 I was wondering if I was getting old.'' That gamin grin. ''At 70, it's all clear, marvelous, a release. You just wait,'' he tells me.

Perhaps it's marvelous for him because he's so successful? But he argues, there are always successful people who ''die young or cut off their ears.'' The difference, he thinks, goes back to the original ''accident,'' that piece of luck that made him so energetic.

''My best friend is Lincoln Kirstein, who is exactly my age. We had the same operation the same

year, same doctor. I was over it in 10 days and he didn't get over it for six months. The doctor explained the difference—'Well, you're an up person.' I saw the rosy lights right away, while he brooded. I said, 'Gee, I'm still alive, isn't that a miracle,' and went right back to work.'' This is not to be taken as an inspiring example of positive thinking, he wants you to know, where ''one wills oneself''—he makes a fist and grits his teeth. ''That's a religious thing, which I don't share. It's just innate. I'm a manic-depressive by nature, and I had a three-year illness when I was at Harvard—they called it a nervous breakdown, and the doctor told me to go home and read whatever I wanted for six months. And once I was out of that, I was perfectly fine. No more depressions. But I'm still manic,'' and he grins.

''Everything is better,'' he assures me again before I leave. ''I'm surprised. I thought that growing old was something you better prepare for and do gracefully. Well, phooey. Graceful or not, you can have fun. I'm free now. I wish you a pleasant 70.''

"I remember my mother used to say, 'Betty, I want you to meet so-and-so and I want you to do bing-bang-boo,' and I'd just do what I want. At an early age! I was a rebel always."

BETTY PARSONS

Betty Parsons has an eye for the new. That's what has made her one of the important art dealers in New York since the forties—she was the first gallery owner to gamble on unknowns like Jackson Pollock, Mark Rothko, Hans Hofmann, Barnett Newman, Clyfford Still, Ellsworth Kelly—and that's what keeps her young. Other eyes that are 80 years old long ago rejected the new as a code they could no longer decipher. Parsons's eyes, though, keep changing, being interested; she keeps falling in love with the unfamiliar, the creative. Her ears too. She went to a concert at the Whitney—Philip Glass, you know that fantastic composer? Yes! She was fascinated! It was like the spheres—the music was trying to get up there! And she wrote a lot of poetry during the concert, in the dark, because the music was so vital and so alive!

She is also an artist, of course, and a gallery full of her found-wood and acrylic sculpture can cause an outbreak of joy, with their child-colors, their improvisational wit, their strong totemic shapes. A week before a one-woman show of her work is to open—it is 10 o'clock in the morning, she is due at her own gallery any minute—an interviewer has just shown up at her door. . . . "This won't take all day?" she asks warily.

Her speech is clipped, fast, emphatic, a stone skipping water, as distinctive as her cheekbones, as the style that has her wrapped in a long, classic navy-blue bathrobe (she has just finished her exercises, breakfast, telephone calls). She leads into the living room—"the place is roaring with pictures" as she says—and perches on a couch, very still, concentrated, no unessential gestures. She perches: Her presence is light—not frail at all but weightless.

She lives alone and has since 1922, when she divorced her husband. There were other men she might have married later, but domestic life is not for her. "I am too high-strung and nervous and I have so much to do." She comes from a "very conservative New York business family"—one imagines Edith Wharton's world updated—and so she married as she was supposed to, but divorced as she was not supposed to, and was from then on unimpeded in her pursuit of art. Since then, she has been in the exciting places at the exciting times—Paris in the twenties when the art world was there, New York when the vitality moved here.

Her great cause is what she calls "the creative approach to life"; it's the antithesis of "the dogmatic, cliché approach, the dreary old suburban idea that you do everything the same way as everyone else. You don't. Everybody does it differently, according to their nature. I remember my mother used to say, 'Now, Betty, I want you to meet so-and-so and do so-and-so, and I want you to do bing-bang-boo'—and I'd never contradict her, because what is the use?—but I'd just do what I wanted. At an early age! I intuitively knew that what was right for my mother, my father and my background was not necessarily right for me. I was just born a kind of rebel."

She did take from her family a habit of longevity: One grandfather lived to 96, a grandmother lived into her late eighties, and both her parents lived to 79. A pretty healthy family, she says, and she herself is "amazingly healthy." She eats everything, but in small quantities, and of course her favorite things are vegetables, cheese and nuts. She likes about two drinks a day, wine, a strong drink occasionally at night when she's tired. She was brought up to be athletic, and she's very grateful for that "because I would much rather have read a book but I was made to play tennis, golf, to dance, to exercise. I love dancing. I don't dance so much now—I haven't got very much time. I do get tired quicker now!" she says, half-astonished. "I mean, I cannot sit up all night and work all day the way I used to. I just can't," she laughs. (She has never really thought much about age, she says, about getting old herself. She supposes she should start thinking about it.)

The word "retirement" does not come up. She is still working a full day, reading through a hefty and motley stack of magazines and journals—about art, politics, literature—reading good novels, lunching with clients, installing a new show every three weeks. Weekends she works at her house on the beach (she calls her studio "the largest playroom on Long Island''). And then she juries shows around the country and travels to openings of her own shows.

She travels easily, she says, and gives no signs of the cautiousness one notices in many older people. She is not afraid for herself, then? ''No. When I have to speak in public, I am always terrified, but then I get into it, and I get interested, and I forget myself. You see''—she grabs the idea—''anything that makes me forget myself, I go for! That old ego, that bloody thing! We need our ego to get around, but boy, if something makes me forget my ego, I go right for it.''

Twice a week, Ms. Parsons says, ''I go to this spiritual exercise class. Your exercise is to surrender. You try to empty yourself so the life force enters. And it's a great help. I've been doing it now for 12, 15 years. Everybody surrenders differently,'' she says with wonder. ''Some people sing, some dance, cry, yell, some turn into monkeys,'' she laughs. ''It's fantastic. You've never heard such sounds. I move around, I dance quite a lot and do a little yelling, but it's a release. It puts you in contact with the universal forces. *I believe in the universal forces,*'' she says as though writing the words large. ''It will help you if you respect them, if you're aware of them.''

Her interest in the class, and in Eastern philosophy, is perhaps her way of approaching ''the mystery of what all this thing is about, living in the world.'' This is her vital interest, this mystery. And it feeds into her receptivity—her zesty appetite—for what is constantly emerging, the new. ''I am as interested in my work now as I was 40 years ago because the creative world is endlessly renewing. I am always fascinated with these new phases. I always tell art students, teachers, to keep open! Even if your specialty is such-and-such a

century, remember that today always has something to say. Don't sit back and say, this is it—the world is always moving, there's always change! Look at nature—there's never a day that's the same as yesterday! A lot of people are mesmerized by nostalgia. I'm rather anti-nostalgia. I'm interested in *today*. I had a terrible history teacher who bored me to death—she just made you remember dates,'' she says, vivid with outrage. ''So I was bored with history and,'' she laughs, ''maybe in a way that was a help. If I'd fallen in love with history, I might not have been so old.''

In the cab going downtown to her gallery, she is saying that her artists like her to write statements about their work to accompany

their shows. She looks in her notebook for an example of such a statement. It occurs to me that her pleasure in being asked—and in her work, in her talent for independence, in being who and what she is—is a pleasure reserved for people of age: Young people muddy such satisfactions with false pride and false modesty and crazy fears. But she's found the statement: '' 'These drawings have to do with light, space and the moment beyond the sound of time'—that's the sort of thing I write. And here's something I always read to students—I think it's Willa Cather: 'What was any art but an effort to make a sheath, a mold in which to imprison for a moment, the shining elusive element which is life itself.' *That's* what I'm looking for,'' she says.

"We walked out broke, but we went out with a good meal and a bottle of wine. That's the way I am."

BARNEY JOSEPHSON

In 1938, in Manhattan, Barney Josephson opened a nightclub called the Café Society with a double bill of Billie Holiday and Jack Gilford. In the next 10 years he would introduce Lena Horne, Sara Vaughan, Zero Mostel, Imogene Coca, Carol Channing; he would present and promote Josh White, Pearl Primus, Mary Lou Williams, Art Tatum. He and his clubs (he opened the Café Society Uptown in 1940), thrived until the days of the House Un-American Activities Committee. As the brother of Leon Josephson, an avowed Communist, Barney was suspect; and only a Communist, it was thought, would

run an interracial club. Blacklisted, he says, ''I was losing my shirt. I'd always taken an ad in the *Billboard* annual, usually a half-page. The last year, though I could ill-afford it, I took a full page. You don't quit under fire. In the middle of the page, I had, 'My head is bloody but unbowed—Barney Josephson.' But eventually, I had to sell.''

For years after that, he says, ''I was Mr. Anonymous.'' He opened a hamburger restaurant called The Cookery, then three others in the next four years. It was too fast, too much. He closed the fourth restaurant after only five months. ''I said to hell with it and asked my wife out to dinner. We were walking on

55th Street. My wife said, 'There's a pretty good restaurant'—it was La Caravelle. We walked out broke, but we went out with a good meal and a bottle of wine. That's the way I am. We had a great evening.''

The way he is, is quick on the recovery. To choose a great evening over an evening of regret is, I cannot help thinking, a clue to staying young. Another is that during those Mr. Anonymous years, Mr. Josephson was not bitter, ''not for myself. I felt frustrated because I wasn't able to do the kind of work I love. We all have to make a living but there's a little more than that: You have to like what you're doing. You have some principles to stand by, and if you can't, you grieve.''

Well, this story has a happy ending. He'd kept the Greenwich Village Cookery running, and then, about 10 years ago, Mary Lou Williams ''walked in begging for work. Jazz was dead, rock was all, and she asked if she couldn't play piano in my place in the evenings.''

The Cookery is now a well-known jazz-restaurant, and its resident star is blues singer Alberta Hunter, 85, whom Josephson manages. If you want to get to Hunter —as do people as disparate as a Newark reporter, the casting director of the *Today* show, Robert Altman (for his movie *Remember My Name*), and Jackie Onassis (for a book on Hunter's life)—you call Josephson.

You will guess him to be fiftyish on the telephone, and will be startled when you meet him, to see a man at the end of his seventies (he was born in 1902). He is trim, natty in a dark-gray pinstripe suit, white-haired; he broke his hip three months ago and walks with a slight limp. He disdains crutches, canes; he hates the term ''senior citizen,'' and he wouldn't consider using ''those discounts—no way, no how, not this old man. Like Alberta says, 'keep me away from those old peo-

ple.' '' He still opens the restaurant every morning, stays all day, breaking in late afternoon to rest before the long evening.

He thinks work is the secret of staying young. ''I never want to quit. Every person should work till he expires.... And you can't be a complainer. You make yourself feel worse, and who cares?'' He laughs, enjoying the truth. ''I learned from my mother: 'You've got to keep doing,' she'd say. 'Like a corkscrew, keep turning.' I once said to her, 'You can bore yourself right into the ground.' 'That's true,' she said, 'but you can sometimes turn yourself way up into heaven.' '' He grins.

Josephson was the youngest of four sons—there were also two sisters, he says. His father was a shoemaker who died before Barney was one year old. His mother worked as a seamstress, an older sister worked, a brother started as an errand boy in a shoe company, learned the business, and started his own successful company.

''My mother impressed on all of us that you do the best you can at the moment. You don't feel too proud to take what you can get, and meanwhile you look for how you can improve yourself. No matter what you may have to do—if you have to be a toilet porter, then you make yourself the best toilet cleaner in America.'' Is there a link between being unspoiled, free of false pride, and being a survivor?

Josephson also believes that being interested ''in other things than self'' makes for youthfulness; being interested in world events (he has commented on the ''lucid analysis'' of the Middle East crisis in this morning's *Times*); being involved in ''trying to make the world a little better than when you came in—what else do you live for?'' He is radiantly proud of his two sons because they are politically active, and carry on the lib-

eral tradition. They are 22 and 19, his sons—his first children, product of his third marriage. He and his wife—one of the two lawyers who represented the Rosenbergs—are separated after 23 years of marriage. ''I'm a single man now. I didn't leave her for another girl,'' he laughs, ''though I have one now. At 78, I have a new love life. What do you think of that?'' It is obvious he thinks it's marvelous. ''She's 55, a professor of speech pathology, I wasn't looking for it but....''

Josephson's life continues to open up rather than narrow. He comes from a long-lived family— one brother died recently at 89; his mother died at 73, ''but remember, that's after raising six kids and working hard—she could have lived to 100, I'm sure of it.'' His brother Leon died at 65—''rather young for our family, but his ordeal really took it out of him.'' Barney went through an ordeal too, of course, but the longevity factor— whatever it may be—was left intact. Maybe it is having a reason to live—''I keep striving to do things,'' he says, ''to get better. What I've always wanted to accomplish was always so much more than what I knew was humanly possible. It's not bad to feel you're never going to attain it—so you feel you've failed, but nevertheless you strive for it—you still don't give up, and you still *do*. I was just reading a review of Flaubert's letters —how many days did it take him to write a page? And even then, probably, it was not to his satisfaction. I pointed that out to my lady friend—imagine how much this man suffered!'' Josephson's still awed.

If Josephson's life continues to open up, it must be because he continues to walk into it. He is now introducing Alberta Hunter to audiences, the first time he's stepped in the spotlight. He takes chances. He took a big chance on Alberta herself, five years ago. "A friend had seen her at a party at Bobby Short's. I didn't know she was around. I called her immediately. She was 82 then, and hadn't even hummed in 20 years, and I told her, 'You're going to be singing in three weeks, so get ready.' She said, 'Oh I don't know if I can sing.' I told her that was my problem. What else could I do? I couldn't ask a woman of 82 to audition.''

His eyes fill when he talks about Alberta ("I cry a lot. Mostly for joy. If I'm moved by a great performance, by something about my boys...I can feel so strongly and so pleased. That's just me. I'm enjoying every tear, I guess.''). The night of her opening, he is remembering, "They could have said,

Barney Josephson is terrific or he's scraping the bottom of the barrel. Well, the first night, she's a smash,'' and the tears come to his eyes. "The second night, before the first show, I go downstairs and say, 'Alberta, when you get to be our age, you know you've got to go one day. On the day you go, you're going out in a blaze of glory, and I'm going to be there, feeling the heat on your right side.' Can you imagine what a wonderful time I'm having, what a joyful couple of years I've had working with her?''

He's already said he must stop —he's talked for over two hours. He gets his camel's hair coat, wraps his Dior silk scarf around his neck, and walks home to rest before the first of tonight's two shows.

ago she was focusing on the right of the elderly and the handicapped to be sexual. Today, she is planning a speech to give the Child Welfare League of America, recommending that foster parents be screened for their sexual attitudes: "The child doesn't have to have additional problems of being slapped on the hands for masturbating,'' she says. If old age is often a matter of getting off the bus, and waving life and change on without you, Dr. Calderone is still walking briskly forward, hoping the bus catches up with her.

She is a vigorous, handsome woman—tall, with plank-straight posture, neat gray hair and a great smile. She volunteers that she's had a facelift. "I have a very young body and I was tired of feeling split—taking my clothes off and feeling about 16 and putting my clothes on and looking 70. Plastic surgery made me feel all of one piece. That's why I did it. And vanity. It's a saving grace, vanity. To me it is part of my own self-respect. I've always enjoyed how I look, and dressing up to my looks, and I must say that at my 75th birthday party —did you see the story in *People*? —I really looked gorgeous. Ha!'' She gives out with these victory cries, mixing triumph and delight.

"My sister said that I was incandescent. There were all the 280 people I loved best...can you imagine? Two men I love, all my friends, I was rich! I was so moved. I was not popular as a girl, and always very shy and ill-at-ease, and here am I at 75 and I feel good about myself and have high self-esteem. I'm still correcting myself, oh yes. I think mostly, at this time, I'm working on keeping up my productivity—I find myself flagging a little bit and I have an awful lot to do. I have 'miles to go before I sleep'....'' (Miles literally as well as figuratively: She logged over 100,000 miles last year, taking in

"I have a very young body and I was tired of feeling split—looking young with my clothes off and looking 70 with my clothes on. That's why I had my face lifted. That, and vanity."

MARY CALDERONE

During the sexually eventful years between 1953 and 1964—the dark ages on one side, the sexual revolution on the other— Mary Calderone was the radical voice within the Establishment prodding for change, progress, sexual justice. As medical director of Planned Parenthood, she called for more and better contraception—at the time there was no Pill, foam, or IUD. She attacked the law forbidding public health services from giving out contraceptives as unfair

to the poor. She suggested—it now seems obvious—that family planning be considered part of medical practice, and included as a subject in medical textbooks. She edited a book on abortion in 1958.

Dr. Calderone, who was born in 1904, did not go on to a docile old age. She is to be found at the offices of SIECUS (Sex Information and Education Council of the U.S.), an organization she co-founded in 1964. She would not dream of retiring. Hell no, she says, she'd die. She has moved on from a concern for the right to sexual information to the right to be sexual. A few years

Israel, Mexico, Sweden, Brazil and Australia.)

She doesn't think there's any magical formula for aging well. "You're born with good genes. . . . My father died at 94." (She is so forceful in her own right, you forget that her father—her hero—was the famous photographer Edward Steichen.) "My aunt died at 96. My mother died of a cancer that she lived with happily for 20 years. You're born lucky, with good genes, and the kind of person who's turned on by life, excited, passionate about everything—beauty, activity, books, people, art, science when I discovered it.

"My father was exactly the same kind of person. He used to tell me that with the right outlook, you don't ever have to grow old. When he retired at 65, he then had two more careers, one in the Navy, photographing in the Pacific, and one at the Museum of Modern Art. And I remember that when my stepmother died—his second wife, the real wife of his life—when she died, he told me that he thought he was now going into his old man phase. And he did. I have not yet gone into my old woman phase. I'm too happy. And the people I know who are most excited by life don't seem to *have* age. Look at some of these musicians! I saw a TV program with Daniel Barenboim, Itzhak Perlman, and Zubin Mehta—Lord! Those people were so turned on! I have never seen such joy and pleasure. They're never going to get old."

Her own life, she says, is a cornucopia; it keeps on spilling over. There is an on-goingness in her history that is especially unusual for her generation. She had two children in her twenties and two more in her forties. She went to college early and medical school late: She took the Planned Parenthood job "and made it exciting. There was always something to fight for, some-

thing to point out to people that was reasonable."

She does not consider herself, though, a fighter. "Quakers don't fight. I would say, more persistent —planned persistence. Because if I saw that the American Medical Association should be at *this* point now, I began taking steps here and there. A lot of patience, rationality —not a lot of angry frustration: That wastes energy and doesn't get you anywhere." She became a Quaker when she was 50, having "looked around for what would be the least trammeling, least rigid religion, the one that interfered with me the least, that would free me. That's just what it did. It gave me strength and it freed me, and there it is at the core of me. Before, I had only me."

Now separated from her husband, "in a friendly way," Dr. Calderone lives alone. She has times of being lonely, she says but she lives at her own pace, eats what she wants, and she likes it. Food is significant to her: People who age badly, she's said, "complain and get crabby and stick to their old clothes and their old food." She, to the contrary, boasts of her "extraordinarily varied diet—I may cook Chinese one night, have sushi another night, spaghetti another night, and try raw squid marinated like seviche another night." She does not drink much—wine, sometimes, but not when she's alone. She has never smoked. Her only physical exercise is to run up subway stairs. She no longer reads a book a day, but she is writing another book, on sexuality and the family. She plans, she says, to concentrate on childhood sexuality for the next five years.

After that? "Well, maybe I'll retire then." She seems to study the possibility for a moment, then whoops at the absurdity of it. "I don't know," she says lightly. "I'm living on borrowed time now. I am

very lucky. I haven't any arthritis except for a little old age arthritis I have low blood pressure, low blood cholesterol. I'm past the heart attack age, the cancer age. Now, I'm in the stroke age—that's one thing I'm afraid of, but there's nothing to do to prevent it." She might "go fine" for the next 20 years. Meanwhile, "There isn't a single experience that I want that I'm denying myself," she says. "Close friendships, intimate friendships, sex, new forms of sex ["new to me" is as far as she will go to explain herself]. I have a little money saved up, I'm in a position where I don't have to retire . . . and I still have a sense of growing. I really meant it when I told *People* that I'm just now becoming the person I was meant to be," she laughs that victory laugh. "But I'll probably say that again in two years."

"If you can only do one thing, like drawing, you keep doing that thing and you don't notice that the years fly by."

AL HIRSCHFELD

Al Hirschfeld is wearing a jumpsuit of dark-blue corduroy, and with his great beard and ferocious eyebrows (the facial equivalent of a "Beware of Dog" sign), he looks like a groovy patriarch. Usually one sees him in a suit, at the theater with his wife Dolly, making sketches of the people on stage; these are notes, in effect, for *The New York Times* drawings that have become a Broadway tradition. One of his sinuous, fast, musical lines can change forever the way you visualize Katharine Hepburn, for instance, or Jack Lemmon, or anyone he pens down.

At 77, (he was born June 21, 1903), Hirschfeld still climbs to his studio on the fourth floor of his Manhattan townhouse. He sits at a barber chair pulled up to a drawing board, near the large window with its north light. Seven days a week, 365 days a year, he is here working. Now, tipping back in his chair, he is saying that he doesn't think you can control aging, or learn from other people's experiences. "It would be great if you could. But you've got to stick your finger in the wet paint and you've got to put your finger on the hot stove and burn it. I can't speak for anyone else. I can barely speak for myself," he says, deadpan.

But for himself, the answer is what he likes to call his "great limitation." Drawing. "I've always drawn. I've never tried to do anything else. I *couldn't* do anything else. And that's very helpful, if you can only do one thing, because you keep doing that thing and you don't notice that the years fly by. That blank piece of paper presents a problem: You invent it, and you solve it to your own satisfaction and you spend a whole lifetime doing that, settling problems that don't exist."

For all that Hirschfeld is work-obsessed, he is not ambitious. There is no gnawing drive for money or success. He seems genuinely perplexed when he asks why people throw themselves into rush-hour traffic and other work-related regimentation. He accepts "money" as probably the right answer—"I guess that's the difference. The motivating force behind most people is this business of earning a living. Most people do things they don't want to do to keep from starving" —but this is an alien thought. Hirschfeld has always done pretty much what he wanted to do. "During the Depression, I couldn't stand what was going on here—it was very depressing," he laughs. "I had a tiny amount of money so I left the country and I stayed away for a long time. And when I came back, I was broke, but so was everybody else."

There is something odd about Hirschfeld, something missing. What is it? Frustration? Hardship experienced as such? Scars of stress and conflict? He describes, rather sadly, a brother who died in his seventies (the other died at 18 in a flu epidemic) as a "harassed fellow most of his life." That is just what the youngest of the three brothers is not.

He was raised in circumstances he now recognizes as "penurious," but "I never thought we were poor." His mother supported the family. "My father was an odd fellow, never had any ambitions. He was a marvelous guy to be around. He loved to ride a bike, and he was an umpire at the ballgame, but basically he was interested in nothing until his seventies, when he latched onto the elderly as a cause. He invented that unhappy phrase, 'senior citizen.' At 92 he gave a lecture at Carnegie Hall saying that government should take care of the elderly, and he jammed the place."

His father lived to 93, his mother to 92. Besides leaving their son an encouraging genetic endowment, they must have made old age seem like child's play to him. I wonder if he has much fear of age. "I have no fear of age, really," he says. "It hasn't hit me yet. It'll probably hit me tomorrow. I still feel pretty much the way I've always felt. I have friends who have some of the disabilities of age—one is partly blind and his hearing is gone, but he's not depressing about it. It's to be expected, like a baby's screaming. I don't know people who are bitter about aging. The people I know are all in creative fields, and all have about the same problem, and it usually has to do with their work, and not with the extraneous things of living. People either accept the limitations of age, or they don't and the ones that do, I find more attractive."

The only thing Hirschfeld has ever done consciously for his health was to quit smoking 10 years ago. Going up and down the four flights of stairs is exercise enough for him. One thing he likes to do besides draw is make candy. He also likes to stay up until three AM reading —Thoreau is his favorite, Dickens, Irish writers. Music, ballet—they enrich his life, but really his life is on his drawing board, and the important thing is "seeing things, being interested in that," and "I always want to draw a little better." A drawing problem will keep him awake at night. He's absorbed by "the mystery of recognition," how lines convey character. "All my life is tied up with people.

I would much rather sit in a cafe in Baghdad and draw or watch the crowds go by and the sweetmeats and camels and the insanity of human beings than sit on the lip of the Grand Canyon and try to draw that. Nature doesn't hold any great interest for me. But the foibles of people, the way they move, their relations one to another, has always interested me. That's the impetus that drives me to the drawing board."

"I have a self-image of eternal youth. I can say fairly easily, 'I'm getting older,' but there's a ha-ha below. I'm playing with the idea. Deep down, you believe there's a fountain of youth in you. . . ."

ELSA LEICHTER

Elsa Leichter, born in 1905, is a small delicious woman with apricot coloring, remarkably plump young skin and a smile like clear water. She is Viennese—very Viennese, she would say ("I was a child of the twenties. I loved love and the Vienna Woods and the Blue Danube and everything that was mushy and very Vienna"), and she came to America in 1938 because of Hitler.

She was 33 years old. She had been married and divorced. She had started medical school, then dropped out because of a romance —she still regrets that choice—and became a social worker. Arriving in New York, she saw that she would need an advanced degree to practice social work, so she fought like hell to win a scholarship for a mas-

ters' program at Case Western Reserve. By 1941, she was back in New York with a job at Jewish Family Service, one of the most-respected agencies in the country.

"I often call myself a second-chance person," she says. "Coming to America, finding meaningful work after giving up medicine, and probably the most important of the second chances was my marriage." In the early forties, she was remarried to a journalist, later head of the German press group to the United Nations, a widower with two sons. There are photographs of her husband with Nehru, with Adlai Stevenson, Willy Brandt.

"My husband was the exciting one in the family," she says, "and I played the little woman at home, and at U.N. parties. My husband used to say, 'You know, no one would know you did anything.'" What she was doing was rising to

the position of director of the group therapy department, which she'd started, and widening her reputation as an excellent training supervisor. By the mid-seventies, in her mid-sixties, she was ready to leave JFS—to concentrate on freelance consulting and teaching—when her husband died. "After 30 years of marriage," she says. "A good hunk of my life. And I thought, I don't want to lose everything all at once, so I will stay at the agency another year—it had become like a second family to me." And then she embarked on what she speaks of as her "German Adventure."

Whatever "nature" means, she says, she thinks she is by nature a sort of adventuress. "I led a very steady life with my husband, but after he died . . . I would like to tell you a little episode," she says. "After he died, I went on a vacation alone. I had broken my ankle before I left. And when I went to Europe, I was limping, and limpingly I walked around a lake in Austria, and I said to myself, 'Now what are you going to do with yourself?' And 'Who are *you* when you have been a *we* for 30 years?' And 'What is there in it for you now, in this period of your life?'

"And I began to have a strong pounding of my heart and even when I tell it now I will come near tears (it is an interesting thing) because the thought came to me (really, I was almost frightened with it—I sat down on a tree trunk) . . . because my question was, 'What do you have now?' And the thought that came to me was *freedom.*

"Then I said, 'Big deal, freedom. So what do you mean by freedom?' (I had a real dialogue with myself.) And then I thought, freedom is that if something comes along—and you cannot at this moment know what it will be—you will be open-armed rather than closed." She swings her arms wide,

245

then folds them self-protectively around herself.

"And that was it, and then I felt better. And soon thereafter, I was sought out by the director of a German psychoanalytic institute: Would I come to Germany and teach a seminar in family therapy? And out of that, just about an enterprise has developed, in many cities, and a whole new life for me. And I said *yes* because I did this"—she opens her arms again, then closes them—"instead of this."

Every summer since, she has traveled to Germany. "I go with packing and unpacking, the changing of trains, the suitcases—it's not that I'm very sophisticated about it. I become a frightened old lady on the airplane. So there's a price to be paid and I'm paying it. And at this point, I let people know, 'You know my age, please come and pick me up at the airport....' I will play the old lady to the hilt to save my energy. If I teach from nine in the morning to six at night, and interview a family in front of an audience for four days in succession ... I give my all to that, and it's a marvelous peak experience every time, so I ask for the comforts that go with being older."

Her friends say she's doing too much; she hears that an awful lot. And every year, she says this will be the last time to Germany. "I pay the price when I come back with a feeling of letdown—the high adventure is there; here is more the regular life with the rent and the checks. But what is very important about the German work is that it is a rounding-out of the most violently disruptive period of my life—leaving Austria.

"If you had asked me 20 years ago about some of the things I've seen in German families from working with them—their losses, their wanderings—I would have said it serves them right. Now I have fantastic friends out of the groups, in every city—exquisite friendships—and it is very meaningful for me to come back with what I have learned in America. I give them American thinking and practice as a gift and they receive it and give it back to me—it's very nourishing. There's been a real reconciliation ... it goes under the chapter of second chances," she says.

Another second chance is going back to the piano after her husband died. She hadn't played in years and then was drawn, powerfully, to the piano on a visit to her sister in Maine. ("What we share, what our mother had," Mrs. Leichter says of her 19-months-younger sister, "is a tremendous ability for enthusiasm.") Since then, she has been taking lessons, practicing an hour and a half a day (there is a Chopin waltz on the piano, a Haydn sonata, Bach inventions ...) and is hoping to buy a Baldwin.

I ask her what else is in her life. Friendships? Yes. They're very important to her. Family—her two stepsons and their families are a gift left to her by her husband ("I'm extremely good friends with them," she says).

"And I have one other thing in life which ..." she laughs hesitantly, "I do have a love relationship. I am still a sexual woman and I think that's probably the most important thing in maintaining vitality—if you feel you can still enjoy sex, which I thought I didn't. In many ways the man doesn't fit my husband-image, but we meet on some levels beautifully and I'm ready to accept this as a gift in life. I was not thinking of it at all, but it came my way again. So this is ... a third chance," she laughs. "And it has built into it something which I think all older people who live alone need, a little bit of a support network—a call in the morning, a call late in the evening."

When she was young, she says, she had an image of herself as an old lady ("I was probably all of 50 in this image") sitting in a rocking chair doing all the reading she could. That's not what age has turned out to be. "I can't say I look forward to what's coming—more frailty ... I was a high-energy person ... But I can't say I'm terribly frightened. I have a self-image of eternal youth. I can say fairly easily, 'I'm getting older,' but there's a ha-ha below. I'm playing with the idea. I don't believe in it fully. Deep down you believe there's a fountain of youth in you—it's almost ridiculous."

She wants to show not only her achievements and the life-affirming part of her, she says, "but also the piece that is messy, chaotic, fearful, with which I have to deal almost daily, and have to get through." She wants, in other words, not to be iconized as someone with all the answers, inhuman, a finished product. She is not a finished product.

PHOTOGRAPHERS AND ARTISTS

ACKNOWLEDGMENTS

The editors wish to thank the following people and organizations who contributed in so many ways to the creation of this book: Margaret Allen; Sandi Burrows; Cynthia Cathcart; Deborah Chase; Richard Cole; James Corcoran; Nancy DeSotto; Donnë Florence; Maureen Footer; Susan Greenstein; Beri Greenwald; Marcel Guillaume; Priscilla Massie; Bronwen Meredith; Metropolitan Life Insurance Company; Musée National d'Art Moderne, Centre Georges Pompidou, Paris; Nissa Simon; Elizabeth Thrasher; United States Department of Labor; Jeffrey Weiss. Thanks go to the special efforts of Carl Barile for his help in the design of this book.

INDEX